Effective Methods for Modern Healthcare Service Quality and Evaluation

Panagiotis Manolitzas
Technical University of Crete, Greece

Evangelos Grigoroudis
Technical University of Crete, Greece

Nikolaos Matsatsinis
Technical University of Crete, Greece

Denis Yannacopoulos
Piraeus University of Applied Sciences, Greece

A volume in the Advances in Medical Diagnosis, Treatment, and Care (AMDTC) Book Series

Medical Information Science
REFERENCE
An Imprint of IGI Global

Published in the United States of America by
Medical Information Science Reference (an imprint of IGI Global)
701 E. Chocolate Avenue
Hershey PA 17033
Tel: 717-533-8845
Fax: 717-533-8661
E-mail: cust@igi-global.com
Web site: http://www.igi-global.com

Library of Congress Cataloging-in-Publication Data

Library of Congress Cataloging-in-Publication Data

Names: Manolitzas, Panagiotis, editor. | Grigoroudis, Evangelos, editor. | Matsatsinis, Nikolaos F., editor. | Yannacopoulos, Denis, 1949- editor.
Title: Effective methods for modern healthcare service quality and evaluation / Panagiotis Manolitzas, Evangelos Grigoroudis, Nikolaos Matsatsinis, and Denis Yannacopoulos, editors.
Description: Hershey, PA : Medical Information Science Reference, 2016. | Includes bibliographical references and index.
Identifiers: LCCN 2015051030| ISBN 9781466699618 (hardcover) | ISBN 9781466699625 (ebook)
Subjects: LCSH: Medical care--Evaluation. | Medicare--Qualtiy.
Classification: LCC RA410.53 .E344 2016 | DDC 362.1068--dc23 LC record available at http://lccn.loc.gov/2015051030

This book is published in the IGI Global book series Advances in Medical Diagnosis, Treatment, and Care (AMDTC) (ISSN: Pending; eISSN: Pending)

British Cataloguing in Publication Data
A Cataloguing in Publication record for this book is available from the British Library.

Advances in Medical Diagnosis, Treatment, and Care (AMDTC) Book Series

ISSN: Pending
EISSN: Pending

Mission

Advancements in medicine have prolonged the life expectancy of individuals all over the world. Once life-threatening conditions have become significantly easier to treat and even cure in many cases. Continued research in the medical field will further improve the quality of life, longevity, and wellbeing of individuals.

The **Advances in Medical Diagnosis, Treatment, and Care (AMDTC)** book series seeks to highlight publications on innovative treatment methodologies, diagnosis tools and techniques, and best practices for patient care. Comprised of comprehensive resources aimed to assist professionals in the medical field apply the latest innovations in the identification and management of medical conditions as well as patient care and interaction, the books within the AMDTC series are relevant to the research and practical needs of medical practitioners, researchers, students, and hospital administrators.

Coverage

- Disease Management
- Alternative Medicine
- Experimental Medicine
- Medical Testing
- Emergency Medicine
- Patient Interaction
- Chronic Conditions
- Cancer Treatment
- Internal Medicine
- Critical Care

IGI Global is currently accepting manuscripts for publication within this series. To submit a proposal for a volume in this series, please contact our Acquisition Editors at Acquisitions@igi-global.com or visit: http://www.igi-global.com/publish/.

The Advances in Medical Diagnosis, Treatment, and Care (AMDTC) Book Series (ISSN Pending) is published by IGI Global, 701 E. Chocolate Avenue, Hershey, PA 17033-1240, USA, www.igi-global.com. This series is composed of titles available for purchase individually; each title is edited to be contextually exclusive from any other title within the series. For pricing and ordering information please visit http://www.igi-global.com/book-series/advances-medical-diagnosis-treatment-care/129618. Postmaster: Send all address changes to above address.

Titles in this Series

For a list of additional titles in this series, please visit: www.igi-global.com

Handbook of Research on Trends in the Diagnosis and Treatment of Chronic Conditions
Dimitrios I. Fotiadis (University of Ioannina, Greece)
Medical Information Science Reference • copyright 2016 • 659pp • H/C (ISBN: 9781466688285) • US $385.00 (our price)

Editorial Advisory Board

Table of Contents

Preface xv

Acknowledgment xviii

Section 1
Healthcare Management and Decision Making

Chapter 1
Health Services Quality and Patient Satisfaction: A Review of the Literature 1
Sofia Xesfingi, University of Piraeus, Greece
Athanassios Vozikis, University of Piraeus, Greece

Chapter 2
High-Performance Work Practices in Healthcare Sector 16
Panagiotis Gkorezis, Open University of Cyprus, Cyprus
Mamas Theodorou, Open University of Cyprus, Cyprus

Chapter 3
Organizational Integration of Decision Analytic Methods in Healthcare Settings 45
Christopher L. Pate, Brook Army Medical Center, USA
Mark D. Swofford, Brook Army Medical Center, USA

Section 2
Operational Research (OR) in Medicine and Health Systems

Chapter 4
Modelling Spatial Medical Data 75
S. Zimeras, University of the Aegean, Greece
Y. Matsinos, University of the Aegean, Greece

Chapter 5
Surgery Operations Modeling and Scheduling in Healthcare Systems 90
Fatah Chetouane, Université de Moncton, Canada
Eman Ibraheem, Université de Moncton, Canada

Section 3
Information Technology (IT) in Health Care

Chapter 6
Examining the Influence of Information Technology on Modern Health Care 110
Edward T. Chen, University of Massachusetts – Lowell, USA

Chapter 7
Geographic Information System Applications in Public Health: Advancing Health Research 137
Sandul Yasobant, Indian Institute of Public Health Gandhinagar, India
Kranti Suresh Vora, Indian Institute of Public Health Gandhinagar, India
Ashish Upadhyay, Indian Institute of Public Health Gandhinagar, India

Section 4
Strategy and Policy

Chapter 8
Strategies for Expanding Access and Improving the Quality of Pharmaceutical Services 168
Marcus Vinícius Dias-Souza, Federal University of Minas Gerais, Brazil

Chapter 9
Hospital Units Merging Reasons for Conflicts in the Human Resources 202
Athanasia Stamatopoulou, Piraeus University of Applied Sciences, Greece
Eleni Stamatopoulou, Ministry of Health, Greece
Denis Yannacopoulos, Piraeus University of Applied Sciences, Greece

Chapter 10
Towards European Modern Societies with Health Systems That Are Able to Add More Years to Life, But Also to Add More Life to Years 228
Androutsou Lorena, University of Thessaly, Greece
Androutsou Foulvia, University of Crete, Greece

Compilation of References 256

About the Contributors 305

Index 313

Detailed Table of Contents

Preface... xv

Acknowledgment..xviii

Section 1
Healthcare Management and Decision Making

Chapter 1
Health Services Quality and Patient Satisfaction: A Review of the Literature...... 1
Sofia Xesfingi, University of Piraeus, Greece
Athanassios Vozikis, University of Piraeus, Greece

Quality of care from the patient's perspective and patient satisfaction are two major multidimensional concepts that are used several times interchangeably. Patient satisfaction is a topic that is important both to medical (health) providers, the patients (consumers) and other third-party stakeholders in the medical care industry; it is, therefore, a dominant concept in quality assurance and quality improvement programmes. Patient satisfaction is an important measure of healthcare quality because it offers information on the provider's success at meeting the expectations of most relevance to the client. The importance of quality in the health care sector has been recognized recently, but it has been accelerated over the past years through the development of quality assurance, quality improvement programmes and patients' agendas. Patients are the ones situated at the front lines of care; therefore their opinion may provide useful insights into the quality of healthcare in different European systems, nevertheless the methodological limitations that should be taken into consideration.

Chapter 2
High-Performance Work Practices in Healthcare Sector.................................... 16
Panagiotis Gkorezis, Open University of Cyprus, Cyprus
Mamas Theodorou, Open University of Cyprus, Cyprus

High-performance work practices are described as human resource management practices that augment organizational performance through enhancing employees' competencies, motivation, commitment and productivity. Last decades have seen an increase in both research and practice on high-performance work practices. Yet, they have only recently received attention in healthcare settings. Nascent empirical studies have shown that high-performance work practices may play a vital role in fostering positive employee, patient and organizational outcomes. Given the problematic and limited environment of healthcare organizations, high-performance work practices are purported to be an effective "medicine" for organizational functioning. Thus, the purpose of this chapter is to delineate human resource management policies and their core high-performance work practices and also highlight their key role in ameliorating healthcare organizations' performance. By doing so, we provide some useful insights from healthcare literature in relation to the underlying mechanisms that account for this relationship.

Chapter 3
Organizational Integration of Decision Analytic Methods in Healthcare Settings..45
Christopher L. Pate, Brook Army Medical Center, USA
Mark D. Swofford, Brook Army Medical Center, USA

Healthcare organizations face a range of external and internal factors that both enable and hinder the organization's ability to provide safe, quality, timely and reliable healthcare services. The accessibility of data coupled with effectively integrated analytic methods can provide healthcare organizations with essential components of a solid framework for improving performance across the full spectrum of organizational contexts. However, data, methods, and a robust information infrastructure are only part of the solution. Healthcare organizations must consider characteristics of the organization and its strategy in order to effectively integrate analytic methods. Conceptual ideas from organizational theory, economics and strategic management can provide structure to the integration process.

Section 2
Operational Research (OR) in Medicine and Health Systems

Chapter 4
Modelling Spatial Medical Data..75
S. Zimeras, University of the Aegean, Greece
Y. Matsinos, University of the Aegean, Greece

Models are sometimes incomplete, especially in scaling data where other information of large regions needs to be predicted by smaller ones. Uncertainty analysis is the process of assessing uncertainty in modelling or scaling to identify major uncertainty sources, quantify their degree and relative importance, examine their effects on model output under different scenarios, and determine prediction accuracy. Especially for large dimensional data where spatial process in regional investigation are difficult to applied due to incompleteness leading us to spatial heterogeneity and non-linearity of our data. Modelling the uncertainty particular in scaling data starts with a general structure (linear most of the time) that explains as accurate as it is the real data and the model is built through adding variables, which are significant or which aid in prediction (hierarchical modelling). Parameter estimation is an important issue for the evaluation of these proposed models. Statistical techniques based on the spatial modelling could be proposed to overcome the problem of dimensionality and the spatial homogeneity between different grains levels based on the neighbourhood structure of the regions with similar characteristics. Investigation of the neighbourhood structure analysis could be applied using kriging or variogram techniques. In this work, we introduce and analyse methodologies for scaling data under uncertainty where incomplete data can be explained by spatial modelling at different scales. Incomplete data of uncertainties in regions involve spatial homogeneity upon neighbourhood structure between regions. The last could be illustrated by using spatial modelling techniques (like spatial autocorrelation, partition functions, and multilevel models). Parameter estimation of these models could be achieved by using stochastic (spatial hierarchical models, kriging, auto-correlation) methods. Comparison between different models could be achieved by considering statistical measures like log-likelihood ratio test. The best model is the one, which explains better the real data.

Chapter 5
Surgery Operations Modeling and Scheduling in Healthcare Systems 90
Fatah Chetouane, Université de Moncton, Canada
Eman Ibraheem, Université de Moncton, Canada

Surgery operations scheduling is a complex task due to operation duration uncertainties and resource sharing and availabilities in healthcare processes. In current health care systems it is important to minimize staff idle time and maintain a high utilization rate for surgery facilities. In the present study a nonlinear mathematical model for surgery scheduling is described, and an approximated linear model is deduced based on a set of assumptions. The linear model is solved using heuristic approach. The objective is to maximize the utilization of operating rooms and the surgery staff. Computational results show that our model improved the surgery schedule and the resources utilization. Our model also showed the potential of adding cases to the schedule due to minimizing the completion time of the schedule.

Section 3
Information Technology (IT) in Health Care

Chapter 6
Examining the Influence of Information Technology on Modern Health Care 110
Edward T. Chen, University of Massachusetts – Lowell, USA

Health care costs continue to rise at a level that far exceeds the rate of inflation. IT will be necessary in the computation and organization of complex algorithms presented in bundled payments and other initiatives. Currently in health care, a patient's medical history is not easily accessible by physicians and other medical personnel. IT can play the pivotal role in rectifying this problem in tracking the record in a universally designed environment. Advanced databases are needed to integrate facilities within health care systems. This chapter is to explore the current framework of Information Technology in the U.S. health care industry and to examine the topic covering the following areas: (a) IT's influence on the Affordable Care Act, (b) the emergence of the Electronic Health Record (EHR), also known as the Electronic Medical Record (EMR), and (c) the integration of databases across health care organizations through advanced systems like Epic.

Chapter 7
Geographic Information System Applications in Public Health: Advancing Health Research 137
Sandul Yasobant, Indian Institute of Public Health Gandhinagar, India
Kranti Suresh Vora, Indian Institute of Public Health Gandhinagar, India
Ashish Upadhyay, Indian Institute of Public Health Gandhinagar, India

Geographic information systems or geographic information science is a combination of computer-mapping capabilities with additional database management/data analysis tools. GIS is widely used in various sectors such as environmental science, urban planning, agricultural applications etc. Public health is another focus area, where GIS has been used for research and practice areas such as epidemic surveillance and monitoring, among others. The journey of use of GIS in public health spans more than a century and GIS application in public health has evolved from the simple maps to the higher level geostatistical analysis and interactive WebGIS in recent times. GIS is an analytical tool which differs from conventional computer-assisted mapping and any statistical analysis programs in its ability to analyze complex data and visual presentation of spatial data. Specialized GIS techniques such as network analysis, location-allocation models, site selection, transportation models, and geostatistical analysis are well established and used in many developed and developing nations. Unfortunately owing to the high cost of licensed software and specialized skills for advanced data analysis, use of these techniques is limited mainly for the research and by few experts. GIS is proved to be useful for various public health practices and research purposes including epidemiological surveys/investigation, implementation research, program/policy decision making and dissemination of information. The advantage of using GIS is that maps provide an added dimension to data analysis, which helps in visualizing the complex patterns and relationships of public health issues, thus many unanswered questions in public health, can be understood well through use of GIS techniques. Use of GIS in public health is an application area still in its infancy.

Wider use of GIS for public health practice such as program planning, implementation and monitoring in addition to building evidence base for the policy making will help reduce inequities in health and provide universal healthcare. Overall, GIS is a helpful and efficient tool especially for public health professionals working in low resource settings. In the future with inclusion of advanced GIS technology like WebGIS can help reach the goal of optimal health care services globally.

Section 4
Strategy and Policy

Chapter 8
Strategies for Expanding Access and Improving the Quality of Pharmaceutical Services 168
Marcus Vinícius Dias-Souza, Federal University of Minas Gerais, Brazil

Pharmaceutical services are among the most accessible healthcare assistance systems worldwide, being provided generally in enterprises like Drugstores and Compounding Pharmacies. Pharmacists are highly accessible healthcare professionals considering also the availability, geographic distribution and location of pharmaceutical enterprises. However, there are several challenges for providing these services for patients with limitations such as low education, difficulties on reaching the Pharmacist, and the need for individualized monitoring (due to the complexity of therapy). Reports of low quality services are growing worldwide, and in order to expand access and improve the quality of pharmaceutical services, Pharmacists must move from being medication dispensers with focus in administrative management to a clinically-oriented practice with a humanistic view. The aim of this chapter is to make an approach on the implementation of effective strategies and ways to improve the quality of Pharmacists' work as specialized healthcare providers.

Chapter 9
Hospital Units Merging Reasons for Conflicts in the Human Resources 202
Athanasia Stamatopoulou, Piraeus University of Applied Sciences, Greece
Eleni Stamatopoulou, Ministry of Health, Greece
Denis Yannacopoulos, Piraeus University of Applied Sciences, Greece

The necessity for the control of expenses of health and the reduction of cost, led the Ministry of Health and the government of Greece to the decision-making for fusions of hospitals units of health following the new tendency of health's policy that prevails also in other countries. The research purpose was to appoint the positive and negative results from the fusions of hospitals. Any changes in the health care system aim at the reduction of expenses, however, they constitute the most frequent causes of conflicts among employees. The Hospital is characterized as a natural space for the growth of conflicts. Despite the oppositions that are recorded as for the positive and negative results, it appears finally that through the fusions, resources have been saved, management systems have been improved but in the same time, conflicts in the labour place between the individuals and the teams recruiting hospitals have been aggravated.

Chapter 10
Towards European Modern Societies with Health Systems That Are Able to Add More Years to Life, But Also to Add More Life to Years 228
Androutsou Lorena, University of Thessaly, Greece
Androutsou Foulvia, University of Crete, Greece

The political context in Europe is changing including health. Among the priorities in seeking to influence the future of healthcare is a renewed attachment to health for all, health in all policies and a better coordination between social and health policy. Health issues are by definition international, and Europe has a duty to extend solidarity to the wider world population, in strategy and in delivery. Ensuring equitable access to high-quality healthcare constitutes a key challenge for health systems throughout Europe. The chapter will emphasise the importance of European public health policies. The chapter will offer a real opportunity to address public health areas and values such as right to access to healthcare into the detailed mechanisms of European policy. The chapter will form a tool for health leaders, to enrich their knowledge in the public health spectrum from a European perspective, to support, promote and improve healthcare access at a national level.

Compilation of References 256

About the Contributors 305

Index 313

Preface

The economic crisis, the increase of poverty and unemployment, and the disorganization of primary health care have increased the demand of health services from public hospitals. Moreover, the economic recession has enforced the development of numerous tools and techniques for the efficiency improvement of health care resources. In studying the relevant literature, it can been easily observed that several scholars have developed modern approaches in order to redesign the health care services, find the optimal number of staff, evaluate the quality of health care services, etc. The main aim of this edited book is to present recent methods, case studies, and literature reviews for the effective evaluation of health care services. The book provides a helpful tool for health policy makers, researchers, and the academic community in general interested in the recent advances in the effective and efficient design of health care services.

The edited book is divided in four sections covering subjects like health care management and decision-making, operational research in medicine and health systems, information technology in health care, as well as strategy and policy in the health care sector.

The first three chapters cover the area of health care management and decision-making. More specifically, the first chapter by Xesfigi and Vozikis presents a comprehensive literature review of health services quality and patient satisfaction. The authors pinpoint that patients' perspective about the quality of health care may provide useful insights into the different European health care systems, nevertheless the methodological limitations that should take into consideration.

In the second chapter, Gkoretzis and Theodorou emphasize the increase in both research and practice on high performance work practices, during the last decades. The scope of the chapter is to delineate human resource management policies and their core high-performance work practices, and also highlight their key role in ameliorating health care organizational performance. By doing so, they provide some useful insights from health care literature regarding the underlying mechanisms that account this relationship.

Pate and Swofford, in the third chapter, describe how decision analytic methods can provide competitive advantages to healthcare organizations if organizational structures and processes are effectively aligned. Furthermore, they outline several key considerations in analytic integration, while they also underscore the idea that the best organizational solution will ultimately be unique to the organization that has chosen to embark on the journey of deliberately considering the integration of analytics throughout the organization. Consequently, this chapter may help readers to define the concept of analytics, identify essential theoretical concepts related to the integration of analytics, and understand the importance of analytic integration in health care settings.

The second section of the book is devoted to operational research in medicine and health systems and presents real world application in the aforementioned area. More specifically, Zimeras and Matsinos, in chapter 4, introduce and analyze methodologies for scaling data under uncertainty, where incomplete data can be explained by spatial modelling at different scales. Through the analysis, they demonstrate that data quality and quantity is very crucial and affect uncertainty in a number of ways. Also, they propose that Kriging via semi-variagram models could be used in order to tackle uncertainty across scales.

In the next chapter Chetouane and Ibraheem elucidate the recent studies on modelling and scheduling of surgery procedures, focusing on the mathematical description of the constraints involved in the surgery planning and scheduling problem. The proposed nonlinear model is then simplified to a linear mathematical program, and a heuristic procedure is presented to solve this simplified model. The proposed approach is tested on an illustrative example, and based on the obtained results the authors show that the scheduling approach can improve the utilization of the resources.

Chapters 6 and 7 refer to the scientific area of information technology in health care. In this context, in Chapter 6 Chen explores the current framework of Information Technology (IT) in the U.S. health care industry and discussed the IT's influence on the Affordable Care Act, the emergence of the Electronic Health Record (EHR), also known as the Electronic Medical Record (EMR), and the integration of databases across health care organizations through advanced systems like Epic.

The following chapter by Yasobant, Vora, and Upadhyay shows how the usage of the Geographic Information Systems (GIS) may be useful in various research purposes, including epidemiological surveys/investigation, implementation research, program/policy decision making, and dissemination of information. Through an extensive literature review, the authors present the history of GIS, the historical pathways of GIS in public health, the different types of GIS, and most importantly, the usage of GIS in public health research and practice.

The last three chapters of the book refer to strategy and policy in the health care sector. More specifically, in Chapter 8, Marcus Vinícius Dias-Souza focuses on strategies for expanding access and improving the quality of pharmaceutical services, considering pharmacists as specialized health care providers.

In Chapter 9, Stamatopoulou, Stamatopoulou, and Yannacopoulos analyze the positive and negative results from the fusion of hospitals. The authors demonstrate that fusions may lead to savings of resources, improvement of management systems, but in the same time, they may result conflicts in the labor place between individuals and teams of hospital organizations.

The last chapter of the book emphasizes the importance of European public health policies. Androutsou and Androutsou demonstrate the important role of national governments and regional authorities in public health services and show that it is necessary for all stakeholders to be actively involved. This chapter may be a useful tool for health leaders, to enrich their knowledge in the public health spectrum from a European perspective, in order to support, promote, and improve health care access.

The edited volume may be used as a text book for courses covering topics like management and strategy, information management and technology, decision making, and operational research in health care services. Health policy makers, researchers, and academics will find this text useful in order to enrich their knowledge in the scientific area of health care services research. We hope that this book will provide a useful resource of ideas, techniques, and methods for additional research on this topic.

The editors of the book would like to express their sincere thanks to all the authors who have devoted considerable time and effort for their comprehensive contributions. We thank also IGI Global and the publishing team for their encouragement and support during the preparation of the book.

Panagiotis Manolitzas
Technical University of Crete, Greece

Evangelos Grigoroudis
Technical University of Crete, Greece

Nikolaos Matsatsinis
Technical University of Crete, Greece

Denis Yannacopoulos
Piraeus University of Applied Sciences, Greece

Acknowledgment

The editors of the book would like to express their sincere thanks to all the authors who have devoted considerable time and effort for their comprehensive contributions. We also thank IGI GLOBAL and the publishing team for their encouragement and support during the preparation of the book.

Panagiotis Manolitzas
Technical University of Crete, Greece

Evangelos Grigoroudis
Technical University of Crete, Greece

Nikolaos Matsatsinis
Technical University of Crete, Greece

Denis Yannacopoulos
Piraeus University of Applied Sciences, Greece

Section 1
Healthcare Management and Decision Making

Chapter 1
Health Services Quality and Patient Satisfaction:
A Review of the Literature

Sofia Xesfingi
University of Piraeus, Greece

Athanassios Vozikis
University of Piraeus, Greece

ABSTRACT

Quality of care from the patient's perspective and patient satisfaction are two major multidimensional concepts that are used several times interchangeably. Patient satisfaction is a topic that is important both to medical (health) providers, the patients (consumers) and other third-party stakeholders in the medical care industry; it is, therefore, a dominant concept in quality assurance and quality improvement programmes. Patient satisfaction is an important measure of healthcare quality because it offers information on the provider's success at meeting the expectations of most relevance to the client. The importance of quality in the health care sector has been recognized recently, but it has been accelerated over the past years through the development of quality assurance, quality improvement programmes and patients' agendas. Patients are the ones situated at the front lines of care; therefore their opinion may provide useful insights into the quality of healthcare in different European systems, nevertheless the methodological limitations that should be taken into consideration.

DOI: 10.4018/978-1-4666-9961-8.ch001

INTRODUCTION

Quality of care from the patient's perspective and patient satisfaction are two major multidimensional concepts that are used several times interchangeably (Raftopoulos, 2005). There has been confusion and controversy in health care as to whether patients are in fact consumers. This confusion may be at the root of the overall service failing of hospitals (Fottler *et al.*, 2002). Using a technical definition, a customer is anyone who has expectations about process operations or outputs (James, 2003); therefore all patients are customers, but not all customers are patients. According to Raftopoulos (2005), the quality of care has a subjective profile as it involves a cognitive evaluation process and an objective determinant which is "care" as an outcome, a process or a structure measure. On the other hand patient satisfaction tends to have an objective profile and determinant which is patient's subjection. If we add the word perceived to both terms (quality and satisfaction) we conclude to an opposite meaning result: perceived quality of care and perceived satisfaction become a totally subjective concept as they are based on patients' own feelings.

A competitive health market is usually quality-oriented, and improving the quality of care service is a continuing challenge to healthcare providers (Tzeng, 2002). According to Bleich *et al.* (2009), consumer satisfaction studies are challenged by the lack of a universally accepted definition of measure and by a dual focus: while some researchers focus on patient satisfaction with the quality and type of healthcare services received, others focus on people's satisfaction with the health system more generally. The key to solving this problem may be for the health care sector to focus on perceived health service quality.

Quality was very popular in the marketing literature where the notion of satisfying the customer was a dominant model of quality of service provided and consumer satisfaction ("Satisfaction with Physician and Primary Care Scale", Hulka *et al.*, 1970; "Patient Satisfaction Questionnaire", Ware and Snyder, 1975; "Client Satisfaction Questionnaire", Larsen, 1979, later transformed to "Patient Satisfaction Scale", e.tc.). Only a few researchers developed a conceptual framework for conceptualization of service quality and patient satisfaction, before validating their scale (Wilde *et al.*, 1983). Measurement of patient satisfaction lacks a conceptual soundness as it reflects dimensions considered important by researchers and not by responders. Further, quality in healthcare has been studied largely from the clinical perspective, excluding the patient's perception of service quality (Gill and White, 2009). The most frequently used theoretical model of consumers satisfaction is the one developed by Parasuraman *et al.* (1988). SERVQUAL was designed to accommodate measurement of service quality across a wide spectrum of services including health care services.

Figure 1. Multi-dimensional hierarchical model of perceived service quality
Source: Dagger et al. (2007)

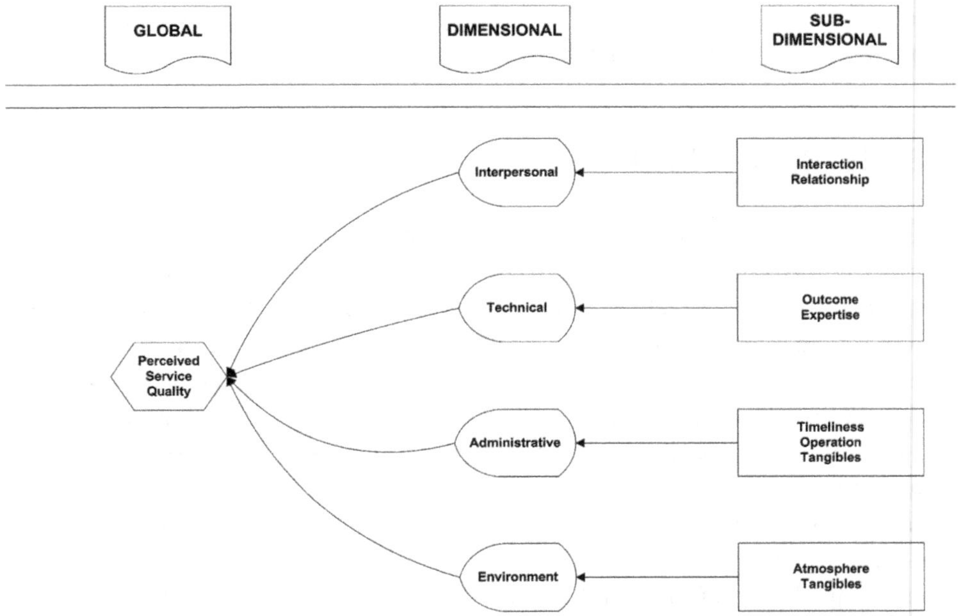

The importance of quality in the health care sector has been recognized recently, but it has been accelerated over the past years through the development of quality assurance, quality improvement programmes and patients' agendas (Raftopoulos, 2005). The stated aims of patient feedback programmes are normally twofold: to monitor performance and to stimulate improvements in the quality of care. These goals are not contradictory, but neither are entirely complementary (Reeves and Secombe, 2007). For example, assessing patient satisfaction can be mandatory for French hospitals since 1998, which is used to improve the hospital environment, patient amenities and facilities in a consumerist sense, but not necessarily to improve care (Boyer *et al.*, 2006).

Patient satisfaction is a topic that is important both to medical (health) providers, the patients (consumers) and other third-party stakeholders in the medical care industry (Ofili, 2014). It is, therefore, a dominant concept in quality assurance and quality improvement programmes (Raftopoulos, 2005). Patient satisfaction is an important measure of healthcare quality because it offers information on the provider's success at meeting the expectations of most relevance to the client (Donabedian, 1983). Recent research has shown than service satisfaction can significantly enhance patients' quality of life (Dagger and Sweeney, 2006) and enable service provides to determine specific problems of customers, on which corrective action can then be taken (Oja *et al.*, 2006) Understanding satisfaction and service quality have, for some considerable time, been recognized as critical to developing service improvement strategies to (Bleich *et al.*, 2009).

ISSUES, CONTROVERSIES, AND PROBLEMS

With the advent of the patient rights movement (Williams, 1994), the debate over the relationship between patient satisfaction as an evaluation of the process of care versus the standard of technical care was well established. As a result, the use of patient satisfaction measures in the health sector became increasingly widespread (Gill and White, 2009). The inaugural quality assurance work of Donabedian (1988) identified the importance of patient satisfaction as well as providing much of the basis for research in the area of quality assurance in healthcare. The desired need for measurement of patient satisfaction has been largely driven by the underlying politics of "new public management" (Hood, 1995) and the concomitant rise in the health consumer movement, with patient satisfaction being the one of the articulated goals if healthcare delivery (Gill and White, 2009). In countries where health systems are largely funded through tax revenue or where access to health is guaranteed by the constitution, surveys of patient satisfaction can give the population an opportunity to express its opinion about an important social programme and hence about the ability of government to deliver on a key obligation (Kruk and Freedman, 2008).

According to Gill and White (2009), there is no consensus on how to best conceptualize the relationship between patient satisfaction and theirs perceptions of the quality if their healthcare. Health sector research into patients' perceptions of the dimensions of service quality (perceived service quality) has been limited (Clemes *et al.*, 2001), yet studies seeking to assess the components of the quality of care in health services predominately continue to measure patient satisfaction (Lee *et al.*, 2006). O'Connor and Shewchuck (2003) emphasized that much of the work on patient satisfaction is based on simple descriptive and correlation analyses with no theoretical framework. They concluded that, with regard, to health services, the focus should be on measuring technical and functional (how care is delivered) quality and not patient satisfaction. Ferris *et al.* (1992) suggest that the behavioral consequences of patient satisfaction should result in betted medical care and improved outcomes, but only if satisfaction correlated primarily with health care of high technical quality.

In a democratic society, claims to health services and conditions that promote health can be seen as assets of citizenship (Mackintosh, 2001). Studies in the developing world have shown a clear link between patient satisfaction and a variety of explanatory factors, among which service quality has been prominent (Rao *et al.*, 2006; Zineldin, 2006). Thus, distinct from clinical and economic goals, we could include public participation in decision making, accountability, and patient satisfaction as key aims of health systems (Kruk and Freedman, 2008). The latter has been studied and measured extensively as a standalone construct and as a component of outcome quality (Heidegger *et al.*, 2006) and continues to be measured as a proxy for the patient's assessment of service quality (Turris, 2005).

As the debates over manage care continues, measuring quality has increasingly become a focus in health care. One approach to measuring quality is the use of a scorecard, which summarizes a critical set of indicators that measure the quality of care. Assuming that one of the primary objectives of a practitioner or organization is to meet patients' needs and expectations, quality indicators that reflect this objective and lead to the desirable outcomes must be selected.

Although patient experience surveys are now widely accepted as valid indicators of healthcare performance, but their usefulness in improving the quality of care at the organizational level has not yet been systematically researched (Reeves and Secombe, 2007), Lin and Kelly (1995) well-articulated the importance of measuring patient satisfaction in the healthcare sector, Hawthorne (2006) believes that patient satisfaction is a multidimensional concept, not yet tightly defined, and part of an apparently yet to be determined complex model, affirming Heidegger *et al.*, (2006), according to whom the concept of satisfaction is complicated, irrespective of the area in which is studied. According to Gill and White (2009), the continued misuse and perpetuation of the inter-changeability of terminology not only compromises the worth of research, it inhibits the possibility of finding much needed answers as how best to conceive and measure health service quality from the patient's perspective.

DISCUSSION

Patient satisfaction is now deemed an important outcome measure for health services, this processes utility rests on a number of implicit assumptions about the nature and meaning of expressions of "satisfaction" since patients may have a complex set of important and relevant beliefs which cannot be embodied in terms of satisfaction (Williams, 1994). Gilbert *et al.* (2004) claim that satisfaction varies depending on the assumptions made as to what satisfaction means. The design of questionnaires by the majority of the investigators, as well as the lack of standardized measures, makes it quite difficult to interpret and compare results across countries. More important, the distribution of scores on patient satisfaction surveys are highly skewed (Ferris *et al.*, 1992).

Figure 2. Framework for health systems performance measures
Source: Kruk and Freedman, 2008

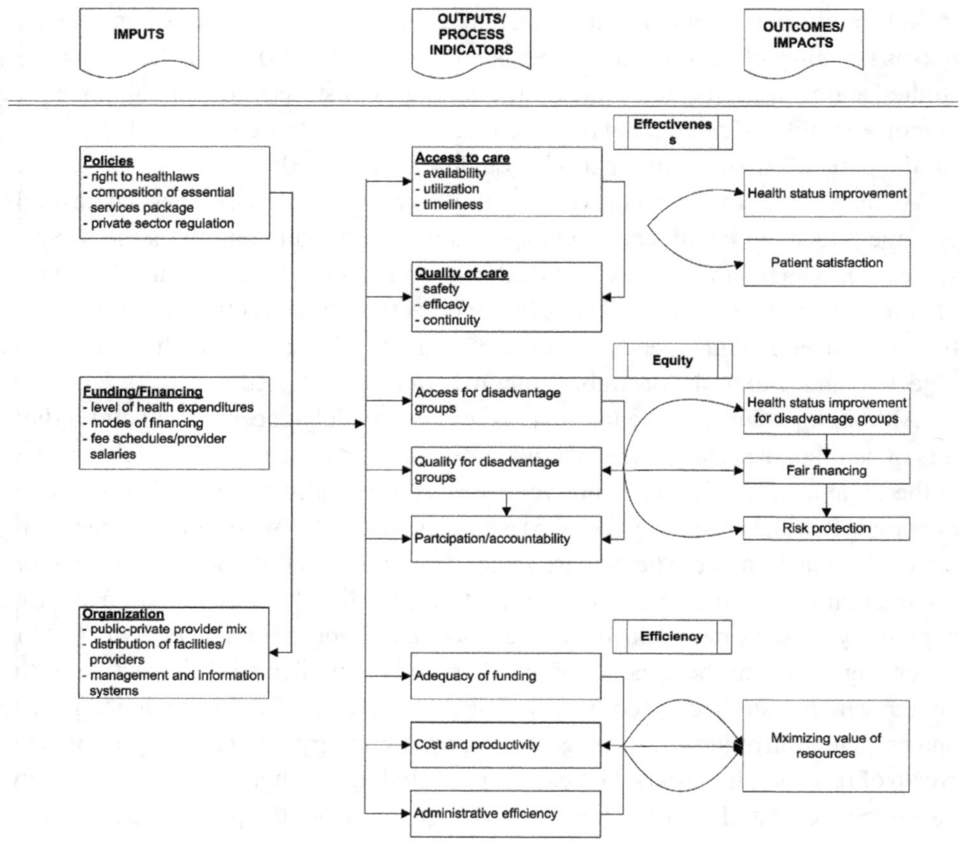

Gill and White (2009) provided a summary of the theories of patient satisfaction in the healthcare. According to Hawthorne (2006), the more recent theories are largely restatements of the five key theories that were published in the 1980s. Those theories were:

1. **Discrepancy and Transgression Theories of Fox and Storms (1981):** If patients' healthcare orientations and provider conditions were congruent then patients were satisfied, if not, then they were dissatisfied.
2. **Expectancy-Value Theory of Linder-Pelz (1982):** Satisfaction is mediated by personal beliefs and values about care as well as prior expectations about care. Pascoe (1983) developed the Linder-Pelz model to take into account the influence of expectations on satisfaction; Strasser *et al.* (1993) further devel-

oped the same model to create a six factor psychological model: cognitive and affective perception formation, multidimensional construct, dynamic process, attitudinal response, iterative, and ameliorated by individual difference.

3. **Determinants and Components Theory of Ware *et al.* (1983):** patient satisfaction is a function of patients' subjective responses to experienced care mediated by their personal preferences and expectations.
4. **Multiple Models Theory of Fitzpatrick and Hopkins (1983):** expectations are socially mediated, reflecting the health goals of the patient and the extent to which illness and healthcare violated the patient's personal sense of self.
5. **Healthcare Quality Theory of Donabedian (1980):** Satisfaction is the principal outcome of the interpersonal process of care.

Gonzales *et al.* (2005) noted that satisfaction questionnaires have been the most commonly used method to survey patient perceptions of healthcare for more than 30 years, but only over the previous five years, had studies tried to ensure that the validity of the instrument was well grounded. Hawthorne (2006) further concluded that of the patient satisfaction literature conducted, none of the instruments reviewed could be considered satisfactory. There is an urgent need for differentiation and standardization of the definitions and constructs for satisfaction and perceived health service quality and their adoption in all future health services research (Gill and White, 2009).

The basic indicator for the level of quality of health services is the consensus of patients about the services provided, known as patient satisfaction. Patient satisfaction surveys typically ask consumers to evaluate the technical quality of the care they receive, the interpersonal aspects of care and the accessibility and availability of services or professionals. On the other hand, the assessment of technical aspects has traditionally been the domain of professionals. According to Raftopoulos (2005), the most consistent predictor of satisfaction is perhaps patient's age with older people being far more satisfied with health care than do younger people. This could be attributed with a halo effect, as elderly patients give socially favorable answers and are not willing to challenge physician and nurse authority. Wirtz and Bateson (1995) argued that it is difficult to distinguish between true correlations and halo effects and that the density of the problem relates to the importance of the service provided.

As core social institutions, health systems also need to be responsive to the needs and demands of the population (Freedman, 2005). Since Andaleeb *et al.* (2007), measuring service quality and satisfaction is very important since a comprehensive model of patient satisfaction has many policy implications in regard to identifying patient needs, developing standards, designing services systems and processes, establishing employee and patient roles in service delivery, enhancing training programmes, managing demand and capacity, and delivering the needed quality of services. Identification of the needs of individuals, whether through formal needs assessment or some surrogate, is an essential first step towards optimizing the use of allocated resources (Asadi-Lari *et al.*, 2004). Basing health care needs on quality of life scores, however, necessarily incorporates several sources of uncertainty due to factors such as age, sex, social class and individual patient's health status. In addition, quality of life tools may fail to distinguish between health problems and the desire to get professional attention (Osse *et al.*, 2000). The optimum approach, perhaps, could be a combination of needs and outcome assessment, preferably at individual levels (Leplege and Hunt, 1997).

There is growing evidence indicating that "quality of life assessment" can be considered as adjuvant to clinical and physiological assessments in many chronic diseases (Goodwin *et al.*, 2003). This approach is postulated to be the "gold standard" in the evaluation of healthcare services and outcome assessment (Asadi-Lari *et al.*, 2004). Patients with better health status have often been shown to be more satisfied with their medical care, but the causal factors in this relation have not been determined (Hall *et al.*, 2003). According to the study of Cheng *et al.* (2006), where the authors investigate what quality and cost factors influence whether patients perceive health care services as expensive, and therefore will recommend a hospital to other patients, they found that quality of care rather than price is the main concern in health care.

Research on health system satisfaction, which is largely comparative, has identified ways to improve health, reduce costs and implement reform (Blendon *et al.*, 2003). The increasing importance of patient experience and the sustained interest in comparing people's satisfaction with the health system across different countries and time periods suggests the need to characterize the relationship between them (Bleich *et al.*, 2009). Research relating global satisfaction ratings with patient experience has revealed strong associations between the two (Young *et al.*, 2000). Yet, to what extent patient experience explains satisfaction with the health care system remains unclear.

Assessing the performance of a health system begins with defining its goals (Kruk and Freedman, 2008). According to World Health Organization, the goal of a health system is the delivery of effective, preventive and curative health services to the full population, equitably and efficiently, while protecting individuals from catastrophic health care costs (WHO, 2000). National health accounts, a record of health sources and uses of health funds, are increasingly being used to assess progressivity of health financing methods (Rannan-Eliya, 2004) and the distribution of government expenditures to different parts of the country and different social groups

(Kruk and Freedman, 2008). According to Iacobuţă (2012), citizens of developed countries have a positive opinion about quality of healthcare in their country while patients' from developing countries evaluate it rather negatively.

CONCLUSION

Patients are the ones situated at the front lines of care (Schoen *et al.*, 2005), therefore their opinion may provide useful insights into the quality of healthcare in different European systems, nevertheless the methodological limitations that should be taken into consideration (Jankauskiene and Jankauskaite, 2011).

REFERENCES

Andalleb, S. S., Siddiqui, N., & Shahjahan, K. (2007). Patient satisfaction with health services in Bangladesh. *Health Policy and Planning*, *2*(4), 263–273. doi:10.1093/heapol/czm017 PMID:17545252

Asadi-Lari, M., Tamburini, M., & Gray, D. (2004). Patients' needs, satisfaction, and health related quality of life: Towards a comprehensive model. *Health and Quality of Life Outcomes*, *2*(1Suppl 32), 1–15. doi:10.1186/1477-7525-2-32 PMID:15225377

Bleich, S. N., Özaltin, E., & Murray, C. J. L. (2009). How does satisfaction with the health-care system relate to patient experience? *Bulletin of the World Health Organization*, *87*(4), 271–278. doi:10.2471/BLT.07.050401 PMID:19551235

Blendon, R. J., Schoen, C., DesRoches, C., Osborn, R., & Zapert, K. (2003). Common concerns amid diverse systems: Health care experiences in five countries. *Health Affairs*, *22*(3), 106–121. doi:10.1377/hlthaff.22.3.106 PMID:12757276

Boyer, L., François, P., Doutre, E., Weil, G., & Labarere, J. (2006). Perception and use of the results of patient satisfaction surveys by care providers in a French teaching hospital. *International Journal for Quality in Health Care*, *18*(5), 359–364. doi:10.1093/intqhc/mzl029 PMID:16931825

Cheng, S.-H., Wei, Y.-J., & Chang, H.-J. (2006). Quality Competition Among Hospitals: The effects of Perceived Quality and perceived Expensiveness on Health Care Consumers. *American Journal of Medical Quality*, *21*(1), 68–75. doi:10.1177/1062860605283618 PMID:16401707

Clemes, M. D., Ozanne, L. K., & Laurensen, W. L. (2001). Patients' perceptions of service quality dimensions: An empirical examination of health care in New Zealand. *Health Marketing Quarterly*, *19*(1), 3–22. doi:10.1300/J026v19n01_02 PMID:11727291

Dagger, T., & Sweeney, J. C. (2006). The effects of service evaluation on behavioral intentions and quality of life. *Journal of Service Research*, *19*(1), 3–19. doi:10.1177/1094670506289528

Dagger, T. S., Sweeney, J. C., & Johnson, L. W. (2007). A hierarchical model of health service quality: Scale development and investigation of an integrated model. *Journal of Service Research*, *10*(2), 123–142. doi:10.1177/1094670507309594

Donabedian, A. (1983). The quality of care in a health maintenance organization: A personal view. *Inquiry*, *20*, 218–222. PMID:6226606

Donabedian, A. (1988). The quality of care: How can it be assessed? *Journal of the American Medical Association*, *260*(12), 1743–1748. doi:10.1001/jama.1988.03410120089033 PMID:3045356

Ferris, L. E., Williams, J. I., Llewellyn-Thomas, H. A., Basinski, A. S. H., Cohen, M. M., & Naylor, C. D. (1992). A guide to direct measures of patient satisfaction in clinical practice. *Canadian Medical Association Journal*, *146*(10), 1727–1731. PMID:1596808

Fitzpatrick, R., & Hopkins, A. (1983). Problems in the conceptual framework of patient satisfaction research: An empirical exploration. *Sociology of Health & Illness*, *5*(3), 297–311. doi:10.1111/1467-9566.ep10491836 PMID:10265564

Fottler, M. D., Ford, R. C., & Heaton, C. P. (2002). *Achieving Service Excellence*. Chicago, IL: Health Administration Press.

Fox, J. G., & Storms, D. M. (1981). A different approach to sociodemographic predictors of satisfaction with health care. *Social Science & Medicine. Part A, Medical Sociology*, *15*(5), 557–564. doi:10.1016/0271-7123(81)90079-1 PMID:6976620

Freedman, L. P. (2005). Achieving the MDGs: Health systems as core social institutions. *Development*, *48*(1), 19–24. doi:10.1057/palgrave.development.1100107

Gilbert, G. R., Veloutsou, C., Goode, M. M. H., & Moutinho, L. (2004). Measuring customer satisfaction in the fast food industry: A cross-national approach. *Journal of Services Marketing*, *18*(4/5), 371–383. doi:10.1108/08876040410548294

Gill, L., & White, L. (2009). A critical review on patient satisfaction. *Leadership in Health Services*, *22*(1), 8–19. doi:10.1108/17511870910927994

Gonzalez, N., Quintana, J. M., Bilbao, A., Escobar, A., Aizpuru, F., Thompson, A., & de la Sierra, E. et al. (2005). Development and validation of an in-patient satisfaction questionnaire. *International Journal for Quality in Health Care*, *17*(6), 465–472. doi:10.1093/intqhc/mzi067 PMID:16100222

Goodwin, P. J., Black, J. T., Bordeleau, L. J., & Ganz, P. A. (2003). Health-related quality-of-life measurement in randomized clinical trials in breast cancer--taking stock. *Journal of the National Cancer Institute*, *95*(4), 263–281. doi:10.1093/jnci/95.4.263 PMID:12591983

Hall, J. A., Milburn, M. A., & Epstein, A. M. (1993). A Causal Model of Health Status and Satisfaction With Medical Care. *Medical Care*, *31*(1), 84–94. doi:10.1097/00005650-199301000-00007 PMID:8417273

Hawthorne, G. (2006). *Review of Patient Satisfaction Measures*. Canberra: Australian Government Department of Health and Ageing.

Heidegger, T., Saal, D., & Nuebling, M. (2006). Patient satisfaction with anaesthesia care: What is patient satisfaction, how should it be measured, and what is the evidence for assuring high patient satisfaction. *Best Practice & Research. Clinical Anaesthesiology*, *20*(2), 331–346. doi:10.1016/j.bpa.2005.10.010 PMID:16850781

Hood, C. (1995). The new public management in the 1980s: Variations on a theme. *Journal of Accounting. Organizations and Society*, *20*(2/3), 93–109. doi:10.1016/0361-3682(93)E0001-W

Hulka, B., Zyzanski, S., Cassel, J., & Thompson, S. (1970). Scale for the measurement of attitudes towards physicians and primary medical care. *Medical Care*, *8*(5), 429–436. doi:10.1097/00005650-197009000-00010 PMID:4920640

Iacobuţă, A. O. (2012). Patients' evaluation of access and quality of healthcare in EU countries: A comparative analysis. *Procedia: Social and Behavioral Sciences*, *62*, 896–900. doi:10.1016/j.sbspro.2012.09.151

Jankauskienė, D., & Jankauskaitė, I. (2011). Access and quality of health care system by opinion of patients in ten European countries. *Management in Health*, *25*(3), 31–39.

Kruk, M. E., & Freedman, L. P. (2008). Assessing health system performance in developing countries: A review of the literature. *Health Policy (Amsterdam)*, *85*(3), 263–276. doi:10.1016/j.healthpol.2007.09.003 PMID:17931736

Larsen, D. L., Attkisson, C. C., Hargreaves, W. A., & Nguyen, T. D. (1979). Assessment of client/patient satisfaction: Development of a general scale. *Evaluation and Program Planning*, *2*(3), 197–207. doi:10.1016/0149-7189(79)90094-6 PMID:10245370

Lee, P.-M., Khong, P., & Ghista, D. N. (2006). Impact of deficient healthcare service quality. *The TQM Magazine*, *18*(6), 563–571. doi:10.1108/09544780610707075

Leplege, A., & Hunt, S. (1997). The problem of quality of life in medicine. *Journal of the American Medical Association*, *278*(1), 47–50. doi:10.1001/jama.1997.03550010061041 PMID:9207338

Lin, B., & Kelly, E. (1995). Methodological issues in patient satisfaction surveys. *International Journal of Health Care Quality Assurance*, *8*(6), 32–37. doi:10.1108/09526869510098840 PMID:10165404

Linder-Pelz, S. (1982). Toward a theory of patient satisfaction. *Social Science & Medicine*, *16*(5), 577–582. doi:10.1016/0277-9536(82)90311-2 PMID:7100990

Mackintosh, M. (2001). Do health care systems contribute to inequalities. In D. A. Leon & G. Walt (Eds.), *Poverty, inequality and health: an international perspective*. Oxford: Oxford University Press.

O'Connor, S. J., & Shewchuk, R. (2003). Commentary – patient satisfaction: What is the point? *Health Care Management Review*, *28*(1), 21–24. doi:10.1097/00004010-200301000-00003 PMID:12638370

Ofili, O. U. (2014). Patient satisfaction in healthcare delivery – a review of current approaches and methods. *European Scientific Journal*, *10*(25), 25–39.

Oja, P. I., Kouri, T. T., & Pakarinen, A. J. (2006). From customer satisfaction survey to corrective actions in laboratory services in a university hospital. *International Journal for Quality in Health Care*, *18*(6), 422–428. doi:10.1093/intqhc/mzl050 PMID:17003077

Osse, B. H., Vernooij-Dassen, M. J., de Vree, B. P., Schade, E., & Grol, R. P. (2000). Assessment of the need for palliative care as perceived by individual cancer patients and their families: A review of instruments for improving patient participation in palliative care. *Cancer*, *88*, 900–911. doi:10.1002/(SICI)1097-0142(20000215)88:4<900::AID-CNCR22>3.0.CO;2-2 PMID:10679661

Parasuraman, A., Zeithanl, V. A., & Berry, L. L. (1988). SERVQUAL: A multiple-item scale for measuring consumer perceptions of service quality. *Journal of Retailing*, *64*(1), 12–40.

Pascoe, G. C. (1983). Patient satisfaction in primary health care: A literature review and analysis. *Evaluation and Program Planning*, *6*(3/4), 185–210. doi:10.1016/0149-7189(83)90002-2 PMID:10299618

Raftopoulos, V. (2005). A grounded theory for patients' satisfaction with quality of hospital care. *ICUs & Nursing Web Journal*, *22*, 1–15.

Rannan-Eliya, R. (2004). *Affordable healthcare: how has Sri Lanka achieved low mortality rates at such low cost?* Sri Lanka: Institute of Policy Studies.

Rao, K. D., Peters, D. H., & Bandeen-Roche, K. (2006). Toward patient-centered health services in india-a scale to measure patient perceptions of quality. *International Journal for Quality in Health Care*, *18*(6), 414–421. doi:10.1093/intqhc/mzl049 PMID:17012306

Reeves, R., & Secombe, I. (2007). Do patient surveys work? The influence of a national survey programma on local quality-improvement initiatives. *Quality & Safety in Health Care*, *17*(6), 437–441. doi:10.1136/qshc.2007.022749 PMID:19064659

Schoen C., Osborn R., Huynh P.T., Doty M. Zapet K., Peugh J. Davis K. (2005). Taking the Pulse of Health Care Systems: Experiences Of Patients With Health problems In Six Countries. *Health Affairs, Supl Web Exclusives*, (W5), 509-525.

Strasser, S., Aharony, L., & Greenberger, D. (1993). The patient satisfaction process: Moving toward a comprehensive model. *Medical Care Review*, *50*(2), 219–245. doi:10.1177/107755879305000205 PMID:10127084

Turris, S. A. (2005). Unpacking the concept of patient satisfaction: A feminist analysis. *Journal of Advanced Nursing*, *50*(3), 293–298. doi:10.1111/j.1365-2648.2005.03392.x PMID:15811108

Tzeng, H. M. (2002). The influence of nurses' working motivation and job satisfaction on intention to quit: An empirical investigation in Taiwan. *International Journal of Nursing Studies*, *39*(8), 867–878. doi:10.1016/S0020-7489(02)00027-5 PMID:12379304

Ware, J. E. Jr, & Snyder, M. K. (1975). Dimensions of patient attitudes regarding doctors and medical care services. *Medical Care*, *13*(8), 669–682. doi:10.1097/00005650-197508000-00006 PMID:1152557

Ware, J. E. Jr, Snyder, M. K., Wright, W. R., & Davies, A. R. (1983). Defining and measuring patient satisfaction with medical care. *Evaluation and Program Planning*, *6*(3/4), 247–263. doi:10.1016/0149-7189(83)90005-8 PMID:10267253

WHO. (2000). *World Health Report: health systems improving performance*. Geneva, Switzerland: World Health Organization.

Wilde, B., Starrin, B., Larsson, G., & Larsson, M. (1993). Quality of Care from a Patient Perspective. A Grounded Theory Study. *Scandinavian Journal of Caring Sciences*, *7*(2), 113–120. doi:10.1111/j.1471-6712.1993.tb00180.x PMID:8248668

Williams, B. (1994). Patient Satisfaction: A Valid Concept? *Social Science & Medicine*, *38*(4), 509–516. doi:10.1016/0277-9536(94)90247-X PMID:8184314

Wirtz, J., & Bateson, J. E. G. (1995). An experimental investigation of halo effects in satisfaction measures of service attributes. *International Journal of Service Industry Management*, *6*(3), 84–102. doi:10.1108/09564239510091358

Young, G. J., Meterko, M., & Desai, K. R. (2000). Patient satisfaction with hospital care: Effects of demographic and institutional characteristics. *Medical Care*, *38*(3), 325–334. doi:10.1097/00005650-200003000-00009 PMID:10718357

Zineldin, M. (2006). The quality of health care and patient satisfaction: An exploratory investigation of the 5Qs model at some Egyptian and Jordanian medical clinics. *International Journal for Quality in Health Care*, *19*(1), 60–99. doi:10.1108/09526860610642609 PMID:16548402

KEY TERMS AND DEFINITIONS

Patient Satisfaction: A measure of the extent to which a patient is content with the health care which they received from their health care provider.

Quality Assurance: Activities and programs intended to assure or improve the quality of care in either a defined medical setting or a program.

Quality of Care: The degree to which health services for individuals and populations increase the likelihood of desired health outcomes and are consistent with current professional knowledge.

Chapter 2
High-Performance Work Practices in Healthcare Sector

Panagiotis Gkorezis
Open University of Cyprus, Cyprus

Mamas Theodorou
Open University of Cyprus, Cyprus

ABSTRACT

High-performance work practices are described as human resource management practices that augment organizational performance through enhancing employees' competencies, motivation, commitment and productivity. Last decades have seen an increase in both research and practice on high-performance work practices. Yet, they have only recently received attention in healthcare settings. Nascent empirical studies have shown that high-performance work practices may play a vital role in fostering positive employee, patient and organizational outcomes. Given the problematic and limited environment of healthcare organizations, high-performance work practices are purported to be an effective "medicine" for organizational functioning. Thus, the purpose of this chapter is to delineate human resource management policies and their core high-performance work practices and also highlight their key role in ameliorating healthcare organizations' performance. By doing so, we provide some useful insights from healthcare literature in relation to the underlying mechanisms that account for this relationship.

DOI: 10.4018/978-1-4666-9961-8.ch002

INTRODUCTION

Contemporary business environment has become increasingly complex, turbulent, and competitive. As a result, organizational survival and prosperity is highly dependent on the effective utilization of potential resources. One of the most valuable resources of each organization relates to its human resources. For this reason, the past decades have witnessed a wide interest in human resource management and their policies and practices. One of the central tenets of human resource management concerns the fundamental role of employee emotions, attitudes and behaviors in enhancing organizational performance. The basic idea behind this ideology is that human resources comprise a source of competitive advantage (Barney, 1991; Wright & McMahan, 1992) and thus it is of utmost importance for organizations to develop and implement such bundles of contemporary human resource management practices that will increase employee performance and, in turn, will lead to higher levels of organizational performance. In the extant literature these practices are often called as high-performance work practices (HPWPs).

Not surprisingly, the vital role of such practices in fostering important outcomes also applies to healthcare organizations. Healthcare organizations have to cope with intensive competition, high operational costs, and limited resources. Even more, they are knowledge-intensive organizations with different professional groups which must be effectively coordinated. In light of these challenges, healthcare organizations strive to minimize costs and maximize effectiveness and service quality. In this pursuit, HPWPs constitute a useful tool for enabling healthcare organizations to achieve their goals.

Oddly, the related literature lacks of substantial theoretical and empirical studies that will point to the effectiveness of such practices. Therefore, the aim of the present chapter is twofold: first, to describe human resource management policies along with some key HPWPs and second, to provide a review of extant empirical evidence regarding the effect of HPWPs on employee and organizational outcomes in the healthcare industry.

HUMAN RESOURCE MANAGEMENT AND HIGH PERFORMANCE WORK PRACTICES

Human resource management constitutes a contemporary approach to managing people. Despite the burgeoning interest in human resource management from both academics and practitioners, the literature lacks a universally agreed definition.

Boxall and Purcell defined human resource management as *all those activities associated with the management of employment relationships in the firm* (2003, p. 1). Human resource management is consisted of a set of core policies namely human resource planning, recruitment and selection, training and development, rewards, performance management, employment relationships, health and safety.

In the extant literature, some scholars have considered human resource management as a contemporary label for describing personnel management policies and activities whereas others as a new, more strategic, approach to manage people in the workplace (Beardwell & Claydon, 2007). As regards the latter, which is the dominant approach, one of its core foundations relate to the fact that human resources constitute one of the major competitive advantages of each organization. Put differently, they comprise the most valuable organizational assets. Human resource management policies and practices should be integrated into the overall business strategy, demonstrating thus a more strategic role of human resource management often called as strategic human resource management. Even more, a key concept of this human resource management approach is the pivotal role of bundles of human resource management practices in facilitating the accomplishment of strategic goals.

Following this approach, various human resource management researchers have highlighted the vital role of human resource management policies and practices in engendering positive organizational outcomes. One of the most seminal studies pertains to Huselid (1995) who demonstrated the effect of human resource practices on both employee outcomes (turnover and productivity) and organizational outcomes (financial performance). In addition, MacDuffie (1995) showed that assembly plants which integrated a bundle of human resource management practices into their strategy presented greater productivity and quality compared to those that adopted more traditional practices. Likewise, subsequent empirical research (Delaney & Huselid, 1996; Delery & Doty, 1996; Huselid, Jackson, & Schuler, 1997, Ostroff & Bowen, 2000) provided further empirical insights into the relationship between various HPWP and performance outcomes.

This positive impact is attributed to the so called high performance work practices (HPWP) which are also referred to as high performance work systems or high involvement work practices. Evans and Davis (2005) defined HPWP as *an integrated system of HR practices that are internally consistent (alignment among HR practices) and externally consistent (alignment with organizational strategy) that include selective staffing, self-managed teams, decentralized decision making, extensive training, flexible job assignments, open communication and performance-contingent compensation* (p. 759-760). In this sense, strategic human resource management posits that these practices promote combined effects through mutually reinforce one another and, as a result, augment organizational performance (Dyer & Reeves, 1995).

Therefore, these HPWP aim at acquiring, developing, motivating and retaining the human capital of each company and organization which in turn will enhance organizational performance (Combs, Liu, Hall, & Ketchen, 2006). In order to offer further insights and elucidate the underlying mechanisms that account for the relationship between HPWPs and organizational performance, scholars have accentuated three core processes namely, knowledge and skills, motivation and commitment, and employee relationships.

As regards the former, HPWPs are predicated on human capital theory (Becker, 1975) which postulates that such practices are likely to increase organizational performance through enhancing employees' repertoire of knowledge and skills. In other words, HPWPs foster and cultivate employees' knowledge and skills and employees have the appropriate "tools" (e.g. problem solving, creative work behavior) to cope with work issues and demonstrate improved individual performance which leads to organizational performance.

Additionally, a second mechanism that associates HPWPs with organizational performance lies in the higher levels of employees' motivation and commitment. In this sense, organizations that implement HPWPs result in developing a long-term relationship with their employees and, as a consequence, the latter demonstrates elevated levels of motivation and commitment which, in turn, increase organizational performance (Tsui, Pearce, Porter, & Tripoli, 1997). Hence, commitment-oriented human resource practices nourish such an organizational culture and climate that augments employee motivation and thus contribute to organizational performance (Gittell, Seidner, & Wimbush, 2010). More recently, researchers have emphasized the importance of employee-employee relationships in explaining the linkage between HPWPs and organizational performance (Evans & Davis, 2005; Gant, Ichniowski, & Shaw, 2002; Gittell et al., 2010). Relationships among employees are considered to play an important role in promoting increased organizational performance. In part, this is attributed to the concept of organizational social capital. Organizational social capital is defined "as a resource reflecting the character of social relations within the organization" and *is realized through members' levels of collective goal orientation and shared trust, which create value by facilitating successful collective action* (Leana & Van Buren 1999, p. 538). Such a capital may benefit organization and increase their performance through facilitating employees' access to various resources and enabling knowledge sharing (Levin & Cross, 2004).

HIGH PERFORMANCE WORK PRACTICES IN ORGANIZATIONS

Recently, based on extant research over the last 20 years Posthuma and his colleagues (Posthuma, Campion, Masimova, & Campion, 2013) provided a coherent taxonomy of HPWPs. They separated numerous HPWPs into some basic categories, each of which includes a variety of practices. Based on this taxonomy and extant research, this chapter attempts to delineate core human resource management policies by focusing on some of the most salient HPWPs.

Job and Work Design

Job and work design is a core activity of human resource planning and encompasses practices that relate to specific elements of jobs and relationships between jobs as well as the organizational structure (Posthuma, et al., 2013). Job and work design has its roots in early motivational theories such as Herzberg's two-factor theory (1966) and the job characteristics model developed by Hackman and Oldham (1975, 1976). Regarding the former, Herzberg argued that there are some, intrinsic in nature, factors related to work (called motivators) that promote need for achievement, recognition, advancement and growth. As such, he noted that in order to facilitate employees' motivation and satisfaction job should be designed in enriched forms compared to more simplistic types of design. Building on the aforementioned theory, Hackman and Oldham posited that there are five core job characteristics (skill variety, task identity, task significance, autonomy and job-based feedback) that will lead to positive psychological states (meaningfulness, responsibility for work outcomes, knowledge of the results of the work) which, in turn, will enhance personal and work outcomes (motivation, satisfaction, performance and low absenteeism and turnover). High performance job and work design practices include among others job enlargement and enrichment, job rotation, self-managed work teams and decentralized participative decision making.

Job Enlargement and Enrichment

Job enlargement refers to the horizontal expansion of an employee's job by adding more different tasks whereas job enrichment involves the vertical enhancement of a job by offering more responsibilities and control in relation to conducting the tasks (Chung & Ross, 1977). Both job enlargement and enrichment are likely to increase employees' self-efficacy in terms of carrying out broader and proactive work tasks

(Parker, 1998). Although some authors have proposed the positive relationship between job enlargement and employee responses (Hulin & Blood, 1968), the majority of empirical studies regarding work redesign has addressed the pivotal role of job enrichment in triggering positive employee outcomes. For instance, research has shown that job enrichment has been associated with higher job satisfaction, involvement, loyalty and performance, as well as lower turnover and absenteeism (Fried & Ferris, 1987; Niehoff, Moorman, Blakely, & Fullerm, 2001; Orpen, 1979; Yang & Lee, 2009).

Job Rotation

Job rotation represents an important tool for organizations in order to reorganize and redesign work. Job rotation describes the official movement of employees from one job to another during a specific time period. This technique is of pivotal importance because it enhances employees' motivation and learning. In regard to the former, job rotation augments employees' motivation through alleviating their boredom, triggering their interest for their job and nourishing their social relationships (Kaymaz, 2010; Ortega, 2001). Concerning the latter, job rotation provides employees with the opportunity to conduct a variety of tasks and, even more, to garner further knowledge in relation to the overall production process (Allwood & Lee, 2004). On this basis, researchers have shown that job rotation has an effect on career-related outcomes such as, salary and promotion, perceptions of skill acquisition as well as positive affect (Campion, Cheraskin, & Stevens, 1994). Last, job rotation has been shown to be related to both job satisfaction and organizational commitment (Ho, Chang, Shih, & Liang, 2009).

Self-Managed Work Teams

Self-managed work teams have the power and authority to set goals, determine schedules and, in general, manage their own processes and function. Self-managing teams provide some important benefits in relation to the organizational operation because they promote allocation of decision making and employees' empowerment. Thus, they can also help organizations to cope with the present turbulent and competitive business environment. In this sense, extant research has argued that such teams enhance job satisfaction, organizational commitment, labor productivity, employee creativity and mitigate turnover (Cohen & Bailey, 1997; Cordery, Wright, & Wall, 1997; Glassop, 2002; Paulus, 2000)

Decentralized Participative Decisions

Decentralized participative decisions represent a delegation of decision making empowering, thus, employees. Providing employees with the opportunity to participate in decision making enhances their motivation through satisfying their needs of human development and growth. In addition, employee participation in decision making leads them to develop a sense of psychological ownership that is they act as if the organization belongs to them (Han, Chiang, & Chang, 2010). Extant research has also demonstrated that participative decision making has an effect on core employee outcomes including satisfaction, commitment and performance (Bakan, Suseno, Pinnington, & Money, 2004; Locke, Alavi, & Wagner, 1997; Mayer & Schoorman, 1998; Schweiger & Leana. 1986; Skott-Ladd, Travaglione, & Marshall, 2006).

Recruiting and Selection

Recruitment and selection constitutes one of the core human resource management policies. Research on such issues has received significant attention in the last decades (Breaugh, 2008). In general, recruiting and selection practices relate to the methods employed by organizations in order to select the most suitable individual for each vacancy based on the job and organizational fit. Such practices are of utmost importance because hired individuals and both their skills and abilities along with their work attitudes and behaviors largely determine the overall organizational performance. For example, researchers have revealed that such practices have a positive effect on organizational performance (Takeuchi, Lepak, Wang, & Takeuchi, 2007) through fostering a high level of collective human capital and emboldening a high degree of social exchange. Also, Michie and Sheehan (2005) indicated that recruitment and selection practices are positively associated with labor productivity. In the literature, there is a host of contemporary and innovative recruiting and selection practices. Some of the most important include employment tests or structured interviews, hiring selectivity or low selection ratio and specific and explicit hiring criteria.

Employment Tests or Structured Interviews

Both employment tests and structured interviews comprise two dominant selection tools that facilitate the effective staffing procedure. Regarding the former, there are various tests such as, ability, aptitude, intelligence and personality tests. Such types of employment tests have been substantially used in organizational context

(Furnham, 2008). Ability tests refer to those tests that attempt to measure already obtained individual skills and abilities whereas aptitude tests emphasize individual's potential to conduct specific tasks (Beardwell & Calydon, 2007). Moreover, intelligence tests measure the mental capacity of an individual whereas personality tests aim at measuring personality characteristics that relate to job performance such as, neuroticism, consciousness, self-esteem, generalized self-efficacy. In most cases, employment tests are supplementary of interviews. In fact, interviews have been positively correlated with some of the aforementioned tests (Campion, Palmer, & Campion, 1998; Campion et al., 1994). Interview constitutes the most widely used selection tool worldwide (Nikolaou, 2011). Salgado (1999; as cited in Robertson & Smith, 2001) demonstrated that highly structured interviews show higher predictive validity compared to those with little predetermined structure.

Hiring Selectivity or Low Selection Ratio

Selective hiring or low selection ratio is concerned with rigorous and sophisticated selection procedures. This method has been proposed as an important tool for organizations in order to recruit talented individuals and thus obtain a source of competitive advantage (Boxall, 1996; Marchington & Grugulis, 2000). In a similar mode, scholars (Thorsteinson & Ryan, 1997) argued that such a method also provides other symbolic facets namely the participants who are hired after a difficult selection process will be more attracted to the organization because they are likely to perceive themselves as members of an elite organization.

Specific and Explicit Hiring Criteria

By its nature, recruitment and selection is a manifold and complex process. As such, it is essential for contemporary organizations to design their staffing procedures in a specific way. In this vein, determining specific and explicit hiring criteria offers some important advantages. That is, it facilitates the effective fit between the applicant and the organization. Put differently, utilizing the job analysis tool, hiring criteria should be aligned not only with the specific job requirements but also with organizational goals, strategies, policies and practices (Olian & Rynes, 1984). In addition, specific hiring criteria enhance the possibility of attracting the most suitable human capital for each vacancy. Taken together, using specific and explicit hiring criteria enhances the overall effectiveness of the recruitment and selection process.

Training and Development

Training and development are two important factors that help organizations to cope with the fast-changing, turbulent and competitive business environment. Training is described as *the act, process or method by which one acquires any type of functional skill or ability that is required to perform a specific job* (Taormina 1997, p. 31) whereas development is the process of *becoming increasingly complex, more elaborate and differentiated, by virtue of learning and maturation* (Beardwell & Calydon 2007, p. 266). HPWPs that relate to the training and development encompass those that ameliorate employees' competencies in relation to both their present and future jobs (Posthuma et al., 2013). Training extensiveness and cross-functional or multi-skill training are, among others, some of the core HPWPs.

Training Extensiveness

The extensiveness of training programs that aim to develop knowledge, skills, and abilities are of utmost importance. Extensiveness of training involves *the depth of training required in order to ensure that trainees acquire appropriate levels of knowledge and skill proficiency by the end of training* (Day, Blair, Daniels, Kligyte, & Mumford, 2006, p. 383). Empirical research has demonstrated that extensive training contributes to organizational performance (Wan, Ong, & Kok, 2002) and innovation (Shipton, West, Dawson, Birdi, & Patterson, 2006).

Cross-Functional or Multi-Skill Training

Given the need for a competitive flexible and decentralized organizational environment, cross-functional and multi-skill training have emerged as effective human resource management tools. As such, compared to the single skill approach both aforementioned training methods nourish equipped employees with a much broader range of skills that are essential to cope with contemporary organizational context (Johnson, 2000; McGuinness & Bennett, 2006). Moreover, such training processes enhance employees' skills and broaden their repertoires of knowledge and experiences and therefore improve organizations' competitive advantages that emanate from their human resources. For instance, multi-skill training is likely to improve service quality in service industries such as, hospitality and healthcare (Chen & Wallace, 2011; Nandan & Agarwai, 2012).

Compensation and Benefits

Compensation and benefits refer to the direct and indirect rewards that organizations and companies offer to the employees in exchange of their work. The present group of practices is important because it motivates employees in order to demonstrate the desired behavior which, in turn, will lead to the achievement of organizational goals. In addition, most authors have considered tangible and financial rewards as synonymous to the general term of rewards. However, it is important to note that this category includes not only financial but nonfinancial rewards as well. In fact, given the current financial crisis and the limited organizational environment nonfinancial may comprise a strong catalyst of effective employee motivation and performance. Paired together, we focus on both financial and nonfinancial rewards namely pay for performance and verbal recognition.

Pay for Performance

Linking employees' pay to performance has long been proposed as an effective method to motivate them and enhance their performance. The influence of this method is attributed to two general mechanisms. More specifically, authors (Gerhart & Rynes 2003; Rynes, Gerhart, & Parks, 2005) argued that there two potential effects: first there is the potential for an "incentive effect", that is, the impact of pay for performance on employees' performance, and, second, there is the potential for a "sorting effect", namely the effect of pay for performance on the workforce processes through attracting and retention of appropriate human resources.

Verbal Recognition

Recognition has been proposed as a motivational factor from the two-factor theory of motivation (Herzberg, 1966). In addition, other scholars have highlighted the important effect of recognition on employees' motivation (McGregor, 1960; Porter & Lawler, 1968; Vroom, 1964). Although employee recognition *has not been systematically conceptualized nor has it been subject to a satisfactory theoretical integration* (Brun & Dugas, 2008, p. 716) its positive role is indisputable. Recognizing employees' contribution to organizational performance has been associated with core outcomes such as, organizational commitment and involvement, job satisfaction and turnover (Abualrub & Al - Zaru, 2008; Appelbaum & Kamal, 2000; McNeese - Smith, 1997; Romzek, 1985; Saunderson, 2004). Verbal recognition constitutes not only a costless but an effective way of motivating and rewarding employees (Goode et al., 1993). In addition, one of the core advantages of this reward pertains to the fact that supervisors and middle managers can easily satisfy employees' need for recognition without necessarily the formal involvement of top management (Appelbaum & Kamal, 2000).

Performance Management and Appraisal

Performance management has received a wide array of definitions in the management literature (Buchner, 2007). Armstrong (1998) termed performance management as a *strategic and integrated approach to delivering sustained success to organizations by improving the performance of the people who work in them and by developing the capabilities of teams and individual contributors* (p. 7). This definition attempts to cover not only organizational attempts to measure individual and team performance but also the important issue of aligning such performance with organizational strategies (Zhang & Li, 2009). Recent research (Farndale, Hope-Hailey, & Kelliher, 2010) has shown that contemporary performance management practices foster employees' perceptions of both organizational justice and commitment. Two of the most widely used and core practices are appraisal based on objective results and involving employees in setting appraisal objectives.

Appraisal based on Objective Results

Performance appraisal comprises a substantial and widely researched topic in human resource management. Appraisal systems aim at assessing employees' performance based on a variety of criteria and indicators. It is a formal process that is usually implemented by the human resource department on an annual basis. Due to the inherently high levels of subjectivity and complexity of such procedures it often turns out that it is beneficial for organizations to make appraisal more objective. That is, to set objective results based on which employees will be assessed. This will probably eliminate potential complaints and mitigate employees' perceptions of organizational injustice.

Involving Employees in Setting Appraisal Objectives

As noted above, organizations may benefit from developing objective appraisals. Even more, organizations often involve employees in setting appraisal objectives. The basic logic behind such processes pertains to the improved understanding and agreement between employees and employer. More specifically, it is logical that employees who participate in setting the appraisal objectives demonstrate a clearer understanding of what is assessed and, further, they experience higher levels of psychological ownership and agreement against these objectives. In parallel, those employees who are involved in determining such goals feel that their organizations listen to their views and opinions and, thus, they feel greater levels of job meaningfulness and satisfaction and organizational commitment. Employee attitude surveys and job security are two key HPWPs which are of utmost importance for organizational functioning.

Employee Relations

Employee relations are a core human resource management policy that emphasizes the relationships between employer and employees. Such processes are critical for the effective management of organizations because they enable them to cultivate and form a trusting and ethical environment combined with a productive culture and climate. When such elements are found in the organization, employees are likely to exhibit positive attitude and behavior (Chuang & Liao, 2010; Cullen et al., 2003; Kim & Wright, 2011).

Employee Attitude Surveys

Employee attitude surveys have long been offered as an effective practice for assessing their perceptions and attitudes vis-à-vis work-related issues (Kraut, 2006; Rogelberg, Luong, Sederburg, & Cristol, 2000). In fact, in the last decades there has been a burgeoning use of these surveys (Mueller, Voelkle, & Hattrup, 2011). Given the importance of assessing employees' attitudes towards a host of workplace elements such as, their job, peers, supervisors or organization, such surveys comprise a useful tool for organizational development, organizational decision making and, in general, human resource management.

Job Security-Emphasis on Permanent Jobs

In the context of contemporary flexible employment relations employees often worry about their stability and job continuity (Loi, Ngo, Zhang, & Lau, 2011). Thus, job (in)security constitutes a critical factor that affects employees' emotions, attitudes and behaviors. In the extant literature job security has been separated into two important facets namely perceived job (in)security and the actual job loss. Most the studies address the former which describe as *a psychological state in which workers vary in their expectations of future job continuity within an organization* (Kraimer, Wayne,

Liden, & Sparrowe, 2005, p. 390). In this vein, several researchers have reported the detrimental impact of job insecurity on core employee outcomes such as, job stress, well-being, organizational commitment, job satisfaction and performance (Ashford, Lee, & Bobko, 1989; De Witte, 1999; Iversen & Sabroe, 1988; Kinnunen & Natti, 2004; Mohr, 2000; Sverke & Hellgren, 2002).

HPWP IN HEALTHCARE ORGANIZATIONS

Like other contemporary firms, healthcare organizations aim at maximizing their effectiveness. Nevertheless, in the healthcare industry effectiveness is -to a great extent- dependent upon improving patients' health and avoiding deaths (West, Guthrie, Dawson, Borrill, & Carter, 2006). Even more, healthcare industry presents some particular characteristics that influence the organizational operation and effectiveness. For example, contemporary healthcare organizations are faced with a plethora of challenges such as, intensive competition, limited financial resources, staff shortages, brain drain and work intensification. Furthermore, there is a large and multi-professional workforce and a plethora of stakeholders (government, insurance organizations, media, management, patients, e.t.c.) (Hyde, Sparrow, Boaden, & Harris, 2013). In this problematic context, healthcare organizations struggle to provide enhanced patient care quality and ameliorate their effectiveness.

Toward this end, recent theoretical and empirical research in healthcare settings has highlighted HPWPs as an effective tool for dealing with aforementioned issues and promoting higher performance outcomes. In this sense, numerous empirical studies have shown the positive role of HPWPs in producing both employee and organizational outcomes. Regarding the former, several scholars have reported the relationship of HPWPs with individual outcomes including job satisfaction, organizational commitment, social identification and organizational citizenship behavior (Boselie, 2010; Harmon et al., 2003; Young, Bartram, Stanton, & Leggat, 2010). As such, implementing HPWPs like those that were previously described is likely to lead healthcare organizations to create a workforce that likes and enjoys its job (job satisfaction), feels committed and high levels of identification with the organization (organizational commitment and identification) and displays discretionary behavior beyond its formal job requirements which nevertheless promotes effective organizational functioning (organizational citizenship behavior).

In parallel, scholars have shown the influence of HPWPs on core organizational outcomes. For instance, West and his colleagues (2002, 2006) have provided some of the most seminal findings. In their studies, they revealed that, after controlling for prior mortality and other factors such as the ratio of doctors to patients, these practices are related to patient mortality. Consequently, these studies showed that above and beyond the influences of a host of significant control variables, HPWPs that focus, among others, on training, decentralized decision making, teams, and job security are likely to be effective in relation to high-quality healthcare. That is, such practices are likely to *be mutually reinforcing and coherent as an interconnected system, and therefore produce the behaviors* and therefore *lead to the provision of high quality health care and, as a consequence, lower patient mortality* (West et al., 2006, p. 996).

Combining, though, both individual and organizational outcomes, most empirical studies have attempted to clarify the impact of HPWPs on organizational outcomes using employee outcomes as a core intervening mechanism. For example, in a nine-hospital study researchers have indicated that the strength of relational coordination among healthcare professionals (doctors, nurses, physical therapists, social workers, e.t.c.) mediated the relationship between HPWPs and both quality and efficiency outcomes for their patients (Gittell et al., 2010). In a similar mode, scholars (Bartram, Karimi, Leggat, & Stanton, 2014; Bonias, Bartram, Leggat, & Stanton, 2010) demonstrated that HPWPs positively affect quality of care through the mediating role of psychological empowerment. In addition, Lee, Lee and Kang (2012) showed that HPWPs are likely to lead to employee engagement which in turn may improve customer satisfaction and loyalty. Along this line of reasoning, Baluch, Salge and Piening (2013) have elucidate the relationship between HPWPs and patient satisfaction using employees' civility towards patients (namely the extent to which employees treat patients with courtesy, dignity and respect) as an underlying mechanism.

Furthermore, drawing on the aforementioned relationship between HPWPs and both employee and organizational outcomes, scholars have attempted to explain the boundary conditions that may affect the role of HPWPs in engendering positive outcomes. For example, a recent study (Fan, Cui, Zhang, Zhu, Härtel, & Nyland, 2014) showed that the use of HPWPs augment employees' subjective well-being and mitigate their levels of burnout. However, they also revealed that both organizational-based self-esteem and the physician-nurse relationship moderated the aforementioned associations. That is, employees with higher levels of organizational-based self-esteem presented a stronger relationship between HPWPs and these two specific outcomes. In addition, physician-nurse relationship influenced the relationship between HPWPs and subjective well-being. Relatedly, scholars (Zhang, Zhu, Dowling, & Bartram, 2013) reported a significant effect of HPWPs on work engagement and emotional exhaustion. Yet, this impact is dependent on employee perceptions about the employee-employer relationship. More specifically, employee perceptions about the economic nature of the relationship with the employer affects the possibility that such practices will result in emotional exhaustion whereas the social nature influences the possibility that HPWPs will lead to work engagement.

SOLUTIONS AND RECOMMENDATIONS

Human resource management policies and practices comprise a relatively contemporary tool for organizations in order to cope with the current complex, unpropitious and problematic environment. In this respect, recent voluminous empirical studies have delineated the salutary role of HPWPs in stimulating positive outcomes and dampening negative ones. These outcomes are of utmost importance because they nurture an organizational environment which fosters employees' development, motivation, commitment and positive relationships and, in turn, enhances key organizational outcomes such as, performance, effectiveness and productivity. Therefore, it is essential that academics and practitioners should be directed towards a better understanding of such HPWPs and their potential effect on both employee and organizational outcomes in the healthcare context.

Yet, despite recent studies on HPWPs in healthcare organizations, more theoretical and empirical research is needed. This dearth may be explained by the fact that there are still some problems that can hamper the theoretical adoption and practical implementation of such practices. First, at a theoretical level the extant literature employs a great number of different terminologies (high-commitment work practices, high involvement work systems, e.t.c.) and further there is a lack of a specific and concise bundle of such work practices (Posthuma et al., 2013). Although recent attempts have attempted to provide a coherent taxonomy regarding HPWPs (Posthuma et al., 2013), additional work needs to be done and particularly in the context of healthcare industry.

Another pertinent issue relates to the synergistic effect of specific work practices which reinforce one another. Namely, aligning different HPWPS that have the appropriate matching and coordination is purported to promote better results compared to the piecemeal implementation of these practices (e.g. Becker & Gerhart, 1996; MacDuffie, 1995). Therefore, an additional challenge for both healthcare academics and professionals is to corroborate the usefulness of integrating specific bundles of HPWPs in relation to core organizational outcomes.

In a similar sense, scholars (Boselie, Dietz, & Boon, 2005) have argued that the incorporation of contingency factors that pertain to critical issues such as, organization's environment its strategy or its systems is essential for increasing the validity of existing results. In this context, the idea of an effective bundle of HPWPs should not solely focus on the formation of an amalgam of practices. Rather, it is also the architecture of such processes which should *suit the changing needs of the organization and contribute to the achievement of organizational flexibility or longevity* (Purcell, 1999, p. 38). Combined, it is of utmost importance for theoretical development and empirical evidence as regards HPWPs to examine potential contextual and boundary conditions that may impair the positive role of HPWPs in the operation and effectiveness of healthcare organizations.

Last, practitioners have lagged behind academic interest. Many organizations still refrain from implementing HPWPs due to environmental threats, government regulations, or political factors (Johns, 1993). Even more, organizations may be skeptical about the usefulness of such contemporary practices or the elevated cost that may bring about (Cappelli & Neumark, 2001). As a result, given the limited and problematic healthcare context, organizations are reluctant to adopt HPWPs which may potentially raise their costs. However, based on the aforementioned promising empirical results on many industries and on healthcare organizations, the latter should implement HPWP that will strengthen their operation (McAlearney, Garman, Song, McHugh, Robbins, & Harrison, 2011).

FUTURE RESEARCH DIRECTIONS

Despite the recent increasing empirical evidence on the relationship between HPWPs and organizational outcomes there still some issues which need to answered in order to provide some more compelling and holistic findings. As noted above, there is a lack of an integrated and concise bundle of HPWPs that will emerge as a useful tool for ameliorating healthcare organizations' operation and effectiveness. Toward this end, future studies could attempt to examine pertinent HPWPs which will fit healthcare environment and its specific contextual circumstances.

Furthermore, some fruitful avenues for future research could aim at investigating both potential underlying mechanisms (mediators) that may provide a better understanding of the relationship between HPWPs and organizational outcomes and boundary conditions (moderators) that may constrain or facilitate this effect. Extant theoretical and empirical studies have highlighted three core mechanisms that associate HPWPs with organizational outcomes. As noted above, HPWPs are likely to trigger employees' knowledge and skills, their motivation and commitment, and also facilitate the development of productive employee relationships. Viewed in this light, future research could examine various pertinent constructs that will advance our understanding of the intervening factors that explain the effect of HPWPs on core organizational outcomes in the healthcare industry. At the same time, there is also a need to investigate the conditions under which HPWPs are related to both employee and organizational outcomes. Thus far, prior empirical studies in healthcare literature have largely neglected the investigation of potential moderating factors that may influence the direction or magnitude of the relationship between HPWPs and key outcomes (see Bartram et al., 2009, for an exception). This stream of research will offer valuable and holistic insights about the universality of these relationships.

An additional area for further research pertains to the important role that leadership plays in determining employees' emotions, attitudes and behaviors. In this vein, future research might address the interaction between HPWPs and contemporary leadership styles in accounting for higher levels of organizational outcomes. Several researchers have proposed that the leadership style of managers is a key factor in affecting employees' perceptions and interpretations of the work environment and climate (Kozlowski & Doherty, 1989; Richardson & Vandenberg, 2005). As a consequence, several positive leadership styles including transformational, ethical, authentic and empowering may support formal HPWPs in order to be effectively diffused and adopted by employees which sequentially will lead to better organizational outcomes.

In a similar vein, culture may also offer a fertile ground for future research directions. Following the seminal categorization of Hofstede (1991), future studies could examine the influence of HPWPs on employee attitudes and behaviors across various levels of cultural values such as power distance, reduction uncertainty or individualism. Moreover, scholars (Lawrence & Lorsch, 1987; Robert et al., 2000) have argued that culture may facilitate or hinder the adoption and implementation of a specific strategy or management practices. Thus, it is essential that future empirical studies might incorporate elements of national and organizational culture when examining HPWPs.

CONCLUSION

HPWPs encompass a wide range of human resource management practices which cover policies such as, recruitment and selection, training and development, performance management, rewards and employee relations. These practices are perceived as integrated bundles that reinforce one another and therefore demonstrate synergistic effects on positive outcomes. In this respect, when organizations implement a bundle of these practices which have the appropriate fit they are likely to enhance, among others, organizational performance.

For the above reasons, HPWPs have attracted increasing interest among both academics and practitioners. Despite human resource management researchers have long addressed the pivotal role of HPWPs in promoting employee and organizational outcomes, in the healthcare industry a stream of research has only recently focused on their importance in relation to core employee, patient and organizational outcomes. Yet, the nascent findings corroborate its usefulness especially in the contemporary deficient and problematic environment. In fact, HPWPs have emerged as an effective tool for healthcare organizations to cope with their limitations and complexities, provide better service quality and enhance patient satisfaction.

As such, this chapter attempted to describe some of the most core human resources policies and their respective practices including, among others, selective hiring, employment security, self-managed teams, job enrichment, multi-skill training, and verbal recognition and highlight their importance to healthcare organizations. Synthesizing and implementing bundles of these HPWPs may provide healthcare organizations with potential solutions to cope with the contemporary unfavorable environment and will enable them to create a win-win-win situation in which employees will be satisfied with their workplace, patients will experience qualitative services and healthcare organizations will increase their effectiveness.

REFERENCES

AbuAlRub, R. F., & Al-Zaru, I. M. (2008). Job stress, recognition, job performance and intention to stay at work among Jordanian hospital nurses. *Journal of Nursing Management*, *16*(3), 227–236. doi:10.1111/j.1365-2834.2007.00810.x PMID:18324981

Allwood, J. M., & Lee, W. L. (2004). The impact of job rotation on problem solving skills. *International Journal of Production Research*, *42*(5), 865–881. doi:10.1080/00207540310001631566

Appelbaum, S. H., & Kamal, R. (2000). An analysis of the utilization and effectiveness of non-financial incentives in small business. *Journal of Management Development*, *19*(9), 733–763. doi:10.1108/02621710010378200

Armstrong, M., & Baron, A. (1998). *Performance Management: The New Realities*. London: Institute of Personnel and Development.

Ashford, S. J., Lee, C., & Bobko, P. (1989). Content, cause, and consequences of job insecurity: A theory-based measure and substantive test. *Academy of Management Journal, 32*(4), 803–829. doi:10.2307/256569

Bakan, I., Suseno, Y., Pinnington, A., & Money, A. (2004). The influence of financial participation and participation in decision-making on employee job attitudes. *International Journal of Human Resource Management, 15*(3), 587–616. doi:10.1080/09585192.2004.10057654

Baluch, A. M., Salge, T. O., & Piening, E. P. (2013). Untangling the relationship between HRM and hospital performance: The mediating role of attitudinal and behavioural HR outcomes. *International Journal of Human Resource Management, 24*(16), 3038–3061. doi:10.1080/09585192.2013.775027

Barney, J. (1991). Firm resources and sustained competitive advantage. *Journal of Management, 17*(1), 99–120. doi:10.1177/014920639101700108

Bartram, T., Casimir, G., Leggat, S. G., Stanton, P., Bonias, D., & Cheng, C. (2009). *Employee participation as a moderator on the high performance work systems and the perception of quality of care relationship in a large regional Australian health service| NOVA*. The University of Newcastle's Digital Repository.

Bartram, T., Karimi, L., Leggat, S. G., & Stanton, P. (2014). Social identification: Linking high performance work systems, psychological empowerment and patient care. *International Journal of Human Resource Management, 25*(17), 2401–2419. doi:10.1080/09585192.2014.880152

Beardwell, J., & Claydon, T. (Eds.). (2007). *Human resource management: a contemporary approach*. Pearson Education.

Becker, B., & Gerhart, B. (1996). The impact of human resource management on organizational performance: Progress and prospects. *Academy of Management Journal, 39*(4), 779–801. doi:10.2307/256712

Becker, G. S. (1975). *Human Capital*. New York: Columbia University Press.

Bonias, D., Bartram, T., Leggat, S. G., & Stanton, P. (2010). Does psychological empowerment mediate the relationship between high performance work systems and patient care quality in hospitals? *Asia Pacific Journal of Human Resources, 48*(3), 319–337. doi:10.1177/1038411110381667

Boselie, P. (2010). High performance work practices in the health care sector: A Dutch case study. *International Journal of Manpower, 31*(1), 42–58. doi:10.1108/01437721011031685

Boselie, P., Dietz, G., & Boon, C. (2005). Commonalities and contradictions in HRM and performance research. *Human Resource Management Journal, 15*(3), 67–94. doi:10.1111/j.1748-8583.2005.tb00154.x

Boxall, P. (1996). The strategic HRM debate and the resource-based view of the firm. *Human Resource Management Journal, 6*(3), 59–75. doi:10.1111/j.1748-8583.1996.tb00412.x

Boxall, P. F., & Purcell, J. (2003). *Strategy and Human Resource Management.* Basingstoke: Palgrave Macmillan.

Breaugh, J. A. (2008). Employee recruitment: Current knowledge and important areas for future research. *Human Resource Management Review, 18*(3), 103–118. doi:10.1016/j.hrmr.2008.07.003

Brun, J. P., & Dugas, N. (2008). An analysis of employee recognition: Perspectives on human resources practices. *International Journal of Human Resource Management, 19*(4), 716–730. doi:10.1080/09585190801953723

Buchner, T. W. (2007). Performance management theory: A look from the performer's perspective with implications for HRD. *Human Resource Development International, 10*(1), 59–73. doi:10.1080/13678860601170294

Campion, M. A., Cheraskin, L., & Stevens, M. J. (1994). Career-related antecedents and outcomes of job rotation. *Academy of Management Journal, 37*(6), 1518–1542. doi:10.2307/256797

Campion, M. A., Palmer, D. K., & Campion, J. E. (1998). Structuring employment interviews to improve reliability, validity, and users' reactions. *Current Directions in Psychological Science, 7*(3), 77–82. doi:10.1111/1467-8721.ep10773001

Cappelli, P., & Neumark, D. (2001). Do "high-performance" work practices improve establishment-level outcomes? *Industrial & Labor Relations Review, 54*(4), 737–775. doi:10.1177/001979390105400401

Chen, L. C., & Wallace, M. (2011). Multiskilling of frontline managers in the five star hotel industry in Taiwan. *Research and Practice in Human Resource Management, 19*(1), 25.

Chuang, C. H., & Liao, H. U. I. (2010). Strategic human resource management in service context: Taking care of business by taking care of employees and customers. *Personnel Psychology*, *63*(1), 153–196. doi:10.1111/j.1744-6570.2009.01165.x

Chung, K. H., & Ross, M. F. (1977). Differences in motivational properties between job enlargement and job enrichment. *Academy of Management Review*, *2*(1), 113–122.

Cohen, S. G., & Bailey, D. E. (1997). What makes teams work: Group effectiveness research from the shop floor to the executive suite. *Journal of Management*, *23*(3), 239–290. doi:10.1177/014920639702300303

Combs, J., Liu, Y., Hall, A., & Ketchen, D. (2006). How much do high-performance work practices matter? A meta-analysis of their effects on organizational performance. *Personnel Psychology*, *59*(3), 501–528. doi:10.1111/j.1744-6570.2006.00045.x

Cordery, J. L., Wright, B., & Wall, T. D. (1997, April). Towards a more comprehensive and integrated approach to work design: Production uncertainty and self-managing work team performance. In *12th Annual Conference of the Society for Industrial and Organisational Psychology*.

Cullen, J. B., Parboteeah, K. P., & Victor, B. (2003). The effects of ethical climates on organizational commitment: A two-study analysis. *Journal of Business Ethics*, *46*(2), 127–141. doi:10.1023/A:1025089819456

Day, E. A., Blair, C., Daniels, S., Kligyte, V., & Mumford, M. D. (2006). Linking instructional objectives to the design of instructional environments: The Integrative Training Design Matrix. *Human Resource Management Review*, *16*(3), 376–395. doi:10.1016/j.hrmr.2006.05.007

Delaney, J. T., & Huselid, M. A. (1996). The impact of human resource management practices on perceptions of organizational performance. *Academy of Management Journal*, *39*(4), 949–969. doi:10.2307/256718

Delery, J. E., & Doty, D. H. (1996). Modes of theorizing in strategic human resource management: Tests of universalistic, contingency, and configurational performance predictions. *Academy of Management Journal*, *39*(4), 802–835. doi:10.2307/256713

Dyer, L., & Reeves, T. (1995). Human resource strategies and firm performance: What do we know and where do we need to go? *International Journal of Human Resource Management*, *6*(3), 656–670. doi:10.1080/09585199500000041

Evans, W. R., & Davis, W. D. (2005). High-performance work systems and organizational performance: The mediating role of internal social structure. *Journal of Management, 31*(5), 758–775. doi:10.1177/0149206305279370

Fan, D., Cui, L., Zhang, M. M., Zhu, C. J., Härtel, C. E., & Nyland, C. (2014). Influence of high performance work systems on employee subjective well-being and job burnout: Empirical evidence from the Chinese healthcare sector. *International Journal of Human Resource Management, 25*(7), 931–950. doi:10.1080/09585192.2014.876740

Farndale, E., Hope-Hailey, V., & Kelliher, C. (2011). High commitment performance management: The roles of justice and trust. *Personnel Review, 40*(1), 5–23. doi:10.1108/00483481111095492

Fried, Y., & Ferris, G. R. (1987). The validity of the job characteristics model: A review and meta-analysis. *Personnel Psychology, 40*(2), 287–322. doi:10.1111/j.1744-6570.1987.tb00605.x

Furnham, A. (2008). *Personality and intelligence at work: Exploring and explaining individual differences at work*. Routledge. doi:10.4324/9780203938911

Gant, J., Ichniowski, C., & Shaw, K. (2002). Social capital and organizational change in high-involvement and traditional work organizations. *Journal of Economics & Management Strategy, 11*(2), 289–328. doi:10.1162/105864002317474576

Gerhart, B., & Rynes, S. (2003). *Compensation: Theory, evidence, and strategic implications*. SAGE publications.

Gittell, J. H., Seidner, R., & Wimbush, J. (2010). A relational model of how high-performance work systems work. *Organization Science, 21*(2), 490–506. doi:10.1287/orsc.1090.0446

Glassop, L. I. (2002). The organizational benefits of teams. *Human Relations, 55*(2), 225–249. doi:10.1177/0018726702055002184

Goode, C. J., Ibarra, V., Blegen, M. A., Boshart-Yoder, T., Cram, E., Finn, L., & Anderson-Bruner, J. et al. (1993). What kind of recognition do staff nurses want? *AJN The American Journal of Nursing, 93*(5), 64–68. PMID:8488903

Hackman, J. R., & Oldham, G. R. (1975). Development of the job diagnostic survey. *The Journal of Applied Psychology, 60*(2), 159–170. doi:10.1037/h0076546

Hackman, J. R., & Oldham, G. R. (1976). Motivation through the design of work: Test of a theory. *Organizational Behavior and Human Performance*, *16*(2), 250–279. doi:10.1016/0030-5073(76)90016-7

Han, T. S., Chiang, H. H., & Chang, A. (2010). Employee participation in decision making, psychological ownership and knowledge sharing: Mediating role of organizational commitment in Taiwanese high-tech organizations. *International Journal of Human Resource Management*, *21*(12), 2218–2233. doi:10.1080/09585192.2010.509625

Harmon, J., Scotti, D. J., Behson, S., Farias, G., Petzel, R., Neuman, J. H., & Keashly, L. (2003). Effects of high-involvement work systems on employee satisfaction and service costs in veterans healthcare. *Journal of Healthcare Management*, *48*(6), 393–405. PMID:14671948

Herzberg, F. I. (1966). *Work and the nature of man*. Cleveland: World.

Ho, W. H., Chang, C. S., Shih, Y. L., & Liang, R. D. (2009). Effects of job rotation and role stress among nurses on job satisfaction and organizational commitment. *BMC Health Services Research*, *9*(1), 8. doi:10.1186/1472-6963-9-8 PMID:19138390

Hulin, C. L., & Blood, M. R. (1968). Job enlargement, individual differences, and worker responses. *Psychological Bulletin*, *69*(1), 41–55. doi:10.1037/h0025356

Huselid, M. A. (1995). The impact of human resource management practices on turnover, productivity, and corporate financial performance. *Academy of Management Journal*, *38*(3), 635–672. doi:10.2307/256741

Huselid, M. A., Jackson, S. E., & Schuler, R. S. (1997). Technical and strategic human resources management effectiveness as determinants of firm performance. *Academy of Management Journal*, *40*(1), 171–188. doi:10.2307/257025

Hyde, P., Sparrow, P., Boaden, R., & Harris, C. (2013). High performance HRM: NHS employee perspectives. *Journal of Health Organization and Management*, *27*(3), 296–311. doi:10.1108/JHOM-10-2012-0206 PMID:23885395

Iversen, L., & Sabroe, S. (1988). Psychological weil-being among unemployed and employed people after a company closedown: A longitudinal study. *The Journal of Social Issues*, *44*(4), 141–152. doi:10.1111/j.1540-4560.1988.tb02096.x

Johns, G. (1993). Constraints on the adoption of psychology-based personnel practices: Lessons from organizational innovation. *Personnel Psychology*, *46*(3), 569–592. doi:10.1111/j.1744-6570.1993.tb00885.x

Kaymaz, K. (2010). The effects of job rotation practices on motivation: A research on managers in the automotive organizations. *Business and Economics Research Journal*, *1*(3), 69–85.

Kinnunen, U., & Nätti, J. (1994). Job insecurity in Finland: Antecedents and consequences. *European Journal of Work and Organizational Psychology*, *4*(3), 297–321. doi:10.1080/13594329408410490

Kraimer, M. L., Wayne, S. J., Liden, R. C., & Sparrowe, R. T. (2005). The role of job security in understanding the relationship between employees' perceptions of temporary workers and employees' performance. *The Journal of Applied Psychology*, *90*(2), 389–398. doi:10.1037/0021-9010.90.2.389 PMID:15769247

Kraut, A. I. (2006). *Getting action from organizational surveys: New concepts, technologies, and applications*. San Francisco, CA: Jossey-Bass.

Leana, C. R., & Van Buren, H. J. (1999). Organizational social capital and employment practices. *Academy of Management Review*, *24*(3), 538–555.

Lee, S. M., Lee, D., & Kang, C. Y. (2012). The impact of high-performance work systems in the health-care industry: Employee reactions, service quality, customer satisfaction, and customer loyalty. *Service Industries Journal*, *32*(1), 17–36. doi:10.1080/02642069.2010.545397

Levin, D. Z., & Cross, R. (2004). The strength of weak ties you can trust: The mediating role of trust in effective knowledge transfer. *Management Science*, *50*(11), 1477–1490. doi:10.1287/mnsc.1030.0136

Locke, E., Alavi, M., & Wagner, J. (1997). Participation in deci sion-making: An information exchange perspective. In G. Ferris (Ed.), *Research in personal and human re sources management* (Vol. 15, pp. 293–331). Greenwich, CT: JAI Press.

Loi, R., Ngo, H. Y., Zhang, L., & Lau, V. P. (2011). The interaction between leader–member exchange and perceived job security in predicting employee altruism and work performance. *Journal of Occupational and Organizational Psychology*, *84*(4), 669–685. doi:10.1348/096317910X510468

MacDuffie, J. P. (1995). Human resource bundles and manufacturing performance: Organizational logic and flexible production systems in the world auto industry. *Industrial & Labor Relations Review, 48*(2), 197–221. doi:10.1177/001979399504800201

Marchington, M., & Grugulis, I. (2000). 'Best practice'human resource management: Perfect opportunity or dangerous illusion? *International Journal of Human Resource Management, 11*(6), 1104–1124. doi:10.1080/09585190050177184

Mayer, R. C., & Schoorman, F. D. (1998). Differentiating antecedents of organizational commitment: A test of March and Simon's model. *Journal of Organizational Behavior, 19*(1), 15–28. doi:10.1002/(SICI)1099-1379(199801)19:1<15::AID-JOB816>3.0.CO;2-C

McAlearney, A. S., Garman, A. N., Song, P. H., McHugh, M., Robbins, J., & Harrison, M. I. (2011). High-performance work systems in health care management, part 2: Qualitative evidence from five case studies. *Health Care Management Review, 36*(3), 214–226. doi:10.1097/HMR.0b013e3182100dc4 PMID:21646881

McGregor, D. (1960). *The human side of enterprise*. New York.

McGuinness, S., & Bennett, J. (2006). Examining the link between skill shortages, training composition and productivity levels in the construction industry: Evidence from Northern Ireland 1. *International Journal of Human Resource Management, 17*(2), 265–279. doi:10.1080/09585190500405538

McNeese-Smith, D. K. (1997). The influence of manager behavior on nurses' job satisfaction, productivity, and commitment. *The Journal of Nursing Administration, 27*(9), 47–55. doi:10.1097/00005110-199709000-00011 PMID:9300015

Michie, J., & Sheehan, M. (2005). Business strategy, human resources, labour market flexibility and competitive advantage. *International Journal of Human Resource Management, 16*(3), 445–464. doi:10.1080/0958519042000339598

Mohr, G. B. (2000). The changing significance of different stressors after the announcement of bankruptcy: A longitudinal investigation with special emphasis on job insecurity. *Journal of Organizational Behavior, 21*(3), 337–359. doi:10.1002/(SICI)1099-1379(200005)21:3<337::AID-JOB18>3.0.CO;2-G

Mueller, K., Voelkle, M. C., & Hattrup, K. (2011). On the relationship between job satisfaction and non-response in employee attitude surveys: A longitudinal field study. *Journal of Occupational and Organizational Psychology, 84*(4), 780–798. doi:10.1348/096317910X526777

Nandan, D., & Agarwal, D. (2012). Human Resources for Health in India: Urgent Need for Reforms. *Indian Journal of Community Medicine, 37*(4), 205.

Niehoff, B. P., Moorman, R. H., Blakely, G., & Fuller, J. (2001). The influence of empowerment and job enrichment on employee loyalty in a downsizing environment. *Group & Organization Management, 26*(1), 93–113. doi:10.1177/1059601101261006

Nikolaou, I. (2011). Core processes and applicant reactions to the employment interview: An exploratory study in Greece. *International Journal of Human Resource Management, 22*(10), 2185–2201. doi:10.1080/09585192.2011.580187

Olian, J. D., & Rynes, S. L. (1984). Organizational staffing: Integrating practice with strategy. *Industrial Relations, 23*(2), 170–183. doi:10.1111/j.1468-232X.1984.tb00895.x

Orpen, C. (1979). The effects of job enrichment on employee satisfaction, motivation, involvement, and performance: A field experiment. *Human Relations, 32*(3), 189–217. doi:10.1177/001872677903200301

Ortega, J. (2001). Job rotation as a learning mechanism. *Management Science, 47*(10), 1361–1370. doi:10.1287/mnsc.47.10.1361.10257

Ostroff, C., & Bowen, D. E. (2000). Moving HR to a higher level: Human resource practices and organizational effectiveness. In K. J. Klein & S. W. J. Kozlowski (Eds.), *Multilevel theory, research, and methods.*

Parker, S. K. (1998). Enhancing role breadth self-efficacy: The roles of job enrichment and other organizational interventions. *The Journal of Applied Psychology, 83*(6), 835–852. doi:10.1037/0021-9010.83.6.835 PMID:9885197

Paulus, P. (2000). Groups, Teams, and Creativity: The Creative Potential of Idea-generating Groups. *Applied Psychology, 49*(2), 237–262. doi:10.1111/1464-0597.00013

Porter, L. W., & Lawler, E. E. (1968). *Managerial attitudes and performance.* Homewood, IL: Irwin-Dorsey.

Posthuma, R. A., Campion, M. C., Masimova, M., & Campion, M. A. (2013). A high performance work practices taxonomy integrating the literature and directing future research. *Journal of Management, 39*(5), 1184–1220. doi:10.1177/0149206313478184

Purcell, J. (1999). Best practice and best fit: Chimera or cul-de-sac? *Human Resource Management Journal, 9*(3), 26–41. doi:10.1111/j.1748-8583.1999.tb00201.x

Robertson, I. T., & Smith, M. (2001). Personnel selection. *Journal of Occupational and Organizational Psychology*, *74*(4), 441–472. doi:10.1348/096317901167479

Rogelberg, S. G., Luong, A., Sederburg, M. E., & Cristol, D. S. (2000). Employee attitude surveys: Examining the attitudes of noncompliant employees. *The Journal of Applied Psychology*, *85*(2), 284–293. doi:10.1037/0021-9010.85.2.284 PMID:10783544

Romzek, B. S. (1985). The effects of public service recognition, job security and staff reductions on organizational involvement. *Public Administration Review*, *45*(2), 282–291. doi:10.2307/976149

Rynes, S. L., Gerhart, B., & Parks, L. (2005). Personnel psychology: Performance evaluation and pay for performance. *Annual Review of Psychology*, *56*(1), 571–600. doi:10.1146/annurev.psych.56.091103.070254 PMID:15709947

Salgado, J. F. (1999). Personnel selection methods. In C. L. Cooper & I. T. Robertson (Eds.), *International Review of Industrial & Organizational Psychology*. New York: Wiley.

Saunderson, R. (2004). Survey findings of the effectiveness of employee recognition in the public sector. *Public Personnel Management*, *33*(3), 255–275. doi:10.1177/009102600403300302

Schweiger, D. M., & Leana, C. R. (1986). Participation in decision making. *Generalizing from laboratory to field settings, 147*, 166.

Scott-Ladd, B., Travaglione, A., & Marshall, V. (2006). Causal inferences between participation in decision making, task attributes, work effort, rewards, job satisfaction and commitment. *Leadership and Organization Development Journal*, *27*(5), 399–414. doi:10.1108/01437730610677990

Shipton, H., West, M. A., Dawson, J., Birdi, K., & Patterson, M. (2006). HRM as a predictor of innovation. *Human Resource Management Journal*, *16*(1), 3–27. doi:10.1111/j.1748-8583.2006.00002.x

Sverke, M., & Hellgren, J. (2002). The nature of job insecurity: Understanding employment uncertainty on the brink of a new millennium. *Applied Psychology*, *51*(1), 23–42. doi:10.1111/1464-0597.0077z

Takeuchi, R., Lepak, D. P., Wang, H., & Takeuchi, K. (2007). An empirical examination of the mechanisms mediating between high-performance work systems and the performance of Japanese organizations. *The Journal of Applied Psychology*, *92*(4), 1069–1083. doi:10.1037/0021-9010.92.4.1069 PMID:17638466

Taormina, R. J. (1997). Organizational socialization: A multidomain, continuous process model. *International Journal of Selection and Assessment*, *5*(1), 29–47. doi:10.1111/1468-2389.00043

Thorsteinson, T. J., & Ryan, A. M. (1997). The effect of selection ratio on perceptions of the fairness of a selection test battery. *International Journal of Selection and Assessment*, *5*(3), 159–168. doi:10.1111/1468-2389.00056

Tsui, A. S., Pearce, J. L., Porter, L. W., & Tripoli, A. M. (1997). Alternative approaches to the employee-organization relationship: Does investment in employees pay off? *Academy of Management Journal*, *40*(5), 1089–1121. doi:10.2307/256928

Wan, D., Ong, C. H., & Kok, V. (2002). Strategic human resource management and organizational performance in Singapore. *Compensation and Benefits Review*, *34*(4), 33–42. doi:10.1177/0886368702034004006

West, M. A., Borrill, C., Dawson, J., Scully, J., Carter, M., Anelay, S., & Waring, J. et al. (2002). The link between the management of employees and patient mortality in acute hospitals. *International Journal of Human Resource Management*, *13*(8), 1299–1310. doi:10.1080/09585190210156521

West, M. A., Guthrie, J. P., Dawson, J. F., Borrill, C. S., & Carter, M. (2006). Reducing patient mortality in hospitals: The role of human resource management. *Journal of Organizational Behavior*, *27*(7), 983–1002. doi:10.1002/job.396

Witte, H. D. (1999). Job insecurity and psychological well-being: Review of the literature and exploration of some unresolved issues. *European Journal of Work and Organizational Psychology*, *8*(2), 155–177. doi:10.1080/135943299398302

Wright, P. M., & McMahan, G. C. (1992). Theoretical perspectives for strategic human resource management. *Journal of Management*, *18*(2), 295–320. doi:10.1177/014920639201800205

Yang, S. B., & Lee, K. H. (2009). Linking empowerment and job enrichment to turnover intention: The influence of job satisfaction. *International Review of Public Administration*, *14*(2), 13–24. doi:10.1080/12294659.2009.10805152

Young, S., Bartram, T., Stanton, P., & Leggat, S. G. (2010). High performance work systems and employee well-being: A two stage study of a rural Australian hospital. *Journal of Health Organization and Management*, *24*(2), 182–199. doi:10.1108/14777261011047345 PMID:20698193

Zhang, M., Zhu, C. J., Dowling, P. J., & Bartram, T. (2013). Exploring the effects of high-performance work systems (HPWS) on the work-related well-being of Chinese hospital employees. *International Journal of Human Resource Management*, *24*(16), 3196–3212. doi:10.1080/09585192.2013.775026

Zhang, Y., & Li, L. (2009, May). Study on balanced scorecard of commercial bank in performance management system. In *Proceedings of the 2009 International Symposium on Web Information Systems and Applications (WISA'09)* (pp. 22-24).

KEY TERMS AND DEFINITIONS

Employee Outcomes: A group of important outcomes that relates to the employee at an individual level.

High-Performance Work Practices: Management practices that form an integrated human resource system and positively affect organizational performance.

Human Resource Management: It is a host of policies and practices that that focus on the successful management of employees.

Human Resource Management Policy: It is the guidelines and principles that determine the actions which will be implemented in order to effectively manage human resources.

Human Resource Management Practice: It is the specific actions and tools that human resource management use in order to implement their policies.

Mediator: It constitutes a variable that explains the relationship between an independent and a dependent variable providing thus the underlying mechanism.

Moderator: It is a variable that influences the direction and the magnitude of the relationship between an independent and a dependent variable.

Organizational Outcomes: A number of core outcomes that pertains to the organizational level and functioning.

Chapter 3
Organizational Integration of Decision Analytic Methods in Healthcare Settings

Christopher L. Pate
Brook Army Medical Center, USA

Mark D. Swofford
Brook Army Medical Center, USA

ABSTRACT

Healthcare organizations face a range of external and internal factors that both enable and hinder the organization's ability to provide safe, quality, timely and reliable healthcare services. The accessibility of data coupled with effectively integrated analytic methods can provide healthcare organizations with essential components of a solid framework for improving performance across the full spectrum of organizational contexts. However, data, methods, and a robust information infrastructure are only part of the solution. Healthcare organizations must consider characteristics of the organization and its strategy in order to effectively integrate analytic methods. Conceptual ideas from organizational theory, economics and strategic management can provide structure to the integration process.

DOI: 10.4018/978-1-4666-9961-8.ch003

INTRODUCTION

The integration of analytics in healthcare settings can be a challenging undertaking for any organization desiring to improve decision making and organizational performance. Yet, effective integration of analytics requires an understanding of the organization, the organization's goals, the organizational structure, and other aspects of an organization's essence. This chapter bridges theoretical and practical lessons related to integration of analytics in healthcare settings.

Chapter Objectives

After completing the chapter, readers will be able to:

1. Define the concept of analytics.
2. Identify essential theoretical concepts related to the integration of analytics.
3. Discuss the importance of analytic integration in healthcare settings.
4. Discuss approaches to improving the integration of analytics in healthcare settings.

BACKGROUND

More than twenty years ago, Drucker observed that healthcare organizations are among the most complex of any organizational form (Drucker, as cited in Golden, 2006). Over these past two decades, changes in the healthcare landscape have only added to the complexity facing healthcare organizations across the full range of organizational forms encountered in the industry. These changes include growth of new technologies, demographic shifts, an aging population, efforts to decrease healthcare costs (Bernstein, Hing, Moss, Allen, Siller & Tiggle, 2003; Lee, 2009), increasing emphasis on accountability (Tabar, 2012), investment in and growth of health information technology, and increased requirements for data monitoring and management (Shortliffe, 2005). In terms of data content, the healthcare industry "is facing a tsunami of health and healthcare related content generated from numerous patient care points of contact, sophisticated medical instruments, and web-based health communities" (Chen, Chiang, & Storey, 2012, p. 1171). Krumholz (2014, p. 1169) notes that "massive repositories of potential knowledge, populated by data from health care visits, devices, administrative claims, and biospecimens, are increasingly available...(yet)...the promise of massive data assets lies not merely in their size, but in the way they are used."

The growth of data does necessarily translate into improvements in organizational decision making in healthcare contexts. In fact, the proliferation and accessibility of data can complicate the decision making process. Creation of an effective decision support framework, which would include specific analytic methods as well as an approach to implementation (Austin & Boxerman, 1998), can enhance decision making and ultimately improve performance in multiple contexts within healthcare organizations. In fact, if knowledge creation and acquisition is "an important requirement for survival" (Davis, 1995, p. 115) and if establishment of effective analytic framework supports knowledge creation, organizations are facing an operational imperative in developing and implementing a robust decision analytic framework.

Organizations face a wide range of related concepts and approaches related to decision support and analytics. Many of these concepts lack definitional consensus and consistency across academic and practitioner-focused publications. Defining decision support as "using an organization's data to aid in management decisions" (Sempeles, as cited in Austin & Boxerman, 1998, p. 310) can provide, however, a starting point for healthcare organizations to begin the process of thinking about the process of integration. Healthcare organizations must understand that a variety of frameworks exist in order to develop an effective analytic framework, yet they must also eschew the Tayloristic notion of "one best way" (Kanigel, 1997, p. 1) in crafting and implementing an analytic framework.

Analytic frameworks also include terms such as business analytics, business intelligence, business intelligence and analytics (BI&A) and business analysis. Although each of may present a slightly different focus, they are ultimately aligned with data, analysis and decision making. For example, Koch (2015) conceptualizes business analysis as a process by which data are transformed into information that is ultimately used for business decisions. Chen, Chiang, and Storey (2012) define BI&A as the "techniques, technologies, systems, practices, methodologies and applications that analyze critical business data to help an enterprise better understand its business and market and make timely business decisions" (p. 1166), whereas Patil and Mishra (2014), define business analytics as an approach that "applies advanced statistical analysis such as simulations and predictions for complex problems at the business unit or organization level" (p. 25).

Conceptualizations of decision support systems can include specific analytic methods as a component, which could be considered a function of a particular system; however, a higher-level perspective of decision support systems may also include system components as well as the functions performed within a particular system (Austin & Boxerman, 1998). This chapter extends the Austin and Boxerman model to explicitly discuss organizational structures and processes as key components to understanding and developing effective, integrated decision support structures and processes. Within every organization, any decision about investment of resources to support and integrate analytic methods within a decision support framework must also be made from the perspective that resources are constrained. Organizations do not have the luxury of unboundless time, physical resources, technology, capital, labor, space and other resources that could potentially be used for business analytic efforts. Second, organizations forego the benefit of the alternative uses of the resources chosen to support analytic efforts. That is, opportunity costs exist for every choice made to invest in business analytic resources and development of a decision support system. Resource constraints necessitate prioritization of efforts.

In today's healthcare environment, a range of advanced analytic methods, such as forecasting, predictive analytics, data modeling and others are considered to be important in meeting organizational goals (Van De Graaf & Cameron, 2013), yet these methods must be considered in the context of the organization that is seeking to meet, sustain, or improve performance objectives.

PERFORMANCE, DECISION MAKING AND INTEGRATION OF ANALYTICS

The performance of healthcare organizations matters. The difference between good and bad performance could be the life or death of a patient, the financial solvency or failure of a community hospital, or the reduction or increase of national healthcare costs. Regardless of the perspective from which the healthcare industry is approached, performance, in at least one of its many dimensions, matters. Although healthcare is a multi-disciplinary field comprised of many types of organizations, and the performance of all healthcare organizations is important, focusing on hospitals as a group of healthcare organizations helps to illustrate the importance of performance. In 2007, hospitals accounted for 31% of total health care spending in the United States, the single largest group of organizations in terms of health care spending (CMS, 2009). Performance data for hospitals are reported by federal and state government entities, non-governmental organizations, industry trade groups, and many private organizations. A simple Google search using the term "hospital performance" returns multiple reports from the Department of Health and Human Services, the Commonwealth Fund, the states of New Jersey, North Carolina, and Pennsylvania, and the private organization HealthGrades. Examination of these different reports reveals great variation in the performance of seemingly similar hospitals.

Presented with such variation, there are two options for interpreting these data: (a) variations in performance are completely random; or (b) variations in performance are not random and can be explained and affected by the actions of organizational leaders. If the first option is chosen (variations in performance are random) then the actions of hospital administrators, clinicians, support staff, and multiple other healthcare professionals make no difference. Despite their best intentions and best efforts, their actions do not affect the performance outcomes of their organizations. When taken to an extreme, this interpretation calls into question the purpose of all of the healthcare administration programs around the country as well as the usefulness of government healthcare agencies that try to improve performance of the various entities that make up our national healthcare system. The alternate interpretation that variations in performance are not random and can be explained, is the view of the vast majority of health care professionals and means that the actions of organizational leaders matter. This is the view embodied by rational organizational theories such as structural contingency theory. Structural contingency theory (sometimes simply called contingency theory) acknowledges the role of organizational leaders and allows room for the idea that their actions may significantly impact organizational performance. As opposed to other major organization theories, which minimize the importance of organizational leaders / actors (population ecology and institutional theory) or attribute their actions to goals other than increasing organizational performance/ efficiency (resource dependence), contingency theory portrays organizational leaders as rational actors who modify the structure of the organization and make decisions to improve performance and achieve stated organizational goals. It is important to note that this does not mean that organizational leaders are prescient or omniscient. Indeed they are "boundedly rational" (March & Simon, 1993), but to the extent that they understand the environment and can identify ways to adapt organizational structure, they will choose the best decision alternative in order to improve performance.

The process of decision making is one of the most critical activities of a healthcare organization. Every leader and individual within the organization faces a spectrum of choices on a daily basis, many of which are routine and many of which are critical and complex (Schoemaker & Russo, 1993). From the hospitality staff that works within the smallest organizational element within a small facility to the CEO of a large healthcare system, decision making is called for at all levels of the organization. All organizations engage in developing decisions, whether the process is structured, unstructured, influenced by pet projects, in isolation of other projects, driven by regulatory requirements, and so on. Lacking the ability to establish a meaningful framework for decision making, organizations may find themselves investing an inordinate amount of time, energy, and resources on solution development without first considering the criteria by which a solution may be developed. Decision making capabilities may be hampered by misalignment of organizational resources, lack of resources, lack of knowledge, and other factors. Further, the very nature of the organization is interwoven with the processes that are critical to enable sound decision making, particularly in healthcare organizations. So then the question becomes, what is the best way to organize in order to ensure sound decision making and high performance?

Theoretical Frameworks for Organizing to Achieve Desired Outcomes

Nearly five decades ago, Avedis Donabedien explicated the general framework of structure – process – outcome as a way to improve quality in healthcare (Donabedian, 1978; Donabedian, 1966). In general, Donabedian's framework emphasizes the interdependence between organizational structure and organizational process in the context of achieving quality healthcare outcomes. His work emphasizes the need to match structure to process in order to achieve desired outcomes or to improve existing outcomes. Similar to structural contingency theory, Donabedian's framework focuses on performance (i.e., outcomes) and assumes that organizational leaders as rational actors make decisions and change the organization in order to improve performance.

Although the structure-process-outcome framework was originally developed in the context of quality – it has broader applications as a robust framework to think about how an organization can achieve its desired outcomes, in this case good decisions that allow an organization to achieve its stated goals and objectives. Thus structure and process are inseparably linked as the organization's structure provides the framework to support the processes of organizational analysis and decision making. Key structural considerations include strategic linkages/alignment, location and organization of analytics and decision support, assignment of responsibility and authority, management of data and information systems/technology, training/education of the organization on chosen analytic methods and tools, and structures to enable the synchronization and prioritization of projects/major decisions. Key process considerations include the process to synchronize and prioritize projects/major decisions, matching of analytic methods with types of projects/decisions that have to be made, presenting information in a uniformed and consistent manner, keeping leaders in touch with operations, monitoring process and managing change.

In order to develop the right combination of structure and process to produce desired outcomes, organizational leaders must understand the basic principles of organizational design and fully integrate the structures and processes related to analysis and decision making into the organization.

Organizational Design and Organization Structure

Similar to the way phylogeny manifests itself in physiology, the basic concepts of organizational design result in the tangible visages of organizational structure. In its simplest form, organizational design has two main parts: (a) the division of work and responsibility, and (b) the coordination of the work assigned to different parts of the organization (Charnes & Young, 2012). The combination of these two tasks generates the organizational structure often symbolized in hierarchical organization charts and the position descriptions that normally exist for the individual positions represented by those charts. To illustrate this concept, imagine a very simply business owned and staffed entirely by one person, let's say it is a jewelry making business. The organization chart contains only a single box and all of the work is performed by a single individual. This single individual buys supplies, makes and then sells the jewelry. There is no need to coordinate the various tasks involved because they are all performed by one person who essentially coordinates the tasks internally. Now imagine a very large manufacturing company with hundreds or thousands of employees grouped by functional departments directed by a central headquarters and supported by logistic, financial, and human resource departments. As you can probably imagine, the organizational chart is very large and personnel perform many different jobs with widely varying functions. In order to produce the desired product on a consistent basis with high quality, this large organization requires various people, offices, and teams to coordinate the work that is performed and ensure that all of the employees are working cooperatively toward the common goal of producing the company's product to standard and with efficiency.

Analysis and decision making in organizations must be structured in a similar manner. Organizational leaders must identify the activities required for good analysis and decision making and then divide these activities into separate jobs/tasks, assign these tasks to persons or work units within the organization, and then coordinate the performance of these tasks in order to achieve the desired outcomes. Ultimately a systematic approach for organizational analysis and decision making is required to overcome common organizational limitations such as the limited complexity of individuals, lack of strategic alignment, the bounded rationality of decision makers, and effectively deal with the complexity of healthcare organizations and the healthcare industry in general.

Structural contingency theory provides useful principles that may be employed in the organizational design process. Contingency theory was developed in the 1960s to study questions related to organizational performance (Lawrence & Lorsch, 1967;

Thompson, 1967; Woodward, 1965). Often referred to as structural contingency theory, it contains the basic paradigm that organizational performance depends on an organization's ability to fit its structure to contingencies that reflect the situation of the organization (Donaldson, 2001). Underlying this paradigm are three basic assumptions: (a) there is no one best way to organize for every situation; (b) different ways of organizing are not equally effective for a given situation; and (c) for a given situation, the best way to organize depends on the dominant environmental characteristic or contingency (Thompson, 1967). Thus contingency theory is fundamentally different from universalistic theories that associate higher organizational performance to the maximum level of a given environmental or structural variable (Donaldson, 2001). Contingency theory asserts that organizational performance depends upon the degree of fit between environment and organization, which implies that organizations with different structures may perform equally as well in different situations.

One formulation of structural contingency theory, which grew out of industrial organization economics, uses the constructs of complexity, uncertainty, and interdependence to describe the work an organization performs and the constructs of differentiation, centralization, and coordination to describe organizational structure (Scott & Davis, 2007). These constructs are paired together in contingent relationships (complexity with differentiation, uncertainty with centralization, and interdependence with coordination) and performance depends on the degree of "fit" between the two sets of constructs. The basic directional propositions are that greater complexity of inputs requires greater organizational differentiation, greater uncertainty of inputs requires less centralized decision making, and greater interdependence of work processes requires more coordination mechanisms to achieve integration of work effort. Donaldson (1995, 2001) asserts that the most prominent contingencies that must be considered by an organization are environmental stability, organizational size, and strategy. Although not the same as the major contingencies identified by Scott and Davis (2007), the core ideas of the theory remain the same. First, there is a relationship between environmental contingency and structure. Second, as the environment changes the structure of the organization should change as well. Third, performance depends on how well the organizational structure fits the environment.

In the context of organizational analysis and decision making, contingency theory implies that there is not a single best way for healthcare organizations to structure analysis and decision making processes. Rather, healthcare organizations must consider key environmental and organizational variables in order to determine the best way to create strategic alignment, organize analytics, manage information technology and data, synchronize and prioritize the problems that need to be addressed, and match analytic techniques to problems in order to present information to decision makers in an appropriate and consistent manner.

Strategic Alignment

One of the initial coordinating actions organizational leaders must perform is the creation of strategic alignment. Strategic alignment ensures that everyone in the organization is focused on the organization's stated goals and objectives and that these goals and objectives drive decision making and the allocation of resources. By following basic strategic planning and strategy development processes, the organization must develop a general strategy to achieve its stated goals and objectives and then link initiatives and projects throughout the organization to this strategy. When this is done, the basic tenants of the organization's strategy can be used to prioritize projects, proposals and initiatives for decision making and also serve as criteria for making decisions and selecting alternatives. Organizations that fail to create strategic alignment risk wasting resources on non-value added processes and actions, and diffusing the energy of their employees rather than focusing that energy on their stated goals and objectives.

Many options exist for strategic planning and creating strategic alignment and each organization must choose a method to achieve this critical task. Two strategic alignment tools, The Balanced Scorecard and the creation of "True North" metrics, are discussed in the following paragraphs to illustrate the different methods available to healthcare organizations.

The Balanced Scorecard (BSC) is a strategic management system originally proposed by Drs. Robert S. Kaplan and David P. Norton in a 1992 *Harvard Business Review* article (Kaplan & Norton, 1992). The BSC was the result of a yearlong research project Kaplan and Norton conducted in 1990 with twelve leading companies in the area of performance measurement (Kaplan & Norton 1992). The genesis of the BSC was the idea that managers should not have to choose between financial and operational measures. The result was a tool (the BSC) that allows managers to monitor a few critical measures that are linked to the organization's strategic objectives, and balance the need to monitor financial and operational measures. Similar to the ideas expressed in Senge's *The Fifth Discipline: The Art and Practice of the Learning Organization* (1990), the BSC is meant to focus the entire organization on the organization's strategy by using mental models (i.e., strategy maps) to ensure employees embrace a systems perspective. From the BSC perspective, the system components include objectives, measures, and targets allocated to four perspectives: financial, customer, internal business, and innovation and learning (Kaplan & Norton, 1996). Organizations that adopt the BSC as their management system are able to assemble and link many disparate organizational elements and guard against sub optimization (i.e., the idea that achievement in one business area comes at the expense of another business area; Kaplan & Norton, 1992). The effect on an organization is that their management system does not produce countless measures with a control bias – i.e., measures that specify what actions an employee should take. Instead the BSC produces a few high-level measures that put an organization's vision and strategy at the center of the management system. The top level scorecard (Level 1) is then cascaded down through the organization (Levels 2 and 3) and subordinate departments and work units develop their own scorecards with objectives, measures, and initiatives that link back to the top level, organizational scorecard. The result is a highly structured strategic management system that ensures strategic alignment for the organization.

An alternate approach is the creation of "True North" metrics as illustrated by the ThedaCare Medical System in Wisconsin. As an adaptation of the Toyota Management System, ThedaCare developed its own Lean management system for the healthcare environment with a core set of metrics, called "True North" metrics that guide the organization (Toussaint & Gerard, 2010). Executive leadership reviews these metrics on a regular basis and subordinate work units must align their Lean process improvement actions and the measures that they track with "True North." This alignment forces various actors throughout the organization to eliminate practices and improvement actions that do not add value and help the organization achieve its stated goals and objectives (as embodied by the "True North" metrics).

Both the Balanced Scorecard and Lean management systems with "True North" metrics are widely used in healthcare today to achieve strategic alignment. It is not clear if one technique is better, but organizational leaders may want to consider the level of differentiation within their organization, the uncertainty of the work environment, and the need for coordination when selecting a given method. As illustrated by these two examples, a more formal system such as the Balanced Scorecard, may be more appropriate for a larger organization with greater differentiation that results in business units or functional departments that perform significantly different work (such as vertically integrated health system). The more highly differentiated the parts of the organization are, the more difficult it may be for them to all align with a small set of "True North" metrics. A tool such as the Balanced Scorecard may accommodate the greater degree of differentiation and also allow for more formal coordination across the interdependent business units. On the other hand, an approach like ThedaCare's with a set of "True North" metrics may offer greater flexibility for organizations with similar business units (such as a horizontally integrated system) that need to adapt quickly and identify process improvement actions in a constantly changing and complex work environment. Or perhaps both methods may work equally well and the best method depends on the organization's culture, the comfort level and commitment of organizational leaders to the chosen method, and skill with which the organization implements. Regardless, the task of strategic alignment is critical to integrating organizational analysis and decision making in healthcare and must be accomplished to maximize the benefit of the other structure and process choices.

Structural Choices for Organizational Integration of Analysis and Decision Making

Assuming strategic alignment has been accomplished to some degree, organizational leaders should consider other structural factors that facilitate the processes of organizational analysis and decision making. Establishing the right structure will facilitate the examination of problems and issues that are important to the organization, increase the likelihood of producing quality analytic products, and lead to better decision making by organizational leaders. In this section, five key structural considers are presented:

1. How to structure organizational analytics,
2. The management of data and information systems,
3. The assignment of responsibility and decision-making authority,
4. Training and education for members of the organization, and
5. How to enable synchronization and prioritization.

Location and Organization of Analytics and Decision Support

Central to the task of performing analysis are the people that are commonly referred to as analysts. Although many workers perform some type of analysis as part of their jobs, analysts are the employees specifically hired to organize, filter, and analyze organization data in order to produce informational products and decision support tools to facilitate work processes and decision making. Depending on the organization, they may come in different types (financial analysts, clinical workflow analysts, management analysts) with somewhat varying skill sets, but their purpose is essentially the same. The key question for healthcare organizations with respect to their analysts is whether to centralize or disperse them within the organization. Key organizational variables to consider when making this decision are organizational size and differentiation. It is often the combination of these two variables that determines the best way to organize the analytic assets of a given organization. Choices for organizing include a consolidated analytic cell, the decentralization of analysts to departments and work units within the organization, or somewhere in between those two extremes. In order to assess which way may be best for a given organization, leaders may consider the flexibility, responsiveness, and uniformity of the analysis that is produced and the amount of coordination required to produce it.

The first option is to centralize all analytic assets into one location or work unit. Complete centralization minimizes the amount of coordination that has to be performed and facilitates the production of highly uniformed products, which makes it easier for organizational customers and leaders to consume the information being produced. However, complete centralization may limit overall organizational flexibility and responsiveness as analytic requirements all enter one central funnel and require a very effective prioritization process to ensure different parts of the organization are being supported. Additionally, as organizations become more differentiated, the types of analysis and methods required increases and may exceed the abilities of one central analytic cell to satisfy all type requirements.

The second option is to decentralize analysts and embed them in the various departments and work units of the healthcare organization. This essentially does the exact opposite of centralizing the assets. Analysts will be much more responsive to the requirements of their department and work unit leaders, and decentralization allows leaders to hire analysts that are tailored to the department or work unit's specific requirements. However, decentralization creates the greatest coordination burden for the organization as a whole and may lead to the production of a wide variety of analytic products that are hard to make sense of above the department level. Additionally, as the complexity of a problem increases, individual analysts assigned throughout the organization may lack the ability to find and collaborate effectively with other analysts who possess complementary skills.

The final choice, and the one that seems most practical for most healthcare organizations, is to take a hybrid approach with a central analytic cell (or perhaps a couple of main cells) complemented by individual or small groups of analysts with specific functions embedded in various departments and work units. The hybrid approach allows for the standardization of common or frequent types of analysis in order to produce uniformed products that are easily understood and used by the organization. Further, the centralized assets provide robust analytic capabilities that may be brought to bear on the most complex problems, and the centralized assets may be organized into cells based on rough typologies such as business/claims data analysis, financial analysis, and clinical data/decision support analysis. The decentralized analytic assets compliment the centralized cells by providing a high level of responsiveness to departmental and work unit leaders, and can be highly specialized to satisfy specific analytic requirements of a given area. But for any of these structures to work, healthcare organizations need to deliberately manage their information systems and their healthcare data. Defined as "...a team of people established to promote collaboration and the application of business intelligence

(BI) standards and best practices across the organization," the business intelligence community of practice or center of excellence is an emerging conceptualization of this hybrid model (Krakauer, 2012, p. 4).

Management of Data and Information Systems/Technology

In 1991 the Institute of Medicine issued a report outlining the many quality and safety related problems associated with use of paper based medical records and urged the adoption of electronic medical records (IOM, 1991). Although slow at first, the adoption of electronic health records (EHRs) has accelerated with the passage of the Health Information Technology for Economic and Clinical Health (HITECH) Act in 2009, which established requirements and incentives for healthcare organizations to meet various meaningful use rules of certified EHR technology. From 2008 to 2013, the percentage of non-federal acute care hospitals with a basic EHR rose from 9.4% to 59.4% and 94% of hospitals have an EHR classified as a certified EHR under HITECH Act incentive measures (Charles et al., 2014) and 78% of office based physician practices reported having an EHR (Hsiao & Hing, 2014).

The proliferation of electronic systems means that healthcare organizations have more data than ever before, but organizing and effectively using it can be a big problem. A review of several studies examining the benefits of increased EHR usage revealed little evidence that increased use has positively impacted the cost, usage patterns, or quality of health care (Rahurkar et al., 2015). In many cases, healthcare organizations are unprepared and ill-structured to capture, store, organize, and use all of the data from their systems to create information and deliver it to customers to improve organizational decision making. Often the problem is not the systems themselves, but the people that use them who are often overloaded with too much data and information (Wong et al., 2000). Wong and his colleagues (2001) point out that as healthcare organizations change with a greater emphasis on ambulatory care and consolidation into larger and larger systems, there will be a greater demand to simplify the ways which we deliver information. To this end, organizations should consider three basic structural decisions concerning information systems and data in order to facilitate organizational analytic and decision making processes.

The first item to consider is the determination of authoritative data sources. A basic component of any effective information technology governance system, the identification of authoritative data sources ensures that analysts and decisions makers throughout the organization are consistently taking data from the system of record. The proliferation of EHRs and the use of billing, financial, and other management information systems in healthcare organizations increases the possibility that an organization's information systems may disagree about the same piece of information. Data are taken from the source system, often referred to as the System of Record, and then combined with data from another system or re-processed to create a data element or a string of data elements in a different system. It is important for healthcare organizations to identify the authoritative sources for various types of data in order to prevent internal disagreements and the possibility that analytic products contradict each other.

The second consideration is how will the organization store, organize, and make its data available to analysts and decision makers. Often, healthcare organizations work to create transactional systems that enable the performance of patient care or support functions that enable patient care. Making data from these systems available for analysis and decision making is in many cases an afterthought, and can seriously hinder organizational analytic efforts. If possible, healthcare organizations should consider data collection and analysis at the start of any information system project, but when not considered at the outset, organizations must determine how they collect, store, and organize their data on the back end of the project. The last thing an organization wants is to encourage analysts and other secondary users to directly tap into the transactional system and slow down the work that the system was meant to enable. Rather, healthcare organizations should seek to develop the method and then build the infrastructure to extract the data from their transactional systems, store and organize it efficiently in a secure environment and then make it available to analysts and other users throughout the organization.

Once stored and organized, how the data are made available to analysts and users is the final structural consideration that will be discussed here. Beginning with the end in mind, the goal is to develop an environment or mechanism to deliver data and information to analysts and decision makers throughout the organization with a common look and feel. In most cases this is accomplished by selecting and purchasing commercial software designed for this purpose, however some large organizations may possess the resources to develop their own software or system to accomplish this task. Regardless of how it is performed, the importance of delivering data and information in a consistent environment to users throughout the organization cannot be understated. An environment with a common look and feel allows users to focus on the information being presented rather than trying to understand and make sense of the method of presentation itself, and over time will increase information transfer and aid decision making.

Stratification of Responsibility and Authority for Decision Making

Another key structural condition for effective organizational analysis and decision making is the establishment of criteria to stratify the level at which an issue or problem is addressed and who has the authority to make a decision concerning the issue or problem. With most healthcare organizations now aspiring to become so called high reliability organizations (HROs; Weick & Sutcliffe, 2008), employees at all levels of the organization are being encouraged to engage in process improvement in order to increase healthcare quality and patient safety. Recent writings on HRO implementation stress the need for robust process improvement as one of the three basic building blocks of an HRO (Chassin & Loeb, 2013), and organizations are encouraged to adopt improvement processes such as Lean, Six Sigma, and Change Management that are inherently more complex than many traditional process improvement methods used in healthcare. This increased complexity is required to deal with the complex processes involved in providing patient care and address issues from a systems perspective, but some research on HRO theory and complex systems highlights that it is often too much for individuals to identify and deal with system problems (Ruchlin et al., 2004).

On way to deal with more complex issues characterized by increased information processing requirements is to establish rules, programs, and hierarchies and elevate more complex issues to more complex individuals (Galbraith, 1973). Figure 1 provides a graphical depiction of this concept in a healthcare organization with essentially five levels of organizational actors/leaders. At the lowest level are front line staff who are directly engaged in patient care and the other support functions of the healthcare organization. Although many of them are highly educated professionals, as organizational actors and decision makers, they have a relatively low level of complexity with neither the tools nor the broad understanding of the entire

Figure 1. Stratification of organizational analysis and decision making

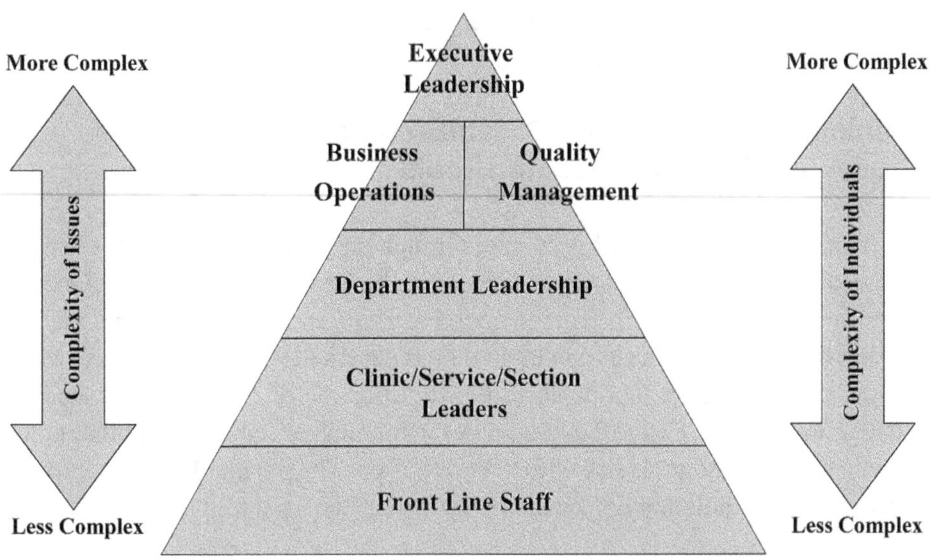

organization and environment that are needed to analyze and make decisions on very complex issues. At the opposite end of the spectrum are the executive leadership of the organization, which are both highly educated professionals and complex organizational actors that are immersed in all aspects of the organization on a daily basis. In between are the different levels of organizational leaders charged with propelling the organization forward toward accomplishment of its stated goals and objectives.

In order to ensure that issues are addressed at the right level and that the complexity of the issue is matched by the complexity of the individual or group of individuals conducting analysis and making decisions about it, the organization must establish rules and/or programs to ensure issues are elevated to the correct organizational actor(s). An example from one healthcare organization that has adopted a Lean management system is the "rule of threes" that it uses to determine if an issue should be elevated from front line workers to division or section management. The "rule of threes" in this organization simply says if addressing the issue requires more than three people, would take more than three days, or would involve more than three changes, then it needs to be elevated. In another healthcare organization, they have the simple rule that individuals in one part of the organization can only address issues that wholly reside within their organizational area. For example, if the Chief of the Department of Surgery needs to address an issue dealing with OR turnover, he has the authority to analyze and make a decision about the issue only if the entire process and the resources to address the issue are within the Department of Surgery. If the issue requires resources from another department or the processes involved cross into another department then he must elevate the issue. No matter what the specific rules an organization chooses, they must develop some method to regulate how issues are analyzed and addressed in order to stratify decision making and ensure the complexity of a given issue is matched by the complexity of the person or persons addressing the issue.

Training/Education of the Organization on Chosen Analytic Methods and Tools

The training and education of personnel throughout the organization goes hand in hand with the stratification of organizational analysis and decision making. Once an organization selects the method or methods that it will use for organizational analysis and decision making, it must train its staff on the methods and tools selected. Much like the previous figure that depicted the stratification of organizational analysis and decision making, Figure 2 depicts how the training and education on the chosen analytic methods and tools should also be stratified. The popular technique process improvement methodology of Lean Six Sigma may be used to illustrate this point.

Figure 2. Training on analytic methods and tools used within the organization

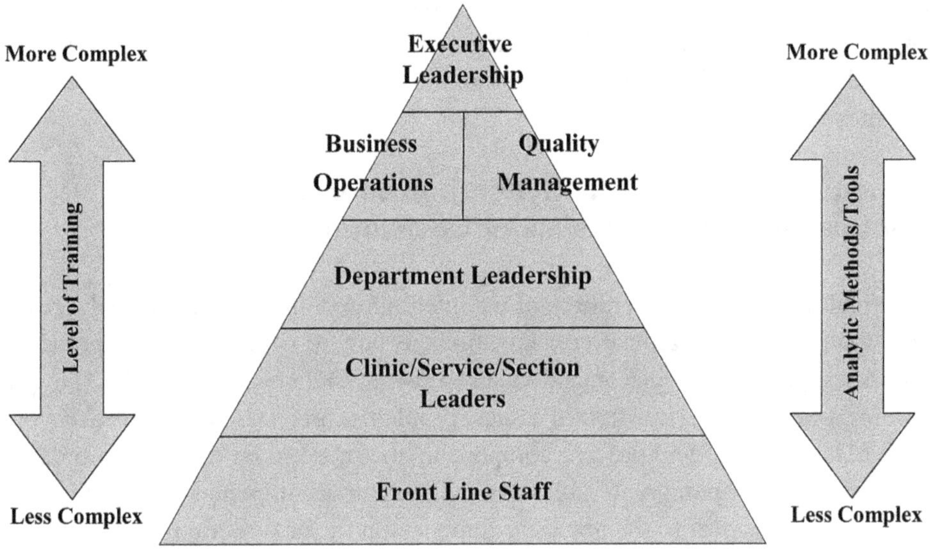

At the highest level, practitioners of this technique become certified Black Belts or Master Black Belts with weeks of formal training and hands on experience with very complex projects that use the entire range of tools in the Lean Six Sigma arsenal. However, organizations that adopt a Lean management system to run and improve their healthcare organization do not need to train every individual in the organization to that level. Nor do they need to treat every problem as a full blown Lean Six Sigma project. Instead, organizational leaders should realize that the Lean Six Sigma methodology includes many different tools, some of which may be used at the lowest levels of the organization to solve very simple problems. Individuals at the front line do not need weeks of formal training to become certified Black Belts. Rather, they need some very basic training in the tools that the organization wants them to apply at that level, and then some basic familiarization training with the entire Lean Six Sigma process so they may be informed consumers of information from more complex projects that may pertain to them or participate as a subject matter expert in a working group that is addressing a more complex issue. Section or department leaders or their administrators may require additional training such as a one-day Yellow Belt course or a Green Belt course that lasts a few days. Finally, individuals responsible for leading, advising, or facilitating multi-disciplinary working groups addressing very complex issues that have been elevated within the organization are the ones that may require Black Belt or Master Black Belt training.

But that is just one example of how training and education on chosen analytic methods and tools may be accomplished for a healthcare organization. Each organization is different and the methods and tools chosen may warrant a different method for determining at what level individuals should be trained. The important take away is that the training and education provided should be specific to the analytic methods and tools chosen and the depth of the training should be appropriate to the complexity of the issues addressed.

Structures to Enable the Synchronization and Prioritization of Projects/Major Decisions

The final structural consideration for the integration of organizational analysis and decision making in healthcare organizations, is how to synchronize and prioritize the issues, problems, projects, and major decisions that need to be made. The synchronization and prioritization of issues, problems, projects, and major decisions have both structural and process components that need to be matched in order to be effective. This paragraph addresses the structural component of this function and then bridges over to the process component in the next section of this chapter.

From a structural perspective, organizational leaders must create an office, section, working group, or recurring forum to continuously synchronize and prioritize the issues that need to be analyzed and then presented for a decision. A suggested method for accomplishing this is to create one or more multi-functional working groups that review the various types of issues, problems, and projects on a recurring basis (weekly, monthly, or quarterly) and then identify a specific office or person to organize and prepare the materials for the recurring meeting. For example, a given healthcare organization may create two multi-functional working groups or committees to review issues, problems, projects that are either clinical or non-clinical in nature. The quality services division would be responsible for organizing the group that reviewed the clinical issues and the business operations division would be responsible for the group that reviewed non-clinical issues. These two groups would be responsible with reviewing projects or analysis efforts that were already underway, discussing newly identified issues that need to be addressed, and then prioritizing all of the identified issues and ensuring that on-going and/or new projects are synchronized. The specific method for reviewing the information, prioritizing issues to address, and synchronizing the various projects is a question of process, but some basic structure must be present on which this process can be overlayed.

Prioritization

The process by which projects are selected is also essential in the alignment of organizational efforts. Project selection refers to the "process where an optimum combination of candidate projects is selected for implementation based on the parameters that are considered the most critical" (Jung & Lim, 2007, p. 55). Given the realities of resource scarcity and opportunity costs, healthcare organizations must selectively choose to deploy analytic efforts for projects that contribute to the goals and objectives of the organization. The process of selecting projects can be complicated by numerous factors within the organization, which include competing interests, hidden agendas among the various stakeholders within the organization, power differentials between organizational elements, lack of leadership, and a host of other factors. Failing to prioritize efforts may not only hinder achievement of goals, but may also result in detrimental outcomes to the organization because resources required to mitigate and perhaps prevent the realized outcomes were used in an alternative capacity. With the ultimate goal of improving performance, prioritization is a necessity in planning integration efforts. Subordinate goals of projection selection may include prioritization of projects that "address serious concerns, (are) aligned with the organizational missions and vision, produce a balance of cost and quality outcomes, (and) engaged stakeholders" (Leininger & Seaman, 2000, p. 28).

In terms of decision analysis integration in healthcare settings, three central ideas are important in prioritization. These ideas include (a) development of evaluative criteria, (b) assessment of evaluative criteria, and (c) assessment of potential projects

Given a set of project options and from a high-level perspective, organizations can conceptualize a project in terms of its potential benefits and costs. A basic way of thinking about the relationship between these two concepts in terms of prioritization is found in the formulaic approach to return on investment (ROI), where:

$$ROI = \frac{BENEFITS(\$) - COSTS(\$)}{COSTS(\$)}$$

In terms of ranking two potential projects that are identical in all ways with the exception of costs and benefits, the project with the higher ROI would be ranked higher. Meredith and Mantel (as cited in Jung & Lim, 2007) also note that other methods of economic analysis such as use of net present value (NPV), internal rate of return (IRR), numerical scoring and the Delphi method can also be used to support prioritization.

One of the biggest challenges with this model is that organizations have specific ideas about what the concepts of benefits and costs actually mean in terms of a particular project. And for a variety of reasons, such as lack of data, ill-defined conceptualizations, and lack of consensus, organizations may face difficulties in assigning dollar values to the basic benefit/cost model. In terms of a framework, operational definitions must be a part of this process. That is, benefits (and costs) must be specifically developed and defined in order to effectively prioritize and, terms that may have multiple meanings, which are aligned with benefits (costs), must be clarified. For example, organizations may consider the improvement on access to care or quality as important benefit-related criteria for a potential project. Each factor must be fully operationalized in such a way that all involved in the analysis of the project have a shared understanding as to meaning and measurement of the concepts. Another critical aspect of the operationalization process is clarification of the perspective being used. Like the perspectives used in cost-of-illness studies (Luce et al., as cited in Segel, 2006), the organization must also consider and clarify perspectives used in smaller-scale, organizational project prioritization. These could include, for example, patient, provider, department, or larger system perspectives. Naturally, each of these concepts must also be linked to the organization's mission, goals and objectives.

Once identified and defined, organizations must answer questions related to the relative importance of the criteria. In many cases, the criteria used to evaluate a project are not all equally important, thus evaluating the relative importance of each criterion provides a way for organizations to properly assess initiatives with recognition of the weight that each criterion carries. In a project that contained the criteria of access to care, impact on clinical proficiency, and impact on quality, the organization could assign percentage weights of 50%, 30%, and 20% to each respectively, reflecting the relative importance of each. The process of weighting criteria results in two important outcomes. First, the process forces the organization to deliberately think about criteria and perhaps engage in dialogue that would not otherwise have occurred in the absence of the weighting process. Second, the process of weighting evaluative criteria contributes to the prioritization process by creating a logical method by which organizations can assess projects.

The final step involves assessment of the proposed initiatives with respect to the criteria. The organization must address how each alternative addressed the evaluative criteria. For instance, in an evaluation of two potential initiatives designed to optimize existing capacity in an organization, an organization could consider partnerships with two different organizations as decision alternatives. With a scale ranging from 1 – 10, for example, the organization would assign scores to each alternative by criteria with higher scores meaning a greater extent to which a particular alternative addresses a specific criterion. The products of the scores and criteria weights are then summed. At this stage a simple comparison can be made between the two alternatives and, if costs are identical, organizations can rank order alternatives. If costs differ between alternatives, the model can easily be extended to including the costs associated with each model. By dividing the summed products into the costs associated with each alternative, organizations can create indices that provide a means of evaluating and ranking decision alternatives over alternatives with different costs. Table 1 presents an example of the model using weights and scores associated with the hypothetical criteria and alternatives presented in this section.

The short discussion on prioritization is designed as a general framework from which we can think of the integration itself. Organizations may be focused on prioritization of deployment of specific business models (Patil & Mishra, 2014) or on the specific types of organizational factors that would contribute to the effectiveness of an integrated decision analytic framework. Here, the focus is on thinking about the goal of effective integration within a particular organization and not prioritization of specific projects within an organization possessing an effective framework for decision analysis. To the extent that organizations are considering changes to an existing system framework, development of an effective decision analytic framework could be considered an operational improvement (OI) type project (Jung & Lim, 2007).

In terms of specific models that could be used for these types of projects, a range of management science techniques are available to healthcare organizations to guide the decision making process. Decision models and techniques containing prioritization components, such as multi-criteria decision analysis, the analytic hierarchy process, scoring models, and other related models are typically found in management science and quantitative analysis texts (e.g., Anderson, Sweeney, & Williams, 2005; Austin & Boxerman, 1995; Lapin & Whisler, 2002; Ozcan, Y.A. 2005; Winston & Albright, 2001).

Structural Linkage and Process Orientation

Scholarly works have long recognized the importance of recognizing and leveraging linkages between organizational design and strategies associated with technology (Davis, 1995); however, no single approach to organizational design and technology integration will be effective across all organizations. Integration of data analytics

Table 1. Sample decision analytic model with multiple criteria and costs

Evaluative Criteria	Weight	Partnership A	Partnership B
Access to care	50%	5	9
Impact on Clinical Proficiency	30%	4	6
Quality	20%	9	8
Weighted Sum		5.5	7.9
Cost ($,000)		15	20
Index		0.37	0.40

does, however, involve decision analytic structures that crosscut typical functional boundaries held by many healthcare organizations (Leininger & Seaman, 2000). In fact, organizations may consider many problems best fielded by team-based structures that include a mix of professional and administrative staff from multiple functional structures within the organization. Key considerations in team-based organizational approaches include (a) systematic, data driven design process from multiple stakeholders and perspectives; (b) clearly defined decision processes, (c) connectedness between interdependent elements of the organization; and (d) shared databases and a common language (Mohrman & Cohen, 1995).

In terms of development and analysis of specific projects, both functional units and team-based structures can enjoy a supportive and effective relationship that encompasses the key considerations of team-based approaches. Design and function of team-based structures viewed as part of an overall decision support framework can also be viewed based upon the goals and objectives of the particular team (Fottler, 2005). For complex projects that involve multiple interdependencies across functional units, the functional units could be charged with providing subject matter experts to support a multidisciplinary, multifunctional process improvement team designed to improve the process that crosscuts the functions. Alternatively, the execution of local, functional level quality improvement projects could conceivably be supported by experts within the functional unit considering the project. In fact, the execution of local-level projects could conceivably be driven at the smallest levels of the organization (Ross, Beath, & Quaadgras, 2013) and supported by a robust functional department staffed by analysts of various specialties (Santacroce, 2014).

Regardless of the organizational structure chosen as the decision analytic support framework, the organization must have a process by which problems are identified and solved within the organization. Here, we differentiate between the approaches to problem identification built into the specific methodologies and the approach used to submit problems within the organizational setting. For example, the Lean Six Sigma methodology includes several problem solving phases, the first of which ("define") requires the analyst to provide details on the nature of the problem, how it is defined, the impact and so on. From on organizational perspective, a key process step is how to submit identified problems to the organizational entity that possesses the skillsets and resources available to provide assistance in resolving the problem. Santacroce (2014, p. 36) proposes the use of a project request form that would include elements such as description, impact, and required analytic skills for requesting and routing support for analytic studies.

To the extent that structure and process changes associated with BI&A integration are viewed as a strategic change initiative, organizations must also consider the specific factors that would support integration efforts. In fact, many of the previously mentioned concepts such as organizational structure and processes are directly related to the findings presented by Kash, Spaulding, Johnson and Gamm (2014) in their qualitative assessment of success factors for change initiatives. These success factors included those are typically found within the management literature (e.g., culture, values, financial resources, and leadership) as well as the finding of service quality (SQ) as a key driver, the latter of which is a unique finding for the healthcare strategic management field (Kash, Spaulding, Johnson, & Gamm, 2014).

Service quality – a concept that refers to the difference between what a customer perceives should be provided and that which is provided (Cho, Kim, Park, & Cho, 2013; Pitt, Watson, & Kavan, 1995) – can be viewed from a variety of perspectives in healthcare, which include patient and internal staff perspectives. If considered from a consumer perspective, SQ is "usually linked to the levels of customer satisfaction" (Cho, Kim, Park, & Cho, 2013, p. 756), which is an essential way of assessing the ability of the healthcare organization to effectively and efficiently provide patient care. From an internal perspective, SQ drivers can be thought of as a diverse set of factors related to the practices, structures, policies, values, norms and culture that exist in the organization as compared to those that should exist from a clinical or administrative staff member's perspective. Although the perspective of the internal staff perspective has primacy with respect to organizational integration, patients are the ultimate beneficiaries of the service system and quality patient care one of the critical end results of high-levels of internal SQ.

From an organizational perspective, both service system and human resource HR practices are essential in achieving high-levels of SQ (Li, Yang, & Wu, 2008). Human resources management practices include those that not only focus on job attitude, but also on service ability (Li, Yang, & Wu, 2008). Job attitudes refer to "...motivation, work value and willingness to abide by or follow company rules, procedures and culture" (p. 971), whereas service ability is defined as "the knowledge required of service personnel in providing services, as well as their technical skills" (p. 971). Not surprisingly, these aspects of HR not only support attainment of the SERVQUAL dimensions of reliability, responsiveness, assurance, and empathy (Cho, Kim, Park, & Cho, 2013), but also strongly support the central ideas that Chassin and Loeb (2013) present when discussing the path that healthcare organizations should take on the journey to becoming a high-reliability organization.

FUTURE RESEARCH DIRECTIONS

Advances in technology, increases in sophistication of business analytic methods, and improved access to data are performance enablers for healthcare organizations;

however, without consideration of the nature of the organization, these potential enablers will be inadequately leveraged to improve decision making and performance of the healthcare organizations.

The education of future healthcare leaders—including physicians, analysts, administrators, nurses, and other professional staff—is a key consideration in the industry's goal to seamlessly integrate and utilize information technology and analytics across the spectrum of activities found within and between healthcare organizations. Because healthcare education plays a substantial role in how managerial functions are approached in practice, research is needed to understand the linkages between the curricular content in higher education settings and integration of analytics in healthcare settings.

From both an academic and managerial perspective, future research should focus on what organizations are doing in terms of analytic integration as well as the outcomes that organizations have achieved in their integration efforts. This body of research should not only focus on internal organizational outcomes (such as retention, turnover, profits, losses, efficiencies, and so on), but should also focus on outcomes associated with patient care. Facing increased resource scarcity, organizations will face mounting pressures to determine the most effective and efficient methods of structuring and integrating analytics to facilitate attainment of organizational goals.

CONCLUSION

Decision support systems and analytic methods can provide healthcare organizations with competitive advantage to the extent that organizational structures and processes are effectively aligned. The concepts of structure and processes embody a wide range of organizational concepts that must be considered in building an effective integration strategy. This chapter has outlined several key considerations in analytic integration while also underscoring the idea that the best organizational solution will ultimately be unique to the organization that has chosen to embark on the journey of deliberately considering the integration of analytics throughout the organization. Clearly one best solution does not exist and tradeoffs will inherently accompany any decision set that the organizational leader chooses.

The growing importance associated with the integration of information systems, analytics, people skills, data, and processes is tied the creation and proliferation of communities of practice (COP) and centers of excellence (COE) in business intelligence and analytics. The ideas presented in the literature behind these communities and centers can provide organizational leaders with a starting point for consideration in integration efforts; however, organizational leaders must temper employment of any particular strategy with organizational realities, particularly those associated with the mission, values, culture, capabilities and resources of the organization. The literature supporting COP and COE development will certainly be consistent with the theories, ideas, concepts and processes presented in this chapter.

In many ways, the process of integration is not unlike any other change process. Organizations may face active and passive resistance to change since the process may be perceived as a threat to the status quo. The integration process may represent the very real potential that the relationships between and the work done by analysts, leaders, and clinical staff could potentially evolve in ways that run counter to the current practice. As such, organizations must be prepared to identify barriers to change and honestly assess the extent to which the organization is prepared to invest the time and resources in integration of analytics. Although many organizations might consider the immediate adoption of principles, techniques, and strategies employed by COPs and COEs as the first step in integration of analytics, an initial assessment of readiness to integrate is even more critical to the success of the effort.

REFERENCES

Anderson, D. R., Sweeney, D. J., & Williams, T. A. (2005). *An introduction to management science: Quantitative approaches to decision making* (11th ed.). Mason, OH: South-Western.

Austin, C. J., & Boxerman, S. B. (1995). *Quantitative analysis for health services administration*. Chicago, IL: Health Administration Press.

Austin, C. J., & Boxerman, S. B. (1998). *Information systems for health services administration* (5th ed.). Chicago, IL: Health Administration Press.

Bernstein, A. B., Hing, E., Moss, A. J., Allen, K. F., Siller, A. B., & Tiggle, R. B. (2003). *Health care in American: Trends in utilization*. National Center for Health Statistics. Retrieved from http://www.cdc.gov/nchs/data/misc/healthcare.pdf

Charles, D., Gabriel, M., & Furukawa, M. F. (May 2014). Adoption of Electronic Health Record Systems among U.S. Non-federal Acute Care Hospitals: 2008-2013. In *ONC Data Brief, no. 16*. Washington, DC: Office of the National Coordinator for Health Information Technology.

Chassin, M. R., & Loeb, L. M. (2013). High-reliability health care: Getting there from here. *The Milbank Quarterly*, *91*(3), 459–490. doi:10.1111/1468-0009.12023 PMID:24028696

Chen, H. C., Chiang, R. L., & Storey, V. C. (2012). Business intelligence and analytics: From big data to big impact. *Management Information Systems Quarterly, 36*(4), 1165–1188.

Cho, I., Kim, J. K., Park, H., & Cho, N. H. (2013). The relationship between organisational culture and service quality through organisational learning framework. *Total Quality Management, 24*(7), 753–768. doi:10.1080/14783363.2013.791100

Davis, D. D. (1995). Form, function, and strategy in boundaryless organizations. In A. Howard (Ed.), *The Changing Nature of Work* (pp. 112–138). San Franciso, CA: Jossey-Bass.

Donabedian, A. (1966). Evaluating the quality of medical care. *The Milbank Memorial Fund Quarterly, 44*(3), 166-206.

Donabedian, A. (1978). The quality of medical care. *Science, 200*(4344), 856-864.

Donaldson, L. (1995). *American anti-management theories of organization: A critique of paradigm proliferation*. Cambridge, UK: Cambridge University Press.

Donaldson, L. (2001). *The contingency theory of organizations*. Thousand Oaks, CA: Sage Publications. doi:10.4135/9781452229249

Fottler, M. D. (2005). Job analysis and job design. In B. J. Fried, M. D. Fottler, & J. A. Johnson (Eds.), *Human resources in healthcare* (2nd ed.; pp. 133–161). Chicago, IL: Health Administration Press.

Galbraith, J. R. (1973). *Designing complex organizations*. Reading, MA: Addison-Wesley Pub. Co.

Golden, B. (2006). Transforming healthcare organizations. *Healthcare Quarterly, 10*(sp), 10–19. doi:10.12927/hcq..18490 PMID:17163111

Hearld, L., Alexander, J., Fraser, I., & Jiang, H. (2008). How do hospital organizational structure and processes affect quality of care? *Medical Care Research and Review, 65*(3), 259–299. doi:10.1177/1077558707309613 PMID:18089769

Hsiao, C. J., & Hing, E. (2014). *Use and characteristics of electronic health record systems among office-based physician practices: United States, 2001-2013. NCHS data brief, no. 143*. Hyattsville, MD: National Center for Health Statistics.

Institute of Medicine (U.S.). (2001). Crossing the quality chasm: A new health system for the 21st century. Washington, DC: National Academy Press.

Jung, J. Y., & Lim, S. G. (2007). Project categorization, prioritization, and execution based on six sigma concept: A case study of operational improvement project. *Project Management Journal*, *38*(1), 55–60.

Kanigel, R. (1997). Taylor-made. *The Sciences*, *37*(3), 1–5. doi:10.1002/j.2326-1951.1997.tb03309.x

Kaplan, R., & Norton, D. (1992). The balanced scorecard: Measures that drive performance. *Harvard Business Review*, *70*(1), 71–79.

Kaplan, R., & Norton, D. (1996). *The balanced scorecard: Translating strategy into action*. Boston: Harvard Business School Press.

Kash, B. A., Spaulding, A., Johnson, C. E., & Gamm, L. (2014). Success factors for strategic change initiatives: A qualitative study of healthcare administrators' perspectives. *Journal of Healthcare Management*, *59*(1), 65–80. PMID:24611428

Koch, R. (2015). From business intelligence to predictive analytics. *Strategic Finance*, *97*(1), 56–57.

Krakauer, J. (2012). *The business intelligence competency center: Enabling continuous improvement in performance management*. Oracle Corporation. Retrieved from www.oracle.com/.../bicc-white-paper-1-2012-148691

Krumholz, H. M. (2014). Big data and new knowledge in medicine: The thinking, training, and tools needed for a learning health system. *Health Affairs*, *33*(7), 1163–1170. doi:10.1377/hlthaff.2014.0053 PMID:25006142

Lawrence, P. R., & Lorsch, J. W. (1967). Organization and environment; managing differentiation and integration. Boston: Harvard University.

Lee, R. L. (2009). *Economics for healthcare managers* (2nd ed.). Chicago, IL: Health Administration Press.

Leininger, C. J., & Seaman, L. H. (2000). Selecting clinical quality improvement projects: Getting a bigger return for your investment. *Topics in Health Information Management*, *20*(3), 27–34. PMID:10747432

Li, J. M., Yang, J. S., & Wu, H. H. (2008). Improving service quality and organisation performance through human resource practices. *Total Quality Management*, *19*(9), 970–985.

March, J. G., & Simon, H. A. (1993). *Organizations* (2nd ed.). Cambridge, MA: Blackwell.

Mohrman, S. A., & Cohen, S. G. (1995). When people get out of the box: New relationships, new systems. In A. Howard (Ed.), *The Changing Nature of Work* (pp. 365–410). San Francisco, CA: Jossey-Bass.

Ozcan, Y. A. (2005). *Quantitative methods in health care management: Techniques and applications*. San Francisco, CA: Jossey-Bass.

Patil, P.R., & Mishra, N. (2014, November). Multipronged approach. *Quality Progress,* 22-29.

Pitt, L. F., Watson, R. T., & Kavan, C. G. (1995). Service quality: A measure of information system effectiveness. *Management Information Systems Quarterly, 19*(2), 173–187. doi:10.2307/249687

Rahurkar, S., Vest, J., & Menachemi, N. (2015). Despite the spread of health information exchange, there is little evidence of its impact on cost, use, and quality of care. *Health Affairs, 34*(3), 477-483.

Ross, J. W., Beath, C. M., & Quaadgras, A. (2013). You may not need big data after all. *Harvard Business Review, 91*(12), 90–98. PMID:23593770

Ruchlin, H., Dubbs, N., & Callahan, M. (2004).The role of leadership in instilling a culture of safety: lessons from the literature. *Journal of Healthcare Management, 49*(1), 47-58.

Santacroce, R. (2014). A case study of a high functioning management engineering department. In J. A. Larson (Ed.), *Management engineering: A guide to best practices for industrial engineering in health care* (pp. 33–39). Boca Raton, FL: CRC Press.

Schoemaker, P. J. H., & Russo, J. E. (1993). A pyramid of decision approaches. *California Management Review, 36*(1), 9–31. doi:10.2307/41165732

Scott, W. R. (1990). Technology and structure: An organizational-level perspective. In P. S. Goodman & L. S. Sproull (Eds.), *Technology and organizations* (1st ed.; p. 109). San Francisco, CA: Jossey-Bass.

Scott, W. R., & Davis, G. F. (2007). *Organizations and organizing: Rational, natural, and open systems perspectives*. Upper Saddle River, NJ: Pearson Prentice Hall.

Segel, J. E. (2006). *Cost-of-illness studies—a primer.* RTI International, RTI-UNC Center of Excellence in Health Promotion Economics. Retrieved from https://www.rti.org/pubs/coi_primer.pdf

Shortliffe, E. H. (2005). Strategic action in health information technology: Why the obvious has taken so long. *Health Affairs*, *44*(5), 1222–1233. doi:10.1377/hlthaff.24.5.1222 PMID:16162567

Tabar, P. (2012). Data analytics: Marrying compliance and strategy. *Long-Term Living: For the Continuing Care Professional, 61*(7), 66-71.

Thompson, J. D. (1967). *Organizations in action; social science bases of administrative theory*. New York: McGraw-Hill.

Van De Graaf, J., & Cameron, A. (2013). Quest for business intelligence in healthcare. *HFM*, *67*(2), 44–48. PMID:23413668

Weick, K. E., & Sutcliffe, K. M. (2007). Managing the Unexpected (2nd ed.). Academic Press.

Winston, S., & Albright, S. C. (2001). *Practical management science* (2nd ed.). Pacific Grove, CA: Duxbury.

Wong, H., Legnini, M., & Whitmore, H. (2000). The diffusion of decision support systems in healthcare: are we there yet?. *Journal of Healthcare Management*, *45*(4), 240-249.

KEY TERMS AND DEFINITIONS

Analytics: An encompassing concept that includes methods, resources, and improvement frameworks, which transform data into information to inform decision making and improve performance.

Decision Support: A concept referring to the collection and use of data within an information technology infrastructure aligned by functions and system types to support decision making.

Integration: The process of addressing and incorporating relevant organizational design features in the introduction and implementation of a new structure or process.

Interdependency: Connectedness between organizational entities, processes, and information technology structures.

Project: An activity with a clearly defined start and end point.

Project Prioritization: The process of selecting and ranking evaluative criteria associated with a potential project.

Section 2
Operational Research (OR) in Medicine and Health Systems

Chapter 4
Modelling Spatial Medical Data

S. Zimeras
University of the Aegean, Greece

Y. Matsinos
University of the Aegean, Greece

ABSTRACT

Models are sometimes incomplete, especially in scaling data where other information of large regions needs to be predicted by smaller ones. Uncertainty analysis is the process of assessing uncertainty in modelling or scaling to identify major uncertainty sources, quantify their degree and relative importance, examine their effects on model output under different scenarios, and determine prediction accuracy. Especially for large dimensional data where spatial process in regional investigation are difficult to applied due to incompleteness leading us to spatial heterogeneity and non-linearity of our data. Modelling the uncertainty particular in scaling data starts with a general structure (linear most of the time) that explains as accurate as it is the real data and the model is built through adding variables, which are significant or which aid in prediction (hierarchical modelling). Parameter estimation is an important issue for the evaluation of these proposed models. Statistical techniques based on the spatial modelling could be proposed to overcome the problem of dimensionality and the spatial homogeneity between different grains levels based on the neighbourhood structure of the regions with similar characteristics. Investigation of the neighbourhood structure analysis could be applied using kriging or variogram techniques. In this work, we introduce and analyse methodologies for scaling data under uncertainty where incomplete data can be explained by spatial

DOI: 10.4018/978-1-4666-9961-8.ch004

INTRODUCTION

Incompleteness of the data in the models, especially when a prediction is taking place leading us to uncertainty analysis, where variability is the important measure during the investigation process (Katz 2002). Many times uncertainty implies error mostly statistical (due the process or the estimation procedures), unreliability, and incompleteness in our data (Funtowwicz and Ravetz 1990, Petersen 2000, Regan et al. 2002, Katz 2002). Especially for large dimensional data where spatial process in regional investigation are difficult to applied and model estimation is difficult to predict due to incompleteness leading us to spatial heterogeneity and non-linearity of our data (Katz 2002, Regan et al. 2002).

Models sometimes involve incomplete data, especially in grain scaling data where various information of large regions needs to be predicted by smaller ones. Uncertainty analysis is the process of assessing uncertainty in modelling or scaling to identify major uncertainty sources, quantify their degree and relative importance, examine their effects on model output under different scenarios, and determine prediction accuracy (Jansen 1998, Katz 2002).

Modelling the uncertainty particular in grain scaling data starts with a general structure (linear most of the time) that explains as accurate as it is the real data and the model is built through adding variables, which are significant or which aid in prediction (hierarchical modelling) (Zimeras and Aykroyd, 1999; Zimeras, 2007). Parameter estimation is an important issue for the evaluation of these proposed models. For example, the GLUE procedure can be used in estimating likelihoods of all possible outcomes for a specific distribution of inputs as well as to acquire behavioral outcomes (Beven and Binley 1992, Wang et al 2012, Huang et al. 2013) based on likelihood measures in evaluating parameters in model's outcomes. Statistical techniques based on the spatial modelling could be proposed to overcome the problem of dimensionality and the spatial homogeneity between different grains levels based on the neighbourhood structure of the regions with similar characteristics. Investigation of the neighbourhood structure analysis could be applied using geostatistical simulation techniques to generate multiple realizations. The realizations should capture the sample statistics, and the conditioning data provide quantitative measure of local and spatial uncertainties (Goovaerts 1998, Goovaerts 2001, Lin et al. 2008a, Lin et al. 2011).

In this work, we introduce and analyse methodologies for scaling data under uncertainty where incomplete data can be explained by spatial modelling at different scales. Incomplete data of uncertainties in regions involve spatial homogeneity upon neighbourhood structure between regions. The last could be illustrated by using spatial modelling techniques (like spatial autocorrelation, partition functions, and multilevel models). Parameter estimation of these models could be achieved by using stochastic (spatial hierarchical models, kriging, auto-correlation) methods. Comparison between different models could be achieved by considering statistical measures like log-likelihood ratio test. The best model is the one, which explains better the real data.

DATA UNDER UNCERTAINTY

Data most of the times are observed incompletely with large and unknown amounts of measurement error or data uncertainty (Dale, 2002).). Moreover, the spatial structures of the data are affected by spatial configurations of the data locations (Diniz-Filho et al., 2003; Fortin and Dale, 2005; Rangel et al., 2006, Lin et al. 2008). Traditional to overcome the problem of incompleteness more data must be collected, method that is expensive due to the dimensionality of the spatial representation of the data.

Incompleteness introduces uncertainty modelling especially in the case of scaling data, where different grains are combined together (Katz, 2002). In grain scaling data, the choice of grain is very important for the analysis of them. For example, as data change with various scales, the spatial patterns and processes based on the changing data may change (Wu and Li 2006, Lin et al. 2008b). Accordingly, measurements made at a scale may miss important information of spatial patterns and processes operating on different scales (Wu and Li 2006, Lin et al. 2008b). Spatial heterogeneity can disappear at spatial resolutions that are too fine or too broad introducing a modification of a pyramid process based on different levels (multi-resolution process). If the grain size is large, spatial heterogeneity can be masked as discontinuities are averaged across the measurement units. Likewise, if the extent is too small, patterns may occur across a wider range than that visible within the spatial bounds of the region (Turner et. al., 1989)

To detect scale-dependent processes and patterns one depends on observation sets or model calculations of fine grain and large extent (Zimeras and Matsinos, 2013, 2012, 2011). Inter-specific interactions may affect the space use of sympatric species at various spatial and temporal scales, ranging from delineation of distribution patterns (scaling effects the distribution of the species inside the cells). For spatial data or images, spatial grain size corresponds to maximum resolution ratio or pixel size (Figure 1).

Grain scaling could be defined as a window process (considering the spatial point process), where the amount of frequencies of data inside the grain is calculated based on the window of analysis (Sivapalan 1995). Based on Cressie (1993), the process is analogous to nearest neighbor distance process (NND). Based on that process investigation of the randomness of the spatial structure is taking place, and at the same time analysis of the spatial homogeneity (clustering) is investigated (Figure 2).

A point process is a process of locations of events taking place in some space *X*. Each event has associated with a mark, taking place in some mark space *Y* (Diggle, 2003; 2003). A point pattern is a set of point locations $\mathbf{s}=\{s_1, s_2,\ldots,s_n\}$ in a specific sub-region A. (Zimeras and Georgiakodis, 2005). The random variable N(A) is the number of events in the set A$\subset$ *X* introducing a random process. The process calculates the distance between point locations **s** with the nearest neighbours (for example dist=s_i-s_j where s_j is the nearest location). We calculate the average of all the distances given by

$$D = \frac{\sum d_i}{n},$$

Figure 1. Grain data based on different scaling

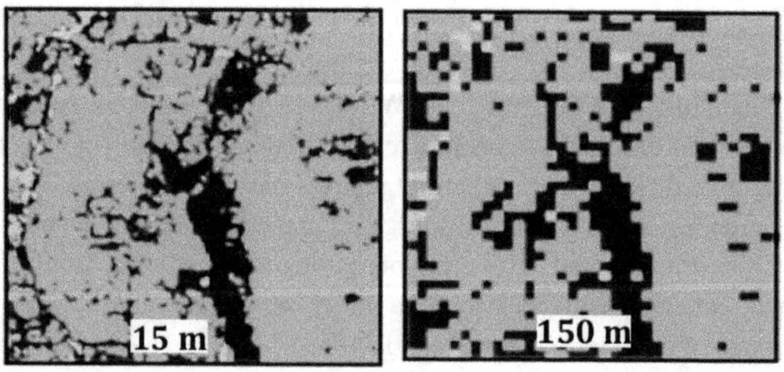

Figure 2. Nearest neighbours distance approach

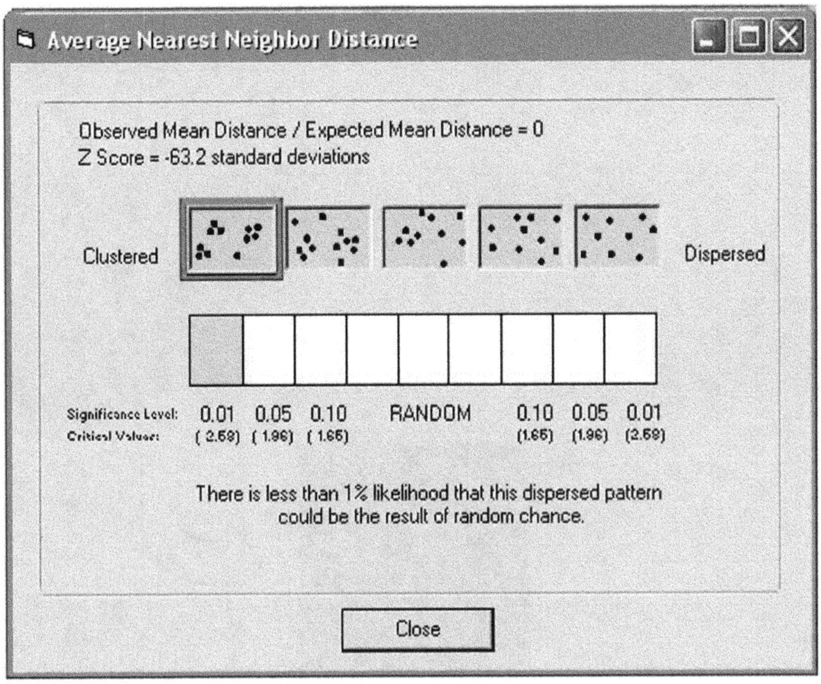

where D is the mean distance and d_i is the calculated distance. The value is compared with a random distribution (for the investigation of the clustering in point process analysis the Poisson distribution or the Binomial distribution is considered) with general form

$$E_d = \frac{1}{2}\sqrt{\frac{D}{n}}.$$

If the mean distance is greater than the distribution value, the data are random otherwise they are clustered. The degree of closeness is given by Diggle (2003):

$$NN = \frac{D}{E_d}$$

with values from 0 to 2.1491 (Cressie, 1993). If NN→0 then the data are clustered, where when NN→2.1491, the data are regular. Considering a lattice region the process is described as before with the only difference the introduction of the windowing process given by Figure 3.

Figure 3. Windowing process based on lattice data system

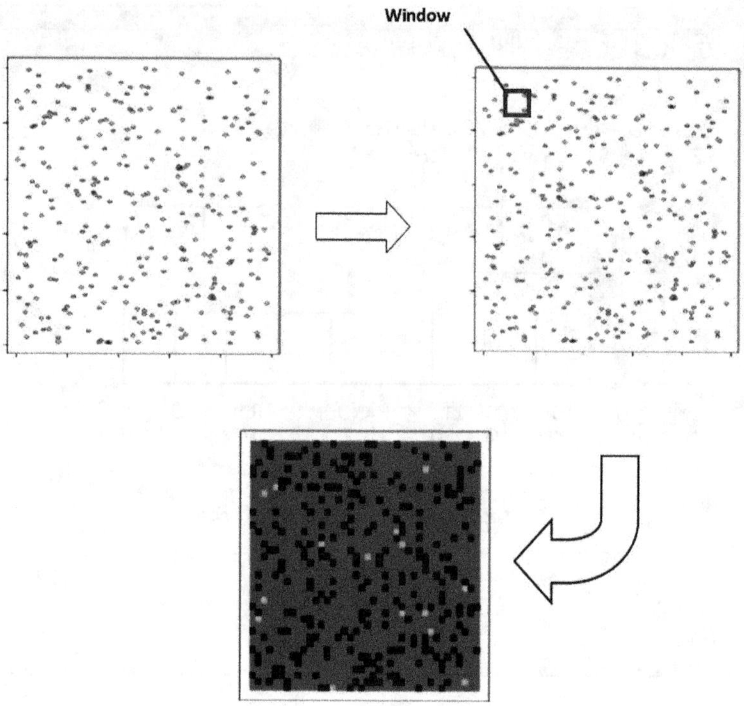

MODEL UNCERTAINTY

Model uncertainty has two basic components, model structure and model parameters (O'Neill and Gardner 1979, Jansen 1998, Katz 2002). Model structure uncertainty is caused by the modelling processes of simplification and formulation. Model simplification is essential to modelling and is the identification and selection of the relationships, and variables that are the most important ones. Moreover, deficient model structures may cause certain levels of error or uncertainty because of simplifying complexity of study systems as well as estimating parameters of the models (Wang et al. 2012, Huang et al. 2013).

Model parameter uncertainty is introduced by the modelling process of parameterization of models (Morgan and Hemion 1990, Klepper 1997, Katz 2002). Model parameterization involves also the estimation and calibration of parameters. Calibration produces a set of optimal parameter values by proposing a selected model outputs to agree with testing data. Model parameter values are built into models and may be fixed or change in space and time. Model parameter uncertainty results from incomplete knowledge about the parameters, and errors in the estimation processes. Uncertainty analysis requires that statistical distributions of parameters be known. However, a common problem in uncertainty analysis is that the accuracy of measurements and/or estimates of parameters are unknown.

Considering that uncertainty models are applied in cases where incomplete data are considered, the choice of the appropriate model most of the times is a difficult and complicate process. Especially when the qualities of the data due to incompleteness are unstable and spatial heterogeneity is appeared causing variability of the system that is investigated (O'Neill and Gardner 1979, Jansen 1998, Regan et al. 2002).

In particular when the data are represented in a lattice system, spatially-indexed structures are associated with geographic regions or areas, where often are presented as aggregated values over an area unit with well defined boundaries. Spatial association among the areal units is specified by defining neighbourhood structure for the areas (regular or irregular) of interest. Examples of such data include a wide variety of problems from disease mapping in counties to modelling air-pollution on a grid. Models described in this section are based on Markov random fields (MRFs). MRFs are a special class of spatial models that are suitable for data on discrete (countable) spatial domains in which a joint distribution of s_i (for i = 1, ..., n, where s_i is the spatial process at spatial unit *i*) is determined by using a set of locally specified conditional distributions for each spatial unit conditioned on its neighbours. MRFs include a wide class of spatial models, such as auto-Gaussian models for spatial Gaussian processes, auto-logistic models for binary spatial random variables, auto-Gamma models for non-negative continuous processes, and auto-Poisson models for spatial count processes (Zimeras and Georgiakodis, 2005; Zimeras 1997). For every grain scale data a proposed MRF model is proposed and a hierarchical (nested) approach is defined for choosing the appropriate model which explains as better as it can the real data. If the starting model fails to include factors of real importance clearly the final model will not include them. In consequence the starting model tends to be very complex, including many unnecessary parameters (Zimeras, 1997). Based on the spatial structure of the lattice data, various models could be introduced (isotropic, anisotropic, n^{th} neighbourhood structure system). To select an appropriate model, based on the above hierarchy, the backward elimination approach could be considered, starting with the most complex model of the MRF family, continuing by dropping parameters and ending with a simple model (Zimeras and Aykroyd, 1999).

In statistical modelling, the basic aim is to define an appropriate family of models and to select the simplest model which adequately describes the data. The approach will be based on hypothesis testing. For each the maximum likelihood ratio test is applied. The critical regions for the comparison tests are based on the x^2 distribution where x_n^2 denotes the (1-α) quantile of the x^2 distribution with n-degrees of freedom with α the required significant level.

The conditional likelihood, l(θ), of the pixel values in one coding set given the values of the pixels in the other coding sets can be obtained by the product of the conditional distributions of the pixel values given the values of their neighbours

$$l(\theta)=\prod_i p(s_i \mid s_{\partial i})$$

where s_i is the point process location, $s_{\partial i}$ is the neighbours of s_i and θ is the set of n model parameters.

The log-likelihood is given by

$$l(\theta)=\sum_i \log\left(p(s_i \mid s_{\partial i})\right),$$

where the log-likelihood conditional function can be expressed as an exponential family model based on the MRF structure. Based on the likelihood function for every proposed model, the likelihood ratio test is computed and hypothesis testing based on the x^2 distribution in considered. If the value from the test is smaller than the value of the x^2 distribution then the proposed model is better.

From probabilistic point of view advanced techniques based on geostatistical analysis could be considered for point estimation approach (Dale, 1999; Diggle, 2003). Therefore, a deterministic model may not be appropriate. If we wish to make predictions at locations for which we have no observations, we must allow for uncertainty in our description as a result of our lack in knowledge. So, the uncertainty inherent in predictions of any property we cannot describe deterministically is accounted for through the use of probabilistic models. Kriging and semi-variagram analysis could be applied for the estimation and prediction of the point location inside the grain scale data especially under uncertainty conditions where data are incomplete. Also these methods could be used to detect spatial correlations between neighbourhood structures. Kriging analysis is spatial point process involves three parameters which can be combined as a spatial linear model with form (Cressie, 1993):

$$Z(s)=m(s)+e(s)+\varepsilon$$

where Z(**s**) is the point process, m(**s**) is a function that explains the characteristics of the point process Z(**s**), e(**s**) is a function that depends on the spatial residuals of the m(**s**) estimation and ε is a Gaussian noise. The main problem is the definition of the appropriate m(**s**) function, which explains better the spatial anomalies (and uncertain regions). For that reason the spatial point structure of the regional area must be considered, where homogeneous and inhomogeneous regions introduces spatial auto-correlation between neighboring structures. In geostatistics, semi-variograms provide a means of quantifying the spatial relationship between the values of the samples (Lin et al. 2001, Lin et al. 2008a). The spatial auto-correlation (semi-variagram) is given by the form for h direction (lag) (Cressie 1993):

$$\gamma(h) = \frac{1}{2} E\left\{\left[Z(s) - Z(s+h)\right]^2\right\}$$

The spatial auto-correlation explains the spatial construction based on the homogeneity of the region. So it could be lead us to the calculation of the spatial residuals. If we combine Z(s) and γ(h) the spatial model becomes

$$Z(s) = m(s) + \gamma(h) + \varepsilon$$

Estimation of the kriging process involves the analysis of the semi-variogram explaining the spatial correlation with distance. A semi-variogram characterised by the following (Figure 4) (Cressie 1993):

Figure 4. Characteristics of the semi-variograms

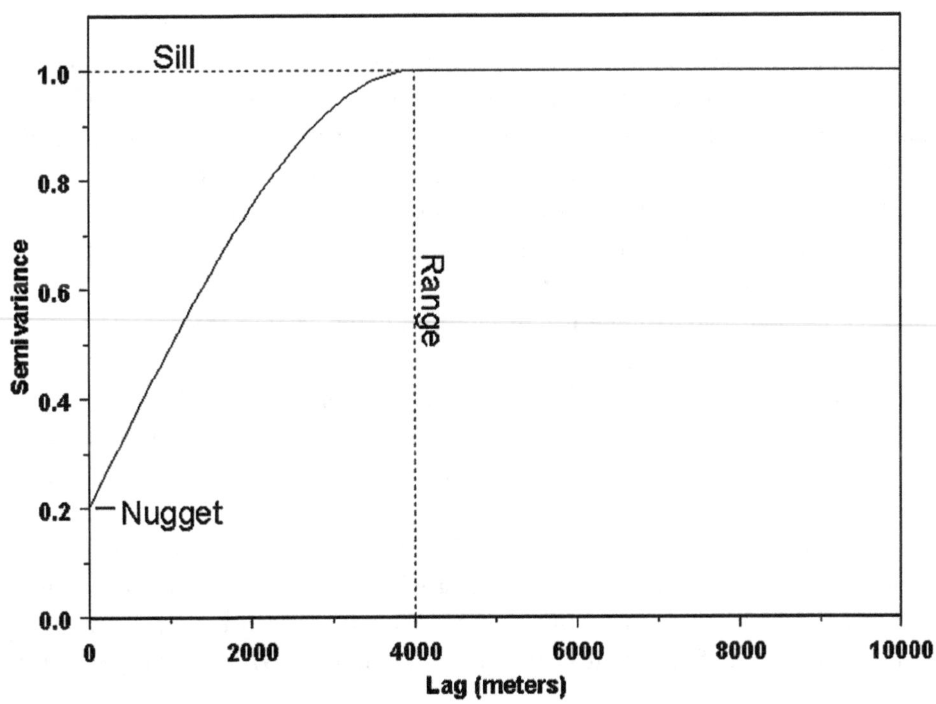

- **Nugget Effects:** Represents variation or measurement error.
- **Sill:** Represent the variance of the random field $\lim_{h \to \infty} \gamma(h)$
- **Range:** Distance at which data are not auto-correlated.

Using h to represent lag distance, a to represent (practical) range, and c to represent sill, the five most frequently used models are:

Nugget $$g(h) = \begin{cases} 0 & \text{if } h = 0 \\ c & \text{otherwise} \end{cases}$$

Spherical $$g(h) = \begin{cases} c\left(1.5\left(\frac{h}{a}\right) - 0.5\left(\frac{h}{a}\right)^3\right) & \text{if } h \le a \\ 0 & \text{otherwise} \end{cases}$$

Exponential $$g(h) = c\left(1 - \exp\left(\frac{-3h}{a}\right)\right)$$

Gaussian $$g(h) = c\left(1 - \exp\left(\frac{-3h^2}{a^2}\right)\right)$$

Power $$g(h) = ch^{\omega}, \quad \text{with } 0 \prec \text{É} \prec 2$$

The nugget model represents the discontinuity at the origin due to small-scale variation. The spherical model actually reaches the specified sill value, *c*, at the specified range, *a*. The exponential and Gaussian approach the sill asymptotically, with *a* representing the practical range, the distance at which the semi-variance reaches 95% of the sill value. These three models are shown below (Figure 5):

The Gaussian model, with its parabolic behavior at the origin, represents very smoothly varying properties. (However, using the Gaussian model alone without a nugget effect can lead to numerical instabilities in the kriging process.) The spherical and exponential models exhibit linear behavior the origin, appropriate for representing properties with a higher level of short-range variability.

However, kriging is an interpolation method which yields the best linear unbiased estimation (BLUE) based on measured data and variograms of the data (Goovaerts 1998, Lin et al. 2001, Lin et al. 2008a). Kriging may produce smoothed data it may capture the local distribution of the data because it yields BLUE (Goovaerts 1998, Lin et al. 2008a). However, kriging provide unbiased estimates with kriging variance. Different to classical interpolation techniques, geostatistical simulation techniques such as Sequential Gaussian Simulation (SGS) based on parametric

Figure 5. Semi-variagram analysis for different proposed nuggets

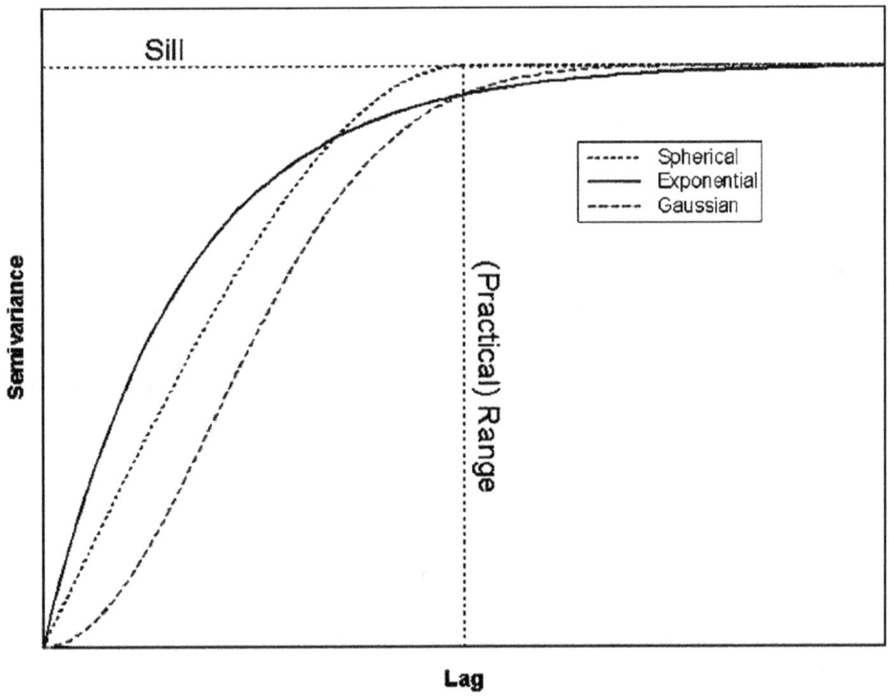

approach or Sequential Indicator Simulation (SIS) based nonparametric approach generate multiple realizations, including an error component (Goovaerts 1996, Lin et al. 2001, Lin et al. 2008a, Lin et al. 2011). However, the aim stochastic simulation is not to minimize error variance but to generate realizations that reproduce statistics while conditioning measured data at their locations (Goovaerts 1998). The statistics of the multiple realizations match those of measured data (conditioning data). Therefore, the multiple realizations can be used to quantify spatial uncertainty from local to global scales.

CONCLUSION

From the previous analysis the following main results can be drawn:

- Data quality and quantity is very critical and affect uncertainty in a number of ways.
- Uncertainty includes incomplete data, especially in spatial modelling at different scales. Incomplete data, spatial differences and statistical modelling

analysis of uncertainties in regions involve spatial connectivity upon neighbourhood structure between regions. The last could be illustrated by using spatial modelling techniques (like spatial autocorrelation, markov random fields models).

- For the spatial connection of the grains where spatial model for every level was applied a hierarchical model selection approach could be considered. Comparison between different models could be achieved by considering statistical measures like log-likelihood ratio test. Finally, a good fitting method was introduced between different grains based on the spatial hierarchical modelling techniques. The best model is the one, which explains best the real data.
- Kriging via semi-variagram models could be used and in fact are good candidates to develop models to tackle uncertainty across scales.

REFERENCES

Beven, K., & Binley, A. (1992). The future of distributed models: Model calibration and uncertainty prediction. *Hydrological Processes*, *6*(3), 279–298. doi:10.1002/hyp.3360060305

Blöschl, G., & Sivapalan, M. (1995). Scale issues in hydrological modelling: A review. *Hydrological Processes*, *9*(3-4), 251–290. doi:10.1002/hyp.3360090305

Cressie, N. A. (1993). *Statistics for Spatial Data* (revised edition). John Wiley & Sons.

Dale, M. R. T. (1999). *Spatial Pattern Analysis in Plant Ecology*. Cambridge University Press. doi:10.1017/CBO9780511612589

Diggle, P. J. (2003). *Spatial Analysis of Spatial Point Patterns* (2nd ed.). Arnold Publishers.

Diniz-Filho, J. A. F., Bini, L. M., & Hawkins, B. A. (2003). Spatial autocorrelation and red herrings in geographical ecology. *Global Ecology and Biogeography*, *12*(1), 53–64. doi:10.1046/j.1466-822X.2003.00322.x

Fortin, M.-J., & Dale, M. R. T. (2005). *Spatial analysis: a guide for ecologists*. Cambridge: Cambridge University Press.

Funtowwicz, S., & Ravetz. (1990). Uncertainty and Quality in Science for Policy. Kluwer Academic Publishers.

Goovaerts, P. (1998). Geostatistical tools for characterizing the spatial variability of microbiological and physico-chemical soil properties. *Biology and Fertility of Soils*, *27*(4), 315–334. doi:10.1007/s003740050439

Goovaerts, P. (2001). Geostatistical modelling of uncertainty in soil science. *Geoderma*, *103*(1), 3–26. doi:10.1016/S0016-7061(01)00067-2

Huang, C.-W., Lin, Y.-P., Chiang, L.-C., & Wang, Y.-C. (2013). *Using CV-GLUE Procedure in Analysis of Wetland Model Predictive Uncertainty*. Submiited.

Jensen, J. B. (2003). Parameter and Uncertainty Estimation in Groundwater Modelling. Aalborg: Aalborg University.

Katz, R. W. (2002). Techniques for estimating uncertainty in climate change scenarios and impact studies. *Climate Research*, *20*, 167–185. doi:10.3354/cr020167

Klepper, O. (1997). Multivariate aspects of model uncertainty analysis: Tools for sensitivity analysis and calibration. *Ecological Modelling*, *101*(1), 1–13. doi:10.1016/S0304-3800(96)01922-9

Lin, Y.-P., Chang, T.-K., & Teng, T.-P. (2001). Characterization of soil lead by comparing of sequential Gaussian simulation, simulated annealing simulation and kriging methods. *Environmental Geology*, *41*(1-2), 189–199. doi:10.1007/s002540100382

Lin, Y.-P., Chu, H.-J., Huang, Y.-L., Cheng, B.-Y., & Chang, T.-K. (2011). Modeling spatial uncertainty of heavy metal content in soil by conditional Latin hypercube sampling and geostatistical simulation. *Environmental Earth Sciences*, *62*(2), 299–311. doi:10.1007/s12665-010-0523-5

Lin, Y.-P., Wu, P.-J., & Hong, N.-M. (2008b). The effects of changing the resolution of land-use modeling on simulations of land-use patterns and hydrology for a watershed land-use planning assessment in Wu-Tu, Taiwan. *Landscape and Urban Planning*, *87*(1), 54–66. doi:10.1016/j.landurbplan.2008.04.006

Lin, Y. P., Yeh, M. S., Deng, D. P., & Wang, Y. C. (2008a). Geostatistical approaches and optimal additional sampling schemes for spatial patterns and future sampling of bird diversity. *Global Ecology and Biogeography*, *17*(2), 175–188. doi:10.1111/j.1466-8238.2007.00352.x

Morgan, M. G., & Henrion, M. (1990). *Uncertainty: A Guide to Dealing with Uncertainty in Quantitative Risk and Policy Analysis*. Cambridge, UK: Cambridge University Press. doi:10.1017/CBO9780511840609

O'Neill, R. V., & Gardner, R. H. (1979). Sources of uncertainty in ecological models. In B. P. M. Zeigles, M. S. Elzas, G. J. Klir, & T. I. Oren (Eds.), Methodology in Systems Modelling and Simulation. North Holland.

Petersen, A. C. (2000). Philosophy of climate science. *Bulletin of the American Meteorological Society*, *81*(2), 265–271. doi:10.1175/1520-0477(2000)081<0265:POCS>2.3.CO;2

Rangel, T. F., Diniz-Filho, J. A., & Bini, L. M. (2006). Towards an integrated computational tool for spatial analysis in macroecology and biogeography. *Global Ecology and Biogeography*, *15*(4), 321–327. doi:10.1111/j.1466-822X.2006.00237.x

Regan, H., Colyvan, M., & Burgman, M. A. (2002). A taxonomy and treatment of uncertainty for ecology and conservation biology. *Ecological Applications*, *12*(2), 618–628. doi:10.1890/1051-0761(2002)012[0618:ATATOU]2.0.CO;2

Turner, M. G., Dale, V. H., & Gardner, R. H. (1989). Predicting across scales: Theory development and testing. *Landscape Ecology*, *3*(3-4), 245–252. doi:10.1007/BF00131542

Wang, Y.-C., Lin, Y.-P., Huang, C.-W., Chiang, L.-C., Chu, H.-J., & Ou, W.-S. (2012). A System Dynamic Model and Sensitivity Analysis for Simulating Domestic Pollution Removal in a Free-Water Surface Constructed Wetland. *Water, Air, and Soil Pollution*, *223*(5), 2719–2742. doi:10.1007/s11270-011-1062-8

Wu, J. (1999). Hierarchy and scaling: Extrapolating information along a scaling ladder. *Canadian Journal of Remote Sensing*, *25*(4), 367–380. doi:10.1080/07038992.1999.10874736

Wu, J., & Li, H. (2006). *Scaling and uncertainty analysis in ecology*. Springer. doi:10.1007/1-4020-4663-4

Zimeras, S. (1997). *Statistical models in medical imaging*. (Ph. D. Thesis). Leeds University.

Zimeras, S. (2007). In E. A. Zoeller (Ed.), *Spatial Pattern Recognition Models with Application in Image Analysis. In Pattern Recognition Theory and Application* (pp. 201–219). Nova Publishers.

Zimeras, S., & Aykroyd, R. G. (1999). Neighbourhood structure estimation of images using hierarchical testing. *Electronics Letters*, *35*(25), 2188–2189. doi:10.1049/el:19991476

Zimeras, S., & Georgiakodis, F. (2005). Bayesian models for medical image biology using Monte Carlo Markov Chain techniques. *Mathematical and Computer Modelling*, *42*(7-8), 759–768. doi:10.1016/j.mcm.2005.09.005

Zimeras, S., & Matsinos, Y. (2011). *Spatial Uncertainty*. Paper presented at the 4th International Conference in Geography and Geology, Corfu, Greece.

Zimeras, S., & Matsinos, Y. (2012). *Bayesian Spatial Uncertainty Analysis*. Paper presented at the 7th IASME/WSEAS International Conference on Energy & Environment (EE '12), Kos Island, Greece.

Zimeras, S., & Matsinos, Y. (2013). Uncertainty analysis in ecological systems System. *International Journal of Systems Biology and Biomedical Technologies*, *2*, 14–24. doi:10.4018/ijsbbt.2013010102

Chapter 5
Surgery Operations Modeling and Scheduling in Healthcare Systems

Fatah Chetouane
Université de Moncton, Canada

Eman Ibraheem
Université de Moncton, Canada

ABSTRACT

Surgery operations scheduling is a complex task due to operation duration uncertainties and resource sharing and availabilities in healthcare processes. In current health care systems it is important to minimize staff idle time and maintain a high utilization rate for surgery facilities. In the present study a nonlinear mathematical model for surgery scheduling is described, and an approximated linear model is deduced based on a set of assumptions. The linear model is solved using heuristic approach. The objective is to maximize the utilization of operating rooms and the surgery staff. Computational results show that our model improved the surgery schedule and the resources utilization. Our model also showed the potential of adding cases to the schedule due to minimizing the completion time of the schedule.

1. INTRODUCTION

Providing efficient healthcare services to patients are gaining an increasing attention over the past few years. Recent budgetary restrictions, prescribed by politics, due to economic changes, led public hospitals to seek and implement methodolo-

DOI: 10.4018/978-1-4666-9961-8.ch005

gies and techniques at their managerial and operational levels, to achieve efficient resource usage, without compromising the quality of their service, risking patient endangerment, or causing additional costs (patient waiting and resources usage costs). Emergency department and surgery department got to be the most critical subsystems in any hospital, due to their role in fulfilling emergent needs. Surgery departments service both urgent and elective surgery procedures, and are linked to referrals from physicians outside the hospital, and/or from other department within, such as the emergency department. The Surgery department is the hospital most expensive center (Health Care Financial Management Association.2005), and due to his linkage to other hospital services (intensive care, preoperative care, post anesthesia care, surgery admission, and recovery units), its impacts the performance of the hospital as whole. To provide an idea of surgery department cost distributions, based on data from statistics Canada collected for the period 2007-2008, the New Brunswick regional health authority expenditures averaged: staff wages (70%), medical and surgical supplies (13%), drugs and medicines (7%), equipment and miscellaneous (10%). When putting these expenditure figures in contrast with the increasing demand in surgery procedures inflicted on the same New Brunswick regional health authority (16% increase over the period from 2005 to 2008), seeking continuous improvement of the operating theatre management becomes critical to ensure quality healthcare delivery for all patients, by keeping a cost-effective, and a flexible scheduling of all surgery demands.

In the same line of thought, this study is aimed, in a first stage, toward the development of a general mathematical programming model (nonlinear) for elective surgery planning and scheduling. During modeling, surgeries are assumed to be of uncertain durations, also operating room, and surgeon preferences are taking into consideration. The two goal of increasing operating room utilization, and reducing surgeon idle times are combined in a single objective formulation. In the second stage of this study, a linear program is extracted from the general model and solved using a simple heuristic approach. Several feasible schedules (no optimal) can be obtained easily using the linear model, providing a flexibility in the decision making process.

The reminder of this chapter starts with a brief background on recent studies on modelling and scheduling of surgery procedures, followed by a mathematical description of the constraints involved in the surgery planning and scheduling problem. The nonlinear model is then simplified to a linear mathematical program, and a heuristic procedure is presented to solve the simplified model. Based on a case study, some results are discussed, with conclusion and future possible extensions.

2. RECENT MATHEMATICAL STUDIES ON SURGERY SCHEDULING

As succinctly defined in (Burke & Riise, 2008), the surgery scheduling problem is to find the optimal allocation of surgeries to operating rooms and days, and their optimal sequence for each day. Objectives are typically tardiness costs (over time), hospitalization costs, intervention costs, operating room utilization, patient's waiting time, patient or personnel preferences, etc. This problem is solved on different time scales, ranging from month-scale admission planning to daily detailed surgery scheduling, using different objectives and constraints. The most common objective is to maximize operating rooms usage (Hans et al., 2008) and staff utilization (Denton et al., 2007). Contributions on surgery scheduling can be classified according to several standpoints and criteria such as: single operating room vs. multiple operating room scheduling; surgery scheduling (not considering sequencing), and vice-versa, or simultaneously sequencing and scheduling (which lead generally to a combinatorial stochastic optimization problem); considering uncertainty, considering costs; and also depending on techniques used to approach the problem whether by using simulation methods, or mathematical optimization methods. For few decades ago mathematical programming models and optimization techniques have frequently used for surgery scheduling (Denton et al. 2007), (Santibáñez et al. 2007), and (Jeroen et al. 2008). A good literature review of surgery scheduling is provided in (Cardoen, B. 2009) and (Cardoen, B. et al. 2010), where authors studied one hundred and twenty four papers on operating room planning and scheduling, and compared their used terminology and primary contributions using several indicators such as: time horizon, accounted uncertainties, analysis and solving methods, patient types, performance metrics (resources, time, quality of care, economic aspects), and decision delineation (discipline, surgeon, patient). The main outcome of their study is an enhanced way to classify existing contribution using the proposed indicators that helps researcher identify manuscripts according to specific research interests. An early, though extensively cited study is described in (Magerlein and Martin. 1978). This citation appears in many succeeding contributions in the field of surgical system scheduling. It provides a comparison of three common surgery scheduling approaches, namely: no blocked (open) booking, blocked booking, admissions scheduling and control system. The conducted comparison is made with regards to operating room performance metrics, service quality, and implementation drawbacks vs. benefits. Blocked and no blocked approaches outperformed admissions control system approach, with regards to the capacity planning stability aspect, while the control system approach outperformed on the managerial and operational flexibility aspect, due its advantage in testing several decision rules for surgery scheduling (first-come-first-serve, longest-cases-first, and shortest-cases-first). The authors discussed the real challenge in surgery scheduling due to the multiple type of uncertainty and imprecision affecting the process, especially surgery procedure durations. Most estimation of surgery durations are based on surgeons' estimates, operating room schedulers' estimates, or historical averages (or a combination of the three). It was advised that accurate estimates are key to achieving quality process analysis and improvements, since lower estimates will result in an overloaded schedule causing cancellations, overtime, and low employee morale, while higher estimates will result in idle times, misused capacity and increased patient waiting times. The variability in surgery durations can also be caused by the fluctuation in surgeon experience and skills. A study on this fluctuation for a two-surgeon team (a responsible and an assistant) is described in (Molina-Pariente, Fernandez-Viagas & Framinan, 2015). A mixed integer linear programming model is proposed for an open surgery scheduling case, with surgeon experience level as an explicit parameter in the model. In addition to uncertainties on surgery durations, uncertainty on downstream resource availabilities (capacity constraints of surgical intensive, and/or post anesthesia care units) are studied in (Min & Yih, 2010b). They formulated thee elective surgery scheduling problem as a stochastic optimization model minimizing patient and overtime costs. Other performance measures were also collected such as: average overtime, average utilization, total number of scheduled patients and cancellations. The solution approach was conducted using sample average approximation method implemented using ILOG, CPLEX software. When compared to a deterministic version of the problem (replacing random variable by their expected value parameters) the stochastic optimization model outperformed the deterministic version by more than 17% in cost reduction. This proves the importance of considering the uncertainties in the modeling and solving of surgery scheduling problems.

Erdogan & Denton (2011) discussed how the design and physical layout of the entire surgical process stages (preoperative, intraoperative and postoperative) complicates the scheduling problem. They based their study on the comparison between two surgical suite designs: one with separate intake and recovery areas; and another with common intake, and recovery areas. Among the complicating factors are duration uncertainties (operative, preoperative and postoperative), variability of patients to be scheduled on a given day (cancelations, no-shows, and emergency add-ons), resource availabilities, and interactions between specialties. Authors discussed the efficiency and limitation of queuing, simulation, mathematical and optimization approaches in addressing these complicating factors. In reference to the interaction between different surgery specialties and units, the joint operating room planning and advanced scheduling problem, where several specialties share a fixed number of operating rooms, and post-surgery beds was studied in (Aringhieri, Landa, Soriano, Tànfani, & Testi, 2015). Using linear programming models, authors exploited the inherent hierarchical interaction between two decision levels: the time block assignment level to surgical specialties, and the patient assignment level to these time blocks. The influence of preoperative preparation tasks, such as sterilization and setting of needed equipment, on the sequencing of elective surgery operations with deterministic durations was also investigated in (Zhao, & Li, 2014), where the surgery sequencing problem is solved using two different approaches: mixed integer nonlinear programming, and constraint programming. Better performance with regards to solution quality and sensitivity to setup tasks where obtained using the constraint programming approach. In (Xiang, Yin, & Lim, 2015) the studied surgery scheduling problem considers nurse schedule constraints (role, specialty, qualification and availability). A mathematical formulation is proposed, and solved using ant colony optimization approach. Despite the resulting complexity of integrating nurse constraints, the obtained results exhibit a shorter completion time, and a balanced resource allocations when compared to those obtained without considering nurse rostering constraints. The problem of scheduling surgical services in a multistage operating room department was also studied in (Saremi, Jula, ElMekkawy & Wang, 2013). Several patient types with stochastic service time and punctual arrivals are considered. Admission is schedule-based, and each patient type is served by a specific specialty (surgeon type). Resource (surgeon) availabilities are restricted by time window constraints. The application of simulation methods enhanced with mathematical programming models improved the appointment scheduling in terms of completion time. Surgeries allocation and sequencing problem for multiple operating rooms and multiple surgical team, was also studied in (Koksalmis, Hancerliogullari & Hancerliogullari, 2014) using a mathematical formulation to minimize the number of unscheduled surgical operations. Adopting an open scheduling strategy, (Bouguerra, Sauvey & Sauer, 2015) studied the case where operating rooms are considered specialized for a given day but multi-functional on the scheduling horizon. The model was solved using heuristic approach, with an objective to maximize operating rooms utilization and to minimize idle time between planned surgeries.

More surgical procedures are now being performed in outpatient procedure centers. These centers are increasingly appealing for their ability to handle specialty procedures in a more accommodating way to patient preferences. These facilities are subjected to similar challenges with regards to surgery booking under uncertainties. Indeed, the problem of optimizing surgical procedure scheduling, in the presence of uncertainty on patient attendance and surgery durations is studied in (Berg, Denton, Erdogan, Rohleder, & Huschka, 2014). A stochastic programming model formulation is used allowing to test exact and heuristic resolution methods. Their study shows that heuristic scheduling methods (easy-to-implement) are more suitable to use in one or both of these cases: overtime costs greater than patient waiting time costs, or procedure duration uncertainty and no-attendance rate for the procedure are directly related. In the same study, the efficiency of double booking, and late-day scheduling of patients with high no-attendance rate, or procedures with high duration variance, is attested to lower waiting, idling, and overtime costs. Generally surgery can be of an elective or emergency type (Encyclopedia of surgery, 2010). This classification is broad and indicates the two essential priority categories for surgery operations. Other classifications such as elective, emergent, urgent can be found in literature (Cardoen, B. et *al.* 2010). Unlike elective surgeries which can be planned off-line, emergency surgeries cannot be planned in advance and must be handled on-line (Yigal, G. et al. 1996). In order to deal with this uncertainty on a daily basis, and to safely handle priority patients, hospitals must reserve a portion of their resource capacity for emergency add-on cases (Guinet and Chaabane. 2003). Lamieri et al. (2008) proposed a stochastic model for operating rooms scheduling where both elective and emergency surgeries were taken into account. Random capacity for emergency surgeries was reserved and the problem was formulated as a stochastic integer model.

Service capacity must be controlled effectively to handle most daily planned elective surgeries, in addition to emergency patients in a cost efficient manner. In (Huh, Liu, & Truong. 2013) this management problem is modelled as a multi-resource allocation scheduling problem in a dynamic and non-stationary environment, where demand and resource availability is continually updated, and patient reneging/no-shows may occur inflicting an additional waiting cost. An overtime cost is also inflicted when elective surgeries exceed available capacity. Authors established patient waitlist equation, and formulated the problem as a Markov decision process, allowing several scheduling algorithms to find the optimal trade-off between over-planning and under-planning for emergency patients. Their study is inspired by optimal control and look-ahead optimization theory. Unlike the common two-priority categories (elective and urgent), Min & Yih (2010a) studied the elective surgery scheduling with several priority categories in a limited capacity surgical facility. Their scheduling policy seeks an optimal trade-off between overtime cost and surgery postponement cost. A stochastic dynamic programming model is formulated to address the problem. Numerical examples point out the importance of taking into account patient priority in the surgery scheduling problem, it also proves that the schedule efficiency doesn't rely only on the total number of patients in a waiting list, but also on the number of patients in each priority category.

3. SURGERY SCHEDULING MATHEMATICAL MODEL

In the following a mathematical model for elective surgery planning and scheduling is proposed to highlight resources constraints and variability of surgical procedure durations. In the following model surgery procedures are assigned to surgery teams according to their specialties. College of surgeons in most hospitals, have different surgery specialties, with at least, one team by specialty. In our model, all surgical procedures are considered confirmed and all resources (medical teams, operating rooms, and equipment) are available over the scheduling horizon. The following notation is used to designate model parameters and variables:

SH: surgery scheduling time horizon
NS: number of elective surgical operations confirmed for scheduling
NR: number of operating rooms considered in the scheduling process
NT: number of surgical teams involved in the schedule plan
***i*:** index for surgical operations, $i \in \{1 \ldots NS\}$
***j*:** index for operating rooms, $j \in \{1 \ldots NR\}$
***k*:** index for surgical teams (not surgical specialties index), $k \in \{1 \ldots NT\}$

Here, the index of surgical team is not used to differentiate between surgical specialties: two different values of index *k* designate two separate teams, albeit they have the same specialty (neurology, dermatology, orthopedic, etc.). To represent an operating room assignment, binary decision variables *X* are used as follows:

***X(i,j)*:** Equals 1 if surgery (*i*) is assigned to room (*j*), and 0 otherwise, $i \in \{1 \ldots NS\}$; $j \in \{1 \ldots NR\}$.

To consider the inherent uncertainty on surgical operation (*i*) durations, let us introduce scheduled beginning and completion times, with duration parameters, as follows:

***Tb(i,j)*:** Scheduled beginning time of operation (*i*) in room (*j*), $i \in \{1 \ldots NS\}; j \in \{1 \ldots NR\}$
***Te(i,j)*:** Scheduled completion time of operation (*i*) in room (*j*), $i \in \{1 \ldots NS\}; j \in \{1 \ldots NR\}$
***D(i)*:** Randomly distributed duration for operation (*i*), $i \in \{1 \ldots NS\}$.

On operation surgery schedule, these variables and parameters are linked by the constraint:

$$Te(i,j)-Tb(i,j)\geq D(i)\cdot X(i,j) \tag{1}$$

In the general case, the duration parameter in constraint (1) is an unknown random variable, making not predictable the respect of this constraint in practice.

An operating room can be idle, active, or undergoing maintenance/cleaning. At the beginning of the scheduling horizon, all operating rooms are assumed to be idle, and ready for use. The cleaning/maintenance duration of an operating room is specific to the surgical room and to the type of surgery completed in it.

Even if cleaning durations can be contained within, relatively accurate, limits, they are assumed to be randomly distributed. Let *M(i, j)* be the random setup-time duration for operating room (*j*), between the two successively scheduled surgeries (*i*) and (*i'*), $i\neq i'\in\{1\ldots NS\};\ j\in\{1\ldots NR\}$. The operating room cleaning constraint is:

$$\min_{i'>i\in\{1,\ldots NS\}}\left[Tb(i',j)-Te(i,j)\right]\geq M(i,j)\cdot X(i',j)\cdot X(i,j) \tag{2}$$

The total idling time *UR(j)* for operating room (*j*), over the entire scheduling horizon *SH*, can be expressed as:

$$UR(j)=\sum_{i=1}^{NS}\left(\min_{i'>i\in\{1,\ldots NS\}}\left[Tb(i',j)\cdot X(i',j)-Te(i,j)\cdot X(i,j)\right]-M(i,j)\cdot X(i,j)\right) \tag{3}$$

The function "min" designates the minimum function. For surgery team allocations, binary decision variables *Y* are used as follows:

Y(i, k): Equals 1 if surgery (*i*) is assigned to team (*k*), and 0 otherwise, $i\in\{1\ldots NS\}$; $k\in\{1\ldots NT\}$. If the beginning and completion times of operation (*i*) by surgical team (*k*) are denoted by *Sb(i, k)* and *Se(i, k)* respectively, then:

$$Se(i,k)-Sb(i,k)\geq D(i)\cdot Y(i,k) \tag{4}$$

Usually, when a surgical team (*k*) performs several surgical procedure over the scheduling horizon, it is required to take a break period *R(i, k)* after completing surgery (*i*) and before starting the next scheduled surgery (*i'*). Such requirement is described by constraint (5).

$$\min_{i'>i\in\{1,\ldots NS\}} \left[Sb(i',k)-Se(i,k)\right] \geq R(i,k)\cdot Y(i',k)\cdot Y(i,k) \tag{5}$$

The break period duration $R(i, k)$ is usually, proportional to the duration of the completed surgical procedure (other criteria can also be considered such as the time of the day the surgery is completed). In this study, the break period duration is assumed to be linearly proportional to the completed procedure duration. This is described by constraint (6), where $i\in\{1\ldots NS\}$; $k\in\{1\ldots NT\}$; a, b real positives.

$$R(i,k)=\left[a+b\cdot D(i)\right]\cdot Y(i,k) \tag{6}$$

In constraints (2), (3) and (5), variables $Tb(i,\ldots)$, $Sb(i,\ldots)$, must be ordered according to their surgical procedure indexes: if surgery (i) precedes surgery (i'), then $Tb(i,\ldots) < Tb(i',\ldots)$ and $Sb(i,\ldots) < Sb(i',\ldots)$. Binary variables are also related in a way that, if $X(i, j)=Y(i, k)$, then equalities: $Tb(i, j)=Sb(i, k)$ and $Te(i, j)=Se(i, k)$, must be both satisfied. Moreover, for each surgical procedure (i), $i\in\{1\ldots NS\}$, the binary variables must respect constraint (7).

$$\sum_{j=1}^{NR}\sum_{k=1}^{NT} X(i,j)\cdot Y(i,k)=1 \tag{7}$$

Similarly to constraint (3), the total idling time $US(k)$ for surgical team (k), over the entire scheduling horizon SH, is expressed by constraint (8).

$$US(k)=\sum_{i=1}^{NS}\left(\min_{i'>i\in\{1,\ldots NS\}}\left[Sb(i',k)\cdot Y(i',k)-Se(i,k)\cdot Y(i,k)\right]-R(i,k)\cdot Y(i,k)\right) \tag{8}$$

The completion date of all tasks associated with room (j) over the scheduling horizon (SH) is $CR(j)$, $j\in\{1\ldots NR\}$. As expressed by constraint (9), this represents the sum of idle, busy, and cleaning period times for room (j).

$$CR(j)=UR(j)+\sum_{i=1}^{NS}\left[D(i)+M(i,j)\right]\cdot X(i,j) \tag{9}$$

Likewise, the completion date of all tasks associated with surgical team (k) over the scheduling horizon (SH) is $CS(k)$, $k\in\{1\ldots NT\}$. As expressed by constraint (10), this represents the sum of idle, busy, and break period times for team (k).

$$CS(k) = US(k) + \sum_{i=1}^{NS} \left[D(i) + R(i,k) \right] \cdot Y(i,k) \tag{10}$$

For optimizing both operating room and surgical team utilization, let α be the weight coefficient, assigned by management team, to the operating room utilization metric in the efficient operation of the system, and β the weight factor indicator for surgical team utilization metric. Based on constraints (3) and (8), these two objectives can be merged into the single objective constraint (11), with $\alpha+\beta=1$.

$$\mathbf{min}\left[\alpha \cdot \mathbf{max}[UR(j)] + \beta \cdot \mathbf{max}[US(k)]\right] \tag{11}$$

The function "max" designates the maximum function. Minimizing surgery completion times is equivalent to minimizing constraint (11) for all defined indexes, $i \in \{1...NS\}; j \in \{1...NR\}; k \in \{1...NT\}$ over the scheduling horizon (*SH*), subject to constraints (1), (2), (4), (5), (6), (7) presented above, and to the constraints (12) to (16) below.

$$\alpha + \beta = 1 \tag{12}$$

$$CR(j) \le SH \tag{13}$$

$$CS(k) \le SH \tag{14}$$

$$D(i) \cong N(\mu_d, \sigma_d) \tag{15}$$

$$M(i,j) \cong N(\mu_m, \sigma_m) \tag{16}$$

In constraint (12), parameters α and β give the model the flexibility to prioritize optimizing operating rooms usage over surgical team and vice versa. A value α =0 means the goal is to maximize surgical staff usage, while β =0 means the goal is to maximize operating room usage. Constraints (15) and (16), describe the normally distributed procedure and room maintenance. The model described above is nonlinear, since it involves products of variables in constraint (7), and nonlinear functions (minimum) in constraints (2), (3), (5) and (8). In the next section, based on the nonlinear model, an approximated linear program is deduced, and a heuristic is defined as a solving method.

4. LINEAR PROGRAMMING MODEL

In the following, few simplifying assumptions are introduced to transform the non-linear model, presented in the previous section, to a linear form that can be solved using linear programming method. Let us assume that a room cleaning duration depends only to the type of surgery performed, and not on room designs or equipment. Thus, constraint (16) is replaced by constraint (17).

$$M(i) \cong N(\mu_m, \sigma_m) \tag{17}$$

When break period durations $R(i, k)$ are independent from surgical teams, and depend only on performed surgical procedures, constraint (6) is replaced by constraint (18).

$$R(i) = \left[a + b \cdot D(i)\right] \tag{18}$$

Assuming that all surgical procedures are indexed based on their order in their assigned resource (room, surgical team) queues constraints (1), (2), (3), (5), (8), (9) and (10), respectively, can be replaced by constraints (19), (20), (21), (22), (23), (24), and (25) correspondingly.

$$Te(i,j) - Tb(i,j) \geq D(i) \tag{19}$$

$$Tb(i+1,j) - Te(i,j) \geq M(i) \tag{20}$$

$$UR(j) = \sum_{i=1}^{NS} [Tb(i+1,j) - Te(i,j) - M(i)] \cdot X(i,j) \tag{21}$$

$$Sb(i+1,k) - Se(i,k) \geq R(i) \tag{22}$$

$$US(k)=\sum_{i=1}^{NS}\left[Sb(i+1,k)-Se(i,k)-R(i)\right]\cdot Y(i,k) \tag{23}$$

$$CR(j)=UR(j)+\sum_{i=1}^{NS}\left[D(i)+M(i)\right]\cdot X(i,j) \tag{24}$$

$$CS(k)=US(k)+\sum_{i=1}^{NS}\left[D(i)+R(i)\right]\cdot Y(i,k) \tag{25}$$

Consequently, the linear program is formulated as minimizing objective (11) subject to constraints (7), (12), (13), (14), (15), (17), and all constraints from (18) to (25).

Many approaches were used in the literature to solve linear program based model for surgery scheduling problem. A branch and price approach is used in (Fei, Chu, Meskens, & Artiba, 2008). The algorithm is based on a column generation approach, where each column represents a schedule for one operating room generated by solving a sub problem of the single operating room case. In (Santibáñez, Begen, & Atkins, 2007), the emphasis is on scheduling surgical blocks considering different surgical specialties. In (Fei, Meskens, & Chu, 2010), the scheduling problem is modeled as two-stage hybrid flow-shop problem and solved using hybrid genetic algorithm. The linear program described above, is solved using a heuristic that is described in the next section.

5. PROPOSED HEURISTIC SOLUTION APPROACH

The solution approach is based on surgery selection rules, programmed using computer codes and spreadsheets (*Microsoft Visual basic, Microsoft Excel*). The selection rules are: *surgical procedure with shortest duration first, surgical procedure with longest duration first, random selection of a surgical procedure*. Schedules obtained using these rules are compared with regards to the objective function (11), and classified based on their resource utilization best score, corresponding to lowest *UR* and *US* value using constraints (21) and (23). For example for the surgical procedure with shortest duration first strategy, the algorithm proceeds iteratively by rearranging the initial list of surgical procedures by increasing durations. The next phase is to update all surgeon and room data to match the produced list. A schedule is computed by screening the ordered list (top-to-bottom) and assigning the earliest start time for a surgical procedure based on its resource availability information. If a resource is not available (room and/or surgical team), the surgery is labeled as unscheduled, and the algorithm move to the next surgical procedure in the list. Two subroutines are used to update surgical team, and room availabilities. These subroutines are constantly accessed and updated by the scheduling algorithm using the scheduling constraints. All durations are entered using mean value and variance using a spreadsheet (*Microsoft Excel*). The schedule computing program is depicted in Figure 1.

Once all surgeries are scheduled according to one strategy (priority rule), the program on Figure 1 restarts again by selecting another strategy. All schedules found

Figure 1. Surgery scheduling algorithm flow chart

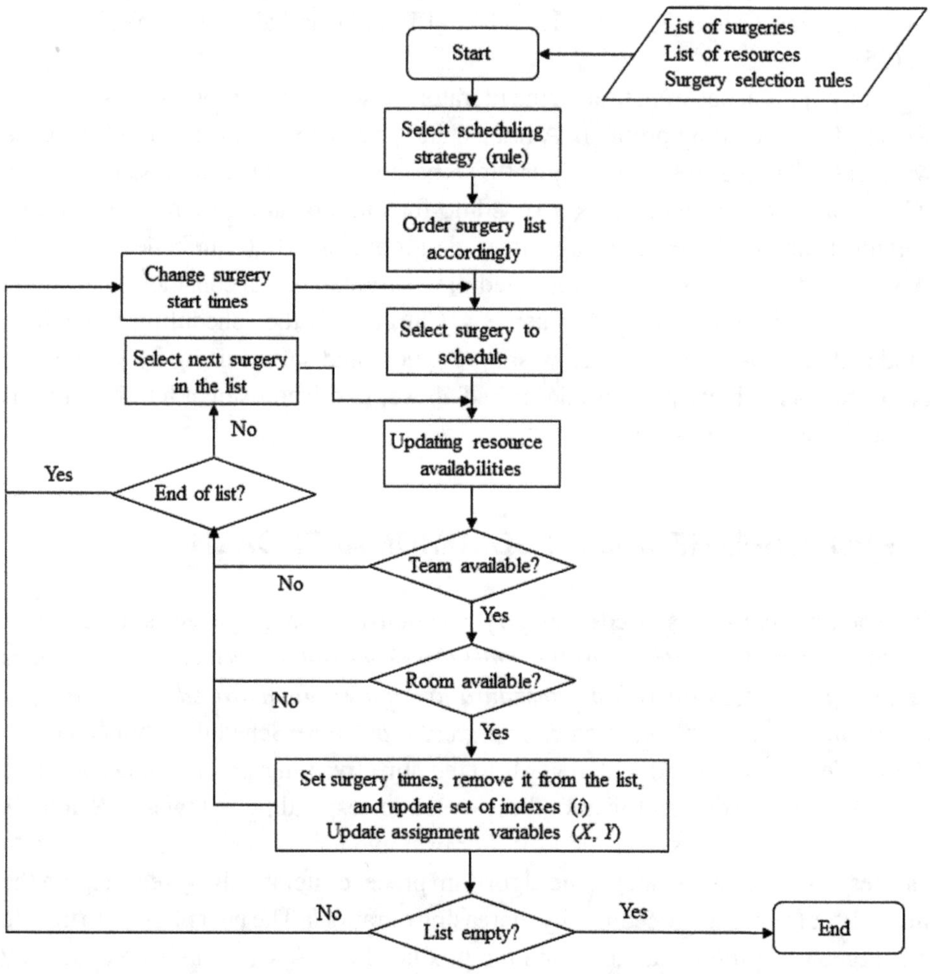

using the three strategies are evaluated with regards to the objective function (11). Although, using priority rules does not find an optimal schedule, the proposed program is flexible, and easy to use and to improve by incorporating other scheduling strategies.

6. ILLUSTRATIVE EXAMPLE

A Canadian public hospital for a town of more than 120,000 people is considered in this example. The increase in surgical demands, results in a longer waiting time to access care. Figure 2 provides a classification of surgical procedures, by wait time, during a six month observation period. Such information is useful for planning elective surgery scheduling. More than 34% of patients waited 3 months to access care, while 22% waited a year or more. The waiting time is expected to increase, while resource are less and less available. In this example, operating room booking clerks are responsible for scheduling patient surgeries, and entering patient information into the hospital computerized system, so a surgical waitlist can be generated. Approximately, 400 new patients are added to the waiting list every month. A schedule is produced every week, and scheduled patients are notified on the surgery date and on the required preoperative tests and diagnosis. The increase in surgical demands with limited resources require the need to improve resources utilization and procedure scheduling.

Figure 2. Classification of performed elective surgeries by wait time, from January to June 2010 (Source: Statistics Canada)

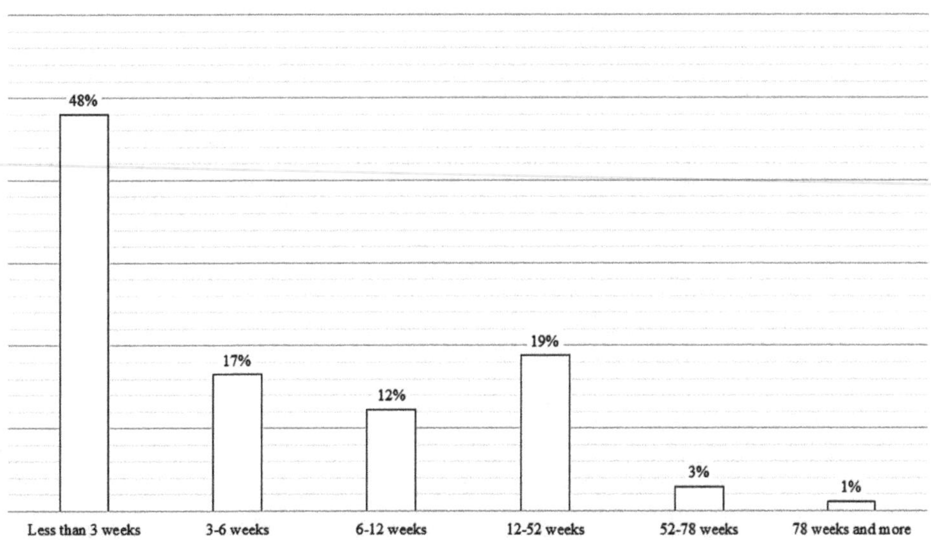

Analyses were conducted for 10 operating rooms shared between 12 surgery teams. Due to the lack of data, surgery procedure durations were considered deterministic. Parameters α and β give are equally set to 0.5, which means that the same importance where given to surgery team and operating room utilizations. To study the effect of time horizon (*SH*) on surgery schedule, a week schedule (5 working days) is determined using two approaches: daily scheduling, where the algorithm is applied on a one-day surgery list; and weekly scheduling, where the algorithm is applied on a one-week surgery list.

7. RESULTS AND DISCUSSION

The make span is defined as the maximum time duration between the start of the first surgery to the completion of the last one in the list (daily or weekly). A comparison between the daily, weekly and actual schedule (used in the hospital) with regards to the make span (in minutes) is provided, for each week day in Table 1.

From Table 1, the heuristic did improve surgery scheduling when compared to the actual schedule, and the make span is reduced. However, the improvement did vary according to the scheduling criteria (weekly vs. daily). The total make span over a week using daily based scheduling is 2420 min, and 2380 min when using weekly based scheduling. The same remark applies for each week day, where the make span varied between 470 min and 480 min for weekly schedule and between 440 min to 520 min for daily schedule. Reducing the make span means better resources utilization, and offers flexibility to integrate add on cases into the off-line schedule with reduced over time cost. Also, a bigger number of scheduled surgeries (*NSS*) reduces patient access waiting time to healthcare services. The proposed

Table 1. Make span (in minutes) and number of scheduled surgeries (NSS)

Day	Actual schedule		Daily based scheduling		Weekly based scheduling	
	NSS	Make span	*NSS*	Make span	*NSS*	Make span
Day 1	31	520	31	480	33	480
Day 2	25	520	25	520	28	470
Day 3	25	480	25	440	30	480
Day 4	28	500	28	460	30	470
Day 5	38	600	38	520	26	480
Total	147	2620	147	2420	147	2380

schedule strategies (daily and weekly) led towards better operating room utilization of and shorter idling periods, when compared with the schedule in use at the hospital. Parameters α and β allow managers to prioritize infrastructure or human resources according to their availability and cost.

8. CONCLUSION

In this study a mathematical model for elective surgery scheduling is proposed. The objective of the model is to improve resource utilizations. After linearization, the proposed model is transformed to a linear mathematical program that is solved using heuristic approach. The program computes different surgery schedules using a set of priority rules using surgery duration length as criteria, or random selection criteria. The program is tested on an illustrative example, and the obtained results show that the scheduling approach improved resource utilizations. In future research, simulation will be used to test the robustness of the proposed approach using random distribution for surgical procedure and room maintenance times. A key strength of simulation is the ability to model the behavior of a system as it develops over time and will allow significant exploration of multiple options. Like this study, most of studies focused on maximizing resource utilizations using mathematical programming models. With the perspective of using discrete event simulation approach, our future focus is toward the dynamic scheduling of add-on cases, by conducting experimentation with different algorithms and discrete event models as initiated in the study by (Dexter, Macario, & Traub, 1999).

REFERENCES

Aringhieri, R., Landa, P., Soriano, P., Tànfani, E., & Testi, A. (2015). A two level metaheuristic for the operating room scheduling and assignment problem. *Computers & Operations Research, 54*, 21–34. doi:10.1016/j.cor.2014.08.014

Berg, B. P., Denton, B. T., Erdogan, S. A., Rohleder, T., & Huschka, T. (2014). Optimal booking and scheduling in outpatient procedure centers. *Computers & Operations Research, 50*, 24–37. doi:10.1016/j.cor.2014.04.007

Bouguerra, A., Sauvey, C., & Sauer, N. (2015, May). *Mathematical model for maximizing operating rooms utilization*. Paper presented at the 15th IFAC/IEEE/IFIP/IFORS Symposium on Information Control Problems in Manufacturing INCOM'2015, Ottawa, Canada. doi:10.1016/j.ifacol.2015.06.068

Burke, E. K., & Riise, A. (2008, August). *Surgery Allocation and Scheduling*. Paper presented at the 7th International Conference on the Practice and Theory of Automated Timetabling, Montreal, Canada.

Cardoen, B., Demeulemeester, E., & Beliën, J. (2009). Operating room planning and scheduling: A literature review. *European Journal of Operational Research, 1016*(10), 14–25.

Cardoen, B., Demeulemeester, E., & Beliën, J. (2010). Operating room planning and scheduling: A literature review. *European Journal of Operational Research, 201*(3), 921–932. doi:10.1016/j.ejor.2009.04.011

Denton, B., Viapiano, J., & Vogl, A. (2007). Optimization of surgery sequencing and scheduling decisions under uncertainty. *Health Care Management Science, 10*(1), 13–24. doi:10.1007/s10729-006-9005-4 PMID:17323652

Dexter, F. (1999). An operation room scheduling strategy to maximize the use of operation rooms. *Anesthesia and Analgesia, 89*(1), 7–20. PMID:10389771

Dexter, F., Macario, A., & Traub, R. D. (1999). Which algorithm for scheduling add-on elective cases maximizes operating room utilization? Use of bin packing algorithms and fuzzy constraints in operating room management. *Anesthesiology, 91*(5), 1491–1500. doi:10.1097/00000542-199911000-00043 PMID:10551602

Erdogan, S. A., & Denton, B. T. (2011). Surgery planning and scheduling. In J. J. Cochran, L. A. Cox, P. Keskinocak, J. Kharoufeh, & J. C. Smith (Eds.), *Wiley Encyclopedia of Operations Research and Management Science*. doi:10.1002/9780470400531.eorms0861

Fei, H., Chu, C., Meskens, N., & Artiba, A. (2008). Solving surgical cases assignment problem by a branch-and-price approach. *International Journal of Production Economics, 112*(1), pp, 96-108.

Fei, H., Meskens, N., & Chu, C. (2010). A planning and scheduling problem for an operating theatre using an open scheduling strategy. *Computers & Industrial Engineering, 58*(2), 221–230. doi:10.1016/j.cie.2009.02.012

Gerchak, Y., Gupta, D., & Henig, M. (1996). Reservation planning for elective surgery under uncertain demand for emergency surgery. *Management Science, 42*(3), 321–334. doi:10.1287/mnsc.42.3.321

Guinet, A., & Chaabane, S. (2003). Operating theatre planning. *International Journal of Production Economics, 85*(1), 69–81. doi:10.1016/S0925-5273(03)00087-2

Hans, E. W., Wullink, G., Van Houdenhoven, M., & Kazemier, G. (2008). Robust surgery loading. *European Journal of Operational Research, 185*(3), 1038–1050. doi:10.1016/j.ejor.2006.08.022

Health Care Financial Management Association. (2005). *Achieving operating room efficiency through process integration.* Technical Report, US National Library of Medicine, National Institutes of Health. *PubMed, 57*(3), 113–119.

Huh, W. T., Liu, N., & Truong, V. A. (2013). Multi-resource allocation scheduling in dynamic environments. *Manufacturing & Service Operations Management, 15*(2), 280–291. doi:10.1287/msom.1120.0415

Koksalmis, E., Hancerliogullari, K. O., & Hancerliogullari, G. (2014, May). *How to schedule surgical operations into operating rooms? An application in Turkey.* Paper presented at the IIE Industrial and Systems Engineering Research Conference, Montreal, Canada.

Lamiri, M., Xie, X., Dolgui, A., & Grimaud, F. (2008). A stochastic model for operating room planning with elective and emergency demand for surgery. *European Journal of Operational Research, 185*(3), 1026–1037. doi:10.1016/j.ejor.2006.02.057

Magerlein, J. M., & Martin, J. B. (1978). Surgical demand scheduling: A review. *Health Services Research, 13*, 418–433. PMID:367987

Min, D., & Yih, Y. (2010a). An elective surgery scheduling problem considering patient priority. *Computers & Operations Research, 37*(6), 1091–1099. doi:10.1016/j.cor.2009.09.016

Min, D., & Yih, Y. (2010b). Scheduling elective surgery under uncertainty and downstream capacity constraints. *European Journal of Operational Research, 206*(3), 642–652. doi:10.1016/j.ejor.2010.03.014

Molina-Pariente, J. M., Fernandez-Viagas, V., & Framinan, J. M. (2015). Integrated operating room planning and scheduling problem with assistant surgeon dependent surgery durations. *Computers & Industrial Engineering, 82*, 8–20. doi:10.1016/j.cie.2015.01.006

Santibáñez, P., Begen, M., & Atkins, D. (2007). Surgical block scheduling in a system of hospitals: An application to resource and wait list management in a British Columbia health authority. *Health Care Management Science, 10*(3), 269–282. doi:10.1007/s10729-007-9019-6 PMID:17695137

Saremi, A., Jula, P., ElMekkawy, T., & Wang, G. G. (2013). Appointment scheduling of outpatient surgical services in a multistage operating room department. *International Journal of Production Economics*, *141*(2), 646–658. doi:10.1016/j.ijpe.2012.10.004

Sciomachen, A., Tànfani, E., & Testi, A. (2005). Simulation models for optimal schedules of operating theatres. *International Journal of Simulation*, *6*, 26–34.

Tyler, D. C., Pasquariello, C. A., & Chen, C. H. (2003). Determining Optimum Operating Room Utilization. *Anesthesia and Analgesia*, *96*(4), 1114–1121. doi:10.1213/01.ANE.0000050561.41552.A6 PMID:12651670

Van Houdenhoven, M., Van Oostrum, J. M., Hans, E. W., Wullink, G., & Kazemier, G. (2007). Improving operating room efficiency by applying bin-packing and portfolio techniques to surgical case scheduling. *Anesthesia and Analgesia*, *105*(3), 707–714. doi:10.1213/01.ane.0000277492.90805.0f PMID:17717228

Van Oostrum, J. M., Van Houdenhoven, M., Hurink, J. L., Hans, E. W., Wullink, G., & Kazemier, G. (2008). A master surgical scheduling approach for cyclic scheduling in operating room departments. *OR-Spektrum*, *30*(2), 355–374. doi:10.1007/s00291-006-0068-x

Wullink, G., Van Houdenhoven, M., Hans, E. W., Van Oostrum, J. M., Van der Lans, M., & Kazemier, G. (2007). Closing emergency operating rooms improves efficiency. *Journal of Medical Systems*, *31*(6), 543–546. doi:10.1007/s10916-007-9096-6 PMID:18041289

Xiang, W., Yin, J., & Lim, G. (2015). A short-term operating room surgery scheduling problem integrating multiple nurses' roster constraints. *Artificial Intelligence in Medicine*, *63*(2), 91–106. doi:10.1016/j.artmed.2014.12.005 PMID:25563674

Zhao, Z., & Li, X. (2014). Scheduling elective surgeries with sequence-dependent setup times to multiple operating rooms using constraint programming. *Operations Research for Health Care*, *3*(3), 160–167. doi:10.1016/j.orhc.2014.05.003

Section 3
Information Technology (IT) in Health Care

Chapter 6
Examining the Influence of Information Technology on Modern Health Care

Edward T. Chen
University of Massachusetts – Lowell, USA

ABSTRACT

Health care costs continue to rise at a level that far exceeds the rate of inflation. IT will be necessary in the computation and organization of complex algorithms presented in bundled payments and other initiatives. Currently in health care, a patient's medical history is not easily accessible by physicians and other medical personnel. IT can play the pivotal role in rectifying this problem in tracking the record in a universally designed environment. Advanced databases are needed to integrate facilities within health care systems. This chapter is to explore the current framework of Information Technology in the U.S. health care industry and to examine the topic covering the following areas: (a) IT's influence on the Affordable Care Act, (b) the emergence of the Electronic Health Record (EHR), also known as the Electronic Medical Record (EMR), and (c) the integration of databases across health care organizations through advanced systems like Epic.

DOI: 10.4018/978-1-4666-9961-8.ch006

INTRODUCTION

The road to change in the health care industry is being paved currently by Health Care Reform. More specifically, the framework of the Patient Protection and Affordable Care Act (PPACA) has held stakeholders in the health care industry accountable for implementing IT modification within their organizations, government bodies, and society as a whole. Health care has an abundance of concentrations, all of which require some form of information technology resource in order for these bodies to achieve the highest service quality of patient care (Rosenbaum, & Margulies, 2011). The purpose of this chapter paper is to explore numerous avenues in the field of health care and to examine the impact that IT has on the U.S. health care industry.

The advancement of information technology in health care is pivotal to the guidelines set in the Patient Protection and Affordable Care Act. As health care organizations have become clinically data driven, the need for information systems and IT is imperative (Vo & Bhaskar, 2012). Analysts in IT departments at hospitals play the role in maintaining and implementing systems. Clinical staff members, such as nurses and physicians, play the role of end users and require the skills needed to effectively operate these systems and forms of technology in order to carry out their clinical duties (Najaftorkaman, Ghapanchi, Talaei-Khoei, & Ray, 2015). Key developments in IT include the transformation of the medical record from paper to digital, the use of mobile devices, and the emergence of integrated health care systems that have the capacity for handling the many complexities that the industry has to offer.

Equally impacted are all U.S. employers who offer health insurance to their employees and the dependents of their employees. While employers attempt to contain the trend of health insurance expense, information systems are needed to pinpoint conditions that prove to be the most costly and implement benefit redesign plans to reduce costs and promote wellness. Employers also keep their staff productive by keeping them healthy. In the same light, information systems help employees examine disease management programs that are geared towards steering employees to engage in healthy behavior and seek preventive care regularly. If health care was once described as being technically challenged when compared with other industries, that notion is being put to rest by the progression of IT in the industry (Vo & Bhaskar, 2012).

For health care to withstand the winds of change, innovation must be at the forefront of the movement. The industry has endured recent developments in IT, but new ideas and expansion in IT staff are imperative for Information Technology to continue to positively impact the health care industry. Ultimately, the goal of a health care organization should be to provide the best possible care to the patient and ensure the well-being of its surrounding community (Ku, Jones, Finnegan, Shin, & Rosenbaum, 2009).

RECENT GOVERNMENT DEVELOPMENTS ON HEALTH CARE IT

The Patient Protection and Affordable Care Act (PPACA) was signed by President Barack Obama on March 3, 2010 and upheld by Congress on June 28, 2012. The act mandates that all Americans are required to be insured with health coverage or pay a penalty to the government beginning in 2014. Another provision includes the expansion of Medicaid to adults whose incomes are at a defined rate at or below the federal poverty limit. Furthermore, the act seeks to decrease the cost of health care (Nussbaum, Tirrell, Wechsler, & Randall, 2010; Rosenbaum, & Margulies, 2011).

Exchanges have been established in the majority of the states either on their own or with the assistance of the Federal Government. The exchanges represent online marketplaces where participants can shop for health insurance plans. The exchanges also provide online resources that allow users to determine their eligibility for a federal subsidy (Carey & Appleby, 2013; Najaftorkaman, et al., 2015).

Healthcare.gov

Many organizations that offer medical insurance as an employee benefit to their staff have adopted online self-service enrollment options. Employees simply log in to an HR system, such as PeopleSoft, and enroll in coverage during their open enrollment period, as new hires, or in lieu of experiencing a qualifying event. Enrolling in coverage through an exchange works in a similar manner. A participant visits Healthcare.gov or a state run exchange and then completes an online application. The system determines the eligibility for Medicaid or a subsidy from the government to offset the full price of commercial insurance coverage. The participant can then enroll in government sponsored or commercial insurance products (Ford, 2013).

Healthcare.gov was scheduled to go live on October 1, 2013 and enrollment in a plan would be effective as of January 1, 2014. However, the website failed. Visitors experienced pages that would not load and were advised through screen prompts to be patient. President Obama's administration announced that the site's issues would be resolved quickly. However, a resolution was not immediately reached and issues began to progressively grow. At this time, the site had been operating at about 43 percent. As a result of strenuous technical maintenance, the site began to operate at 90 percent but not until the beginning of December 2013 (Somashekhar & Sun, 2013).

So what happened? Experts in the field might argue that complex IT systems like the one rolled out with Healthcare.gov are prone to begin with a low level of success upon early stages of operation by end users. In a November 2013 article of *ComputerWorld* magazine, Lev Lesokhin, Senior VP at Cast Software, suggested that the complexity of Healthcare.gov could have been measured in the magnitude of the system's lines of code. Lesokhin estimated this number to be around 500,000. In the same article, author Patrick Thibodeau reports on the findings of Standish Group, a research services organization that specializes in uncovering successes and failures in IT projects. Of the 3,555 government and commercial IT projects from 2003 to 2012 in its database, Standish Group found that 52% were challenged, 41.4% were failures and only 6.4% were considered successful. Ultimately, the researchers came to the conclusion that Healthcare.gov had only a 6.4% chance of being successful. The site was destined to fail at some level (Thibodeau & Gross, 2013).

With enrollments needed to be made at the end of 2013 for a January 1, 2014 effective date, Healhcare.gov had limited time for development and testing phases. Regardless of Standish Group's findings, it is possible that developers did not have adequate time frames to complete testing phases that may have been critical in avoiding the initial failure.

IT in the Accountable Care Organization

Section 3022 of the PPACA introduces a Medicare Shared Savings Program for the Accountable Care Organization (ACO). An Accountable Care Organization is a health care provider that aims at delivering high service quality care and reducing the cost of care. In doing so, the ACO can expect to achieve an incentive in the form of shared Medicare savings (Berwick, 2011).

The ACO model depends greatly on Health Information Technology (HIT). HIT has evolved in the health care industry more and more as data becomes the centerpiece of delivering high service quality care, cost analysis and payment reform. The ACO concept links care and payment risk across multiple organizations and physicians. In order for the model to survive, data sharing will be crucial. The delivery and storage of this data is where technical resources come into play. The ACO portrays a team concept where multiple entities collaborate to achieve financial incentive while providing the best possible care. In order to do so, a patient's Electronic Health

Record (EHR) must be electronically maintained and available across all clinical professionals involved. The EHR concept is at the early stages of development in health care and currently represents limited data sharing capabilities. It is evident that Accountable Care Organizations will be required to invest in IT interfaces that track the patients across the entire episode of care (Bitton & Filer, 2012). Clinical data is at the forefront of the ACO model. As organizations adopt the concept, they will require sophisticated IT resources to share data internally and externally with other acute and post-acute care facilities.

IT in the Patient-Centered Medical Home

The PPACA supports the establishment of the Patient Centered Medical Home (PCMH). The concept of the PCMH is that a single organization delivers comprehensive and primary care to children, youth and adults. This model intends to establish high service quality care for the patient while coordinating specialty care with supporting health care organizations in the community. The structure is such that each patient has a personal physician who leads a team of clinical staff within the PCMH. The clinical staff is responsible for providing ongoing care to the patient (U.S. Department of Health & Human Services, 2014). Ultimately, a medical home should eliminate gaps and foster care coordination that traditional primary care practices may be unable to accomplish. The PPACA supports the concept by making grants available to eligible providers that fit certain PCMH criteria (Epstein, Fiscella, Lesser, & Stange, 2010).

For medical homes to be successful, modern technology should be embraced in the patient to provider relationship. Practices benefit from data analysis and technological communication in the form of decision support systems, electronic registries, systems that facilitate the transition of care, and telehealth (Bates & Bitton, 2010; Fleurant, Kell, Love, Jenter, Volk, Zhang, Bates, & Simon, 2011).

Medical homes rely heavily on the data derived from clinical decision support systems. These are information systems that provide the data needed for clinical staff to analyze patient diagnosis, disease management, illness prevention, and treatment. Decision support systems have been found to be effective in health care organizations that utilize them as a computerized tool. Gurwitz and Wolfstadt (2008) discovered that orders guided by decision support systems were associated with a 90 percent reduction in adverse drug events. The medical home benefits greatly from the system's ability to produce this outcome. In addition, the decision support system can play the role of sending computerized alerts to both the provider and the patient, such as providing notification that a mammogram is due (Gurwitz & Wolfstadt, 2008).

Electronic registries offer clinical staff at medical homes the ability to manage populations with chronic conditions. One technological tool is the Registry Population Manager. This system enables nurses and other clinical staff to identify populations of patients with condition specific criteria. Once the population is identified, the PCMH staff can perform intervention techniques, such as mailings or callings (Fleurant, et al., 2011; Zai, Estey, Lester & Yee, 2008).

Transition of care is important to the PCMH as patients are discharged from acute or post-acute care facilities. Patients should receive post discharge follow up care and medication management from the health professional that typically would be in the form of the patient's personal physician in a medical home setting. Information systems that reconcile a patient's post-discharge and pre-admit electronic medication listing have been evaluated for effectiveness. The tool should allow for smooth transition for a patient's care from the admit facility to the medical home (Bates & Bitton, 2010).

Telehealth is the use of modern telecommunication and electronic information to enable long distance care from the clinician to the patient. Such technologies include video conferencing, email communication, and electronic image transfer. Texas curbs spending by $1 billion by deploying EHRs and telehealth in prisons for the past decade. A telemedicine systems allowed Texas prisons to access healthcare providers at The University of Texas Medical Branch at Galveston in Galveston and Texas Tech University in Lubbock (iHealthBeat, 2011). Telehealth was valued by The Center for Information Technology Leadership at a projected savings across the U.S. of $4.3 billion annually (Bates & Bitton, 2010). Thus, medical homes are at a financially incentivized advantage to adopt telehealth as an option for care. The PPACA's support for the Patient Centered Medical Home is an example of innovation in modern health care. The PCMH's quality of care delivery system should be guided by technological advancements (Krupinski, 2008).

THE ELECTRONIC HEALTH RECORD CONCEPT

In 2009, under the Health Information Technology for Economic and Clinical Health (HITECH) act, the U.S. Department of Health & Human Services released proposed regulations that would support the use to the Electronic Health Record (EHR) in the health care industry. Health care providers would benefit from additional Medicare and Medicaid reimbursement with approved use of the EHR in their practices and facilities. Additional funding for users of EHRs would be provided as well (Blumenthal, 2010).

Ultimately the HITECH act's purpose was to improve care for citizens of the United States and technology was seen as a key component. Laying the groundwork for the EHR adoption would become a guide for health care systems, stand-alone facilities and other providers to use technology in order to optimize care effectively. Providers who could be recognized as "meaningful users" would be incentivized to implement systems that would qualify. The meaningful users of qualifying EHR systems would be required to show use of systems with the following characteristics: electronically capture coded health information, track key clinical conditions, share the information with other providers and patients, and report service quality measures of clinical data and public health information. Proof of these characteristics would help ensure the government's sound investment in the concept (Najaftorkaman, et al., 2015).

The EHR feeds life into a new approach to health care where technology is embraced. Records are kept electronically in virtually all industries and health care, though late in the game, has followed accordingly with the EHR.

The Paper-Based Medical Record

Hospitals and other health care providers in United States have historically kept paper-based medical records of patient files. The information is predominantly hand written which can cause issues of misinterpretation. Generally, paper files can only be stored at the physical location where the patient received the care. In fact, paper files of a patient's medical history are scattered across several locations – from the office of the primary care physician to the specialist's office to the central medical filing stations at the patient's acute care facility. If a physician requires medical history to treat a patient, other providers must be contacted to share this information. The transfer of this information is both time consuming and costly as files are passed on via fax, scan, or mail. In an industry where historical information is essential to provide the best possible care, modern technology possesses the cure for this dated system of paper filing (Schoen, OsbornSquires, Doty, Rasmussen, Pierson, & Applebaum, 2012).

The Electronic Medical Record (EMR)

An alternative to the paper file of a Care Delivery Organization (CDO) for any one particular patient is the Electronic Medical Record (EMR). The EMR is an electronic account of the patient encounter at the CDO. It contains clinical data, decision support, pharmacy data, and more across inpatient and outpatient environments of the CDO.

It is important to note that the EMR does not store data from a patient's encounters at other CDO's, yet it serves as the basis for integrating a centralized record which will be discussed (Holroyd-Leduc, Lorenzetti, Straus, Sykes, & Quan, 2011).

The EMR's environment is the Clinical Data Repository (CDR). The CDR is referred to as a live database of patient information available to all practitioners within a CDO. Controlled Medical Vocabulary (CMV) is stored in the database and is pertinent to the patient encounter. This information must be accurately represented in the database in order for the Clinical Decision Support (CDS) and workflow of the EMR to perform as expected (Hillestad, Bigelow, Bower, Girosi, Meili, Scoville, & Taylor, 2005). The EMR components include clinical documentation, Computerized Provider Order Entry (CPOE), and pharmacy management (Garets & Davis, 2006).

The Electronic Health Record (EHR)

The Electronic Health Record (EHR) is reliant on the EMR being in place first. The EHR represents the environment where multiple stakeholders have access to a patient's medical information. The stakeholders include patients, providers, employers, payers (insurers), and the government. The stakeholders find value in obtaining this information to gain an advantage in accomplishing their purpose. While the EMR is owned by one singular CDO, the EHR is electronically shared and contains data of multiple CDO's within a community, region, state or even an entire country. National Health Information Network (NHIN) standards establish exchanges of data between the EMR to the EHR environment. The EHR environment consists of the stakeholder's and CDO's that rely on the data (Fontenot, 2014; Garets & Davis 2006).

EHR Advantages

Hospitals should predict beneficial outcomes that can be accomplished with the adoption of an EHR system. Advantages of EHR systems are exemplified by the hospital's ability to use the system in order to maintain preventive care measures, reduce operational expenses, pave the way for other forms of technology, and enhance access to data for hospital based research. EHRs can improve adherence rates for routine care and preventive screenings. Electronic alerts notify providers that a patient is due for a preventive screening. The alert system streamlines a process that would have normally been tedious and difficult to organize. The process is necessary and beneficial to the patients' health and well-being as preventive care is essential (Fontenot, 2014).

Treatments have become more effective with the use of EHRs. More patient information is available and easier to access by the nursing staff. One study found a 5% decrease in pressure ulcers after six months of an EHR system implementation (Menachemi & Collum, 2011). Menachemi and Collum (2011) found that the alert system, which is a part of Clinical Decision Support, accounted for an 11.3% appropriate hypertension treatment in primary care.

An initiative in the health care industry in recent years is to reduce "waste." Waste comes in the form of medical errors causing inappropriate costs, using less expensive alternatives of care, or fraud. Unnecessary laboratory and radiology tests are reduced with the presence of an EHR. This allows for the reduction in ancillary expense and the opportunity to fill the time saved performing inappropriate care with appropriate care (Menachemi & Collum, 2012).

An EHR capability that reduces errors in hospital operations is the Computerized Physician Order Entry (CPOE). A CPOE is an information system that is used in the medical field to communicate orders for a patient by a medical practitioner. The practitioner can electronically enter medication instructions, laboratory tests, radiology examinations and physical therapy orders. Prior to the development of this system, orders were written on paper and delivered to nursing, pharmacy and other medical staff. The existence of the CPOE system increases efficiency and reduces errors (Kaushal, Shojania, & Bates, 2003).

Operating expenses are reduced with the placement of an EHR system. The cost of chart pulls is virtually eliminated due to direct accessibility by the end user. Paper costs, previously used for creating paper based files, become almost obsolete. Salaries and wages can be reduced due the reduction in staff needed to perform duties that can be performed by the EHR. Legal expenses reduce as a result of increased communication across providers, adherence to medical guidelines, and reduction in malpractice claims (Mekhjian, Kumar, Kuehn, Bentley, Teater, Thomas, Payne, & Ahmad, 2002).

Hospitals that house research departments benefit from the EHR in that electronically stored data makes it more feasible for researches to collect information needed for studies. Measuring outcomes across a population in particular studies can be performed with ease because EHRs store data across multiple providers amongst numerous regions. The EHR advantages justify the effectiveness of the system. If the systems are implemented and maintained adequately, positive outcomes should be obtained.

EHR Limitations

There are several limitations of the EHR that have been recognized in the health care industry. These limitations include financial issues, changes in workflow, loss in productivity, threats to Protected Health Information (PHI) and others. The costs of implementing an EHR system include software and hardware purchases, overhead and additional salaries associated with converting existing paper based files to electronic, and training expenses for hospital staff. These costs affect both inpatient and outpatient settings in a health care organization. Ongoing maintenance costs include expenses related to regular updates and hardware replacement, salaries and benefits paid to hired technical staff to support the system, and fees paid to consultants and external contractors. Positive financial outcomes of an effective EHR system are shared by the third party insurance payer. The shared savings impact the payer as errors are eliminated and efficiency is improved from a billing standpoint. With the exception of Medicare, the payer does not invest financial resources in the adoption of the EHR. The entire cost is incurred by the health care provider. Thus, the benefit is reaped by the payer.

Loss in productivity can come in the form of medical staff spending non-productive time learning the system as opposed to providing medical care. EHR systems require extensive training for medical staff. Nurses, laboratory and radiology technicians, and other hospital staff are removed from their duties to learn the system. This process can take three months where a portion of the each staff member's worked hours are required for training each month. The productivity can be back filled with replacement staff. However, the replacement factor also leads to additional compensation, sometimes at a much higher hourly rate, which can burden the hospital budget. Because, hospital administrators emphasize the importance of keeping the Full Time Equivalent (FTE) budget on target, replacement can account for an unfavorable option.

EHR's do not offer full protection in terms of patient privacy. As sensitive data is shared electronically over a network, Protected Health Information (PHI) data is at risk of IT security breaches just as credit card data is at risk in the retail industry. Regulations are required for hospital staff with access to PHI. Employees must adhere to the strong guidelines of the Health Insurance Portability and Accountability Act (HIPAA). This represents another challenge for health care organizations that must educate their staff on HIPAA regulations and how they are connected with EHR systems (U.S. Department of Health & Human Services, 2015).

Other limitations and setbacks of the technology can include an overdependence on the technology, increases medical errors if the system is poorly designed or if the employees are not adequately trained, and loss of autonomy for physicians due to system limitations. The limitations can be addressed with strategic planning by hospital administrators. Also, as systems become more mature, limitations are liable to be alleviated.

An EHR Study: Costs and Benefits Analysis

Gundersen Lutheran Medical Center in La Crosse, Wisconsin, was examined in a study of the outcomes demonstrated by one hospital that adopted the EHR. The hospital is a 325 licensed bed trauma center that implemented an inpatient EHR system in November of 2008. For comparison purposes, data were collected one year pre-EHR implementation and one year post-EHR implementation. For purposes of this study, the impact of the CPOE system implementation was considered in the results because of the proximity of the CPOE implementation to that of the EHR and for the reason that CPOE and EHR systems are directly linked in terms of their capabilities (Zlabeck, Wickus, & Mathiason, 2011).

Laboratory tests and radiology examinations were analyzed in the study. The analysis showed that the number of laboratory test per week per hospitalization reduced from 13.9 in the pre-EHR period data to 11.9 in the post-EHR data. Zlabeck, Wickus, and Mathiason (2011) point out that this decrease of 18% in the rate of lab tests begin to show signs of significant trend at month three of the post-EHR period. This leads to the suggestion that the reduction in tests was a result of the CPOE system's implementation. However, the EHR needed to be in place in order for the CPOE system's implementation to occur. Therefore, both systems should be recognized in this performance driven statistic. Similarly, the rate of radiology tests per hospitalization did not show signs of a decrease until month three of the post-EHR period. The number decreased from 2.06 in the pre-EHR period to 1.93 in month 9 of the post-EHR period.

Significant savings were demonstrated in transcription costs. The cost per month decreased from $74,596 to $18,938. This represented an impressive outcome where costs reduced by 74.6% from the pre-EHR period to the post-EHR period. Over the twelve month post-EHR period, total savings calculated to $667,896. This outcome was attributable to the EHR system directly (Zlabeck, Wickus, and Mathiason, 2011).

An obvious positive financial outcome came in the form of cost savings in supplies specifically related to a reduction in paper consumption. The EHR eliminates the need for paper based medical files, therefore this cost savings would generally be expected. The hospital experienced a 26.6% decrease in reams of paper orders, and one hundred and eighteen paper forms were eliminated. The total cost savings decreased in the post-EHR period by a total of $30,351. Medication errors were reduced after the EHR implementation as well. Errors per 1,000 hospital days dropped from 17.9 prior to the EHR system to 15.4 by month nine in the post-EHR period. As was the case with lab tests and radiology exams, the CPOE played a vital role in this outcome (Mekhjian, et al., 2002; Zlabeck, Wickus, & Mathiason, 2011) .

The statistics prove that positive operational and cost benefits were associated with the implementation of the EHR and CPOE systems at Gundersen Lutheran Medical Center. The study also demonstrates that the adoption of the EHR can open doors to other modern formers of Health Information Technology. In this case it led to an effective implementation of the CPOE system (Mekhjian, et al., 2002).

Epic: Judith Faulkner's Systems

Judith Faulkner has built Epic Systems gradually and quietly over several years of development, capitalizing off of an evolving health care environment that has recently adapted to the benefits the EHR. Epic was founded in 1979 in Verona, Wisconsin and is presently becoming the preferred technological system solution for the majority of the stakeholders in the U.S. health care industry. Its clients include dominant health care systems such as Johns Hopkins and Cleveland Clinic (Moukheiber, 2012). Massachusetts-based Partners HealthCare, founded by the prestigious Massachusetts General Hospital and Brigham and Women's Hospital, is currently implementing the system across all of its hospitals – the first of which began in February of 2014 at Newton Wellesley Hospital. In an article in Forbes Magazine, it was determined that 40% of the U.S. population is being stored in an Epic digital record. This share continues to grow as the U.S. health care industry proceeds to become more innovative in the field of technology (Moukheiber, 2012).

Epic develops software for medical groups, hospitals and integrated health care systems. At a lower level, it serves community based hospitals, academic facilities, children's hospitals and health safety net providers (Ku, et al., 2009). The EHR methodology employed by Epic is based on a health care programming language referred to as MUMPS (Massachusetts General Hospital Utility Multi-Programming System). Its products include EpicCare EMR that normalizes care delivery for physicians, EpicCare Inpatient Clinical System that allows for health information sharing across organizations, mobile applications, and portals. Also available is a resource for patients to retrieve the same electronic medical records that are accessed by their physicians. A patient's Personal Health Record (PHR) is portable for both patients and providers alike through an Epic application known as Lucy. Epic also offers PlanLink which is a tool for payers (i.e., insurers) and employers that makes information available via the web (Bloomberg Business Week, 2014; Holroyd-Leduc, et al., 2011; O'Brien, 2006;).

In the era of digitalized health care, security is a strong selling point when it comes to investing in health care IT. Faulkner backs up her product's security status by proclaiming "to the best of our knowledge, in the 32 years we've been in business, there has never been a breach of Epic's data by a hacker" (Freudenheim, 2012). The company's leader stresses the importance of firewalls and security systems that

Epic has in place to protect sensitive and protected data. In fact, Faulkner holds the position of an industry representative on a government panel that examines security issues in health care. Her goal is to assure the protection of the data while still allowing for the flow of information sharing. Such a balance is difficult to reach with success, yet Epic manages to do so strategically. The information sharing can only be shared across providers if they are clients or if they meet certain conditions. Organizations must prove patient consent and have a digital certificate to be presented to other organizations in order to engage in digital information sharing. The benefit of sharing health care data is something the Faulkner sees as a privilege that should be treated accordingly. The Health Insurance Portability and Accountability Act of 1996 mandates the privacy and security of sensitive patient data. Epic's reputation for safeguarding the data increases the effectiveness and marketability of its software products (Freudenheim, 2012; O'Brien, 2006).

USE OF HEALTH CARE IT TO IMPROVE SERVICE QUALITY

Healthcare IT applications in the medical community bring in many strengths of service quality. The strengths, broadly speaking, include user satisfaction, employee productivity, and business performance. Weaknesses include stakeholder issues, regulatory environment, technical issues, and financial issues. Threats include government mandates, third party e-Health and e-Medicine, competition for scarce IT resources and talent, market and competitive pressure, and the threat of government run healthcare. There are opportunities as well. Institutions that are developing effective systems now have the benefit of being early adopters. They can affect change of standards toward those that are beneficial to them since these standards are just now being developed. They can appeal to younger patients searching for locations and healthcare professionals with better service quality. They can gain prestige among peers and increase their own service quality outcomes (Andrews, 2015; Lettieri, Bartoli, & Masella, 2013).

The strength of user satisfaction takes a couple of different forms. First there are now more Internet interactions than ever before. People are used to doing their banking, shopping for products, arranging food deliveries, paying bills, communicating, taking classes, and many other aspects of daily living online. They are often surprised that medical processes are still inaccessible in many facets. This has led to higher patient expectation that can be met with Health IT solutions. People are more tech savvy now as well that makes a more educated and able consumer. People are also beginning to shop for healthcare services and products including both physicians and facilities (Matysiewicz & Smyczek, 2013; Razzaque, Eldabi, & Jalal-Karim, 2013).

The strength of employee productivity is due to labor efficiency and service effectiveness. There is a shortage of health care professionals especially in the general practitioner area. Manual record keeping and searches are a laborious and time consuming process. Health IT can deliver instant information on demand to improve labor efficiency. The accuracy of health IT generated reports will improve the diagnosis and service effectiveness. Employee productivity can be increases by using health IT applications to free up data searching time and to help serve the growing patient need. The strength of business performance centers on using health IT to reduce costs. Health IT applications of efficiencies increase employee productivity and reduce operating costs. Health medical records are stored electronically and can be queried or reported in various customized ways. Business performance can be further increased by reducing malpractice through automatic guards, checks, and alerts (Menachemi, & Collum, 2011; Menon & Kohli, 2013).

Information Systems Guide Management in Health Benefits and Costs

In 2013, employer sponsored health insurance covered about 149 million employees and their dependents. Over the past decade, employer sponsored health insurance costs have trended at a rate much higher than inflation. Data from the 2003 and 2013 versions of the Kaiser Survey of Employer Sponsored Health Benefits depict an 80% increase in the average total insurance premiums and an 89% increase in the average employee contribution to the full premium. In 2003, employers subsidized the full health insurance premium by a very generous 75%. However, as the employee contributions have experienced an upward trend at a higher rate than the total, the employer sponsored subsidy has decreased over the ten year period to 74% (Kaiser Family Foundation, 2013).

The data infer that in an effort to withstand the astronomical spike in health benefit costs, employers have decided to cut benefits and push a higher share of the premium payments onto their employees. As companies seek to both cut costs and remain competitive from a compensation standpoint, they have invested in data warehouses such as Truven Health Analytics and other systems. The investment in these systems is a practice aimed towards organizations empowering themselves with the reporting capabilities needed to analyze data and develop strategies for mitigating the trend of health insurance costs (Vo & Bhaskar, 2012).

Truven Health Analytics offers a product to employers called Advantage Suite, which is a dynamic database that stores in-depth health and Rx claim data of employees and their dependents. Member information is submitted to Truven by the group health and Rx insurance carriers that the employer uses to offer health benefits to its employees. The employer submits job and demographic data that are combined to the claims data by Truven to build a database the employers can use to report on clinical and financial member data. Advantage Suite allows employers to dive into the data of their health benefit costs and utilization. Employers can determine the drivers for substantial increases in trend and develop plans of action to reduce costs. They can identify preventive measures, such as colonoscopy and mammography rates, in their population and compare these measures to norms using a built in benchmarking tool. The tool pulls information using a resource known as MarketScan data, a comparative application that can be industry and demographically adjusted. After interpreting the results, employers can take action to steer their population into healthy behavior and ultimately reduce costs or care related to chronic conditions. Employers can also use the system to develop forecast and budget assumptions on employee health expenses and perform benefit modeling analytics used to measure the cost impact of plan changes.

In a study performed by the Employee Benefit Research Institute (EBRI), Truven data were used to examine the costs of spouses in employer sponsored health plans. The EBRI sought to address the notion that spouses incur higher health costs in employer sponsored health plans. Using Truven Health Analytics MarketScan Commercial Database, researchers were able to analyze claims data of 317,180 couples and 634,360 individual members across multiple employers. The system allowed the researchers to dice the data by geographic location, health status, gender, and age. For the population analyzed, the results showed that the employees (i.e., policy holders) cost $5,430 on average while the spouses averaged $6,609. The findings revealed a 21.7% increase of the spouse cost per member over that of the subscribing employee. A powerful information system allows the end user to uncover the layers by drilling down into the detail to determine the root causes.

By running subsequent reports, Fronstin and Roebuck (2014) found that the majority of the $1,179 difference was due to gender, health status, and other factors. Researchers adjusted their reports to normalize the data and still found that average spouse costs were 7% higher than the average policy holder costs. The end result of the analysis was that, even when adjusting for outliers, spouses still carry a higher cost on average than the policy holding employee.

If an employer performs a similar analysis using a Truven product or a similar system, decisions can be made to reduce employee health costs. The EBRI indicates that the United Postal Service (UPS) applied the same approach to reduce health costs. UPS decided to change its benefit package by only offering coverage to the spouses of its employees who did not have coverage offered to them by their own employer. UPS actually cited the PPACA as the cause of its decision, indicating that the change enabled the company to provide affordable coverage. The PPACA requires employers to offer coverage to dependent children through the age of 26, but does not require coverage to be offered to spouses (Fronstin & Roebuck, 2014).

Were it not for a sophisticated technologically advanced system like Truven's, the analysis would have limitations and perhaps UPS would not be able to place a value on the cost impact of its decision. The investment in information technology by employers can prove to carry a positive return, because the accessible data empowers employers with knowledge that would otherwise be unavailable.

Information Systems Guide Employee Wellness and Productivity

A healthy workforce translates into a productive workforce. In order to remain competitive, an organization must take action in order to keep its workforce healthy and productive. Information systems, like Truven's, allow employers to track clinical measures on employee health to identify areas that can be improved upon. Truven's Advantage Suite data warehouse offers a reporting environment that allows employers to track the effectiveness of disease management programs.

Insurers often enroll members in these disease management programs, which are programs equipped with clinical staff who offer health coaching to members with certain clinical conditions. Using the condition of diabetes as an example, a member with the disease would generally be contacted with reminders to get their periodic exams such as HbA1c and eye tests needed to maintain the well-being of the member. An employer with Truven Advantage Suite could access the reporting environment, set their clinical condition criteria to diabetes, and query on the frequency of periodic exams and the overall health of their members. Because the database offers time constraints, the employer can track the improvement over multiple time periods to analyze trends. If the employer wishes to set parameters on the population within the clinical condition population, subsets can be created limiting the person IDs. The use of subsets is most effective when the analysis calls for an examination on cohorts. If issues are identified, such as an unfavorable rate in HbA1c testing, employers can deliver the results to the insurer and order further intervention (Truven Health Analytics, 2014).

An employer can also use the database to perform home grown analytics on the overall health and wellness of the employee population. For instance, through statistical analysis a company may reveal a portion of their population to have a higher prevalence for mental health conditions, such as depression. That company might decide to establish an employee assistance program for these employees in order for them to have access to counseling on site. HIPAA complicates the communication process, however, if done strategically the wellness initiative can foster a healthy workforce.

IT PROFESSIONS IN HEALTH CARE

Role of the Chief Medical Information Officer (CMIO)

The Chief Medical Information Officer (CMIO) role has recently been gaining popularity in the health care industry. The CMIO is responsible for directing the implementation and maintenance of clinical information systems. Generally, this position is held by a physician. The emergence of the EHR and EMR has added depth to the CMIO role as health care organizations convert to digital record keeping. Responsibilities also include facilitating data warehouse initiatives, physician website and email maintenance, and network security. CMIOs can be partially dedicated to performing direct patient care as attending physicians or fully dedicated to their roles in health care IT (Holroyd-Leduc, et al., 2011).

CMIOs set goals and expectations for IT projects. They also lead the vendor selection process when new systems or technology are requested. For instance, the CMIO would be responsible for the selection process involved for a health care organization to choose Epic Systems to replace an existing system, such a Meditech. Once implemented, the CMIO would then direct plans for training registered nurses and other clinical staff on new information. CMIOs can also chair senior health system committees and information technology committees. Also, CMIOs participate and direct the establishment of information security and that HIPAA regulations are carried out from a systems standpoint. CMIOs lead staff reporting directly to them or collaborate with the organizations internal IT staff to achieve the effective completion of these initiatives (Leviss, Kremsdorf, & Mohaideen, 2006).

Nursing Informatics

The American Medical Informatics Association (AMIA) defines nursing informatics as the "science and practice (that) integrate nursing, its information and knowledge, with management of information and communication technologies to promote the health of people, families, and communities worldwide" (American Medical Informatics Association (AMIA), 2014). Positions in this field are staffed by health care organizations and include Nurse Informaticists and Chief Nursing Informatics Officers. Nursing informatics is expanding and the need for these positions is increasing. The 2014 Healthcare Information and Management Systems Society (HIMSS) Nursing Informatics Survey revealed that there are three areas where nursing informatics add value to an integrated health care system. These areas are the development and implementation of IT systems, optimization of HIT systems, defining context for patient care. The survey indicates that 30 percent of health care organizations support the CNIO position. The role is evolving as that number is expected to grow in subsequent years (Gabriel, Jones, Samy, & King, 2014; Pizzi, 2014).

Clinical Decision Support (CDS)

Clinical Decision Support (CDS) systems provide intelligence that fuels decision making in the health care environment. These decisions benefit clinical staff and patients, enhance the delivery of care, control costs, and increase revenue. CDS system analysts filter information to the health care environment using technical tools such as computerized alerts, reporting platforms, diagnostic support, and clinical guidelines. Ultimately, health care organizations improve from service quality decision support by increasing the quality of care, reducing errors and complications, improving efficiency, and satisfying patients (Kaushal, Shojania, & Bates, 2003; Romano & Stafford, 2011).

Health care organizations staff departments specifically dedicated to CDS. These departments tend to consist of analysts who operate and maintain databases used to provide support for the decisions made within their organizations. One of these systems is Allscripts EPSi. EPSi is a web-based information system that is specific to the health care industry and stores data and analytical tools that guide financial management. CDS analysts operate the system to provide integrated analytics, budget support, and general decision support. EPSi offers multiple modules to organizations that include Budget Manager, Capital Budget Manager, Strategic Product Budgeting, Productivity Manager, Cost Manager, Product Line Analyst, and EPSi Management Dashboard. Budget Manager allows the health care organization to combine payroll and capital budgeting with patient level budgeting so that realistic spending goals and assumptions can be made. Analyst can perform financial modeling using this module's ad hoc report writing resource and flex budget mode (Allscripts, 2014).

Analysts in health care organizations use IT resources, such as EPSi, in order to equip themselves and their organizations with the information needed to determine appropriate investment and allocation of resources. The information system makes this possible. Without the assistance of EPSi and other CDS systems, analysts would not be capable of impacting the health care system. CDS systems have paved the way for business intelligence professions in health care organizations.

CONCLUSION

Health care systems continue to swell into massive heaps of facilities, insurance companies, service organizations, consultants and more. Partners HealthCare consists of entities from acute care facilities to mental health facilities to rehabilitation hospitals and centers. Partners and other Massachusetts based systems, like Steward Health Care and Hallmark Health, base their business models on the concept of integrating care across their systems. IT has played in integral role in effectively coordinating care within any one particular system. What remains to be seen is how effectively IT will integrate all U.S. health care organizations. The Electronic Health Record will be the element that allows organizations to facilitate with one another from a technical sense. Patient information must be properly shared for the betterment of patient care and effectiveness of care delivery by health care professionals. As the adoption of the EHR spreads across the United States in future years, systems will improve their care delivery models and processes.

The government has established itself as a major player in the industry with the passing of the PPACA. President Obama's Health Care Reform has been designed to steer the industry improvement and adoption. As more focus is placed on IT resources within health care organizations, systems should continue to improve and IT departments should expand.

Epic will continue to sweep the nation with its state of the art systems catered to the current need for today's health care environment. Systems that previously controlled the market, such as Soarian and Meditech, will need to improve their products as soon as possible in order to withstand Epic's domination. The emergence of a new entrant into the world of IT systems will be a more likely scenario.

The access to systems will expand for organizations who offer employer sponsored health plans to their employees and the families of their employees. Systems, like Truven, will be adopted by both employers and benefit consultants across the U.S. The return on investment has been demonstrated by the early adopters of these IT systems and more employers will fall in line to cut costs and keep their workforce healthy and productive.

Health care organizations can be for profit or non-profit, acute or non-acute, outpatient or inpatient. Regardless of an organization's disposition, it cannot continue to exist without information sharing and gathering through technological advancements. IT analytical tools provide the business intelligence needed for health care organizations to survive and flourish. It is with these tools that health care professionals strive to fulfill their duties and work for the betterment of the patient in their care.

REFERENCES

Allscripts. (2014). *Solutions that round-out all the elements of financial health.* Retrieved December 1, 2014 from https://www.allscripts.com/en/solutions/acute-solutions/performance-management/performancemanagement.html

American Medical Informatics Association (AMIA). (2014). *Nursing Informatics.* Retrieved December 1, 2014 from http://www.amia.org/programs/working-groups/nursing-informatics

Andrews, R. M. (2015). Statewide hospital discharge data: Collection, use, limitations, and improvements. *Health Services Research, 50*(1), 1273–1299. doi:10.1111/1475-6773.12343 PMID:26150118

Bates, D. W., & Bitton, A. (2010). The future of health information technology in the patient-centered medical home. *Health Affairs, 29*(4), 614–621. doi:10.1377/hlthaff.2010.0007 PMID:20368590

Berwick, D. (2011). Launching Accountable Care Organizations — the proposed rule for the Medicare shared savings program. *The New England Journal of Medicine, 10*(1056), 1–4. PMID:21452999

Bitton, A., Filer, L. A., & Jha, A. K. (2012). Health information technology in the era of care delivery reform. *Journal of the American Medical Association, 307*(24), 2593–2594. doi:10.1001/jama.2012.6663 PMID:22735426

Bloomberg Business Week. (2014). *Company overview of Epic Systems Corporation.* Retrieved December 10, 2014 from http://investing.businessweek.com/research/stocks/private/snapshot.asp?privcapId=6479863

Blumenthal, D. (2010). Launching HITECH. *The New England Journal of Medicine, 362*(5), 382–385. doi:10.1056/NEJMp0912825 PMID:20042745

Carey, M. A., & Appleby, J. (2013). *How do the health law's online exchanges work? What you need to know to get started.* Retrieved December 10, 2014 from http://www.washingtonpost.com/national/health-science/how-do-the-health-laws-online-exchanges-work-what-you-need-to-know-to-get-started/2013/09/16/ef7974c8-1988-11e3-a628-7e6dde8f889d_story.html

Epstein, R. M., Fiscella, K., Lesser, C. S., & Stange, K. C. (2010). Why the nation needs a policy push on patient-centered health care. *Health Affairs, 29*(8), 1489–1495. doi:10.1377/hlthaff.2009.0888 PMID:20679652

Fleurant, M., Kell, R., Love, J., Jenter, C., Volk, L. A., Zhang, F., & Simon, S. R. et al. (2011). Massachusetts e-Health Project increased physicians' ability to use registries, and signals progress toward better care. *Health Affairs (Project Hope), 30*(7), 1256–1264. doi:10.1377/hlthaff.2010.1020 PMID:21734198

Fontenot, S. F. (2014). The affordable care act and electronic health care records: Can technology help reduce the cost of health care? *Physician Executive*, *40*(1), 68–72. PMID:24575706

Ford, P. (2013). *The Obamacare website didn't have to fail. How to do better next time*. Retrieved December 10, 2014 from http://www.businessweek.com/articles/2013-10-16/open-source-everything-the-moral-of-the-healthcare-dot-gov-debacle#p3

Freudenheim, M. (2012). Digitizing health records before it was cool. *The New York Times*. Retrieved December 10, 2014 from http://www.nytimes.com/2012/01/15/business/epic-systems-digitizing-health-records-before-it-was-cool.html?pagewanted=all&_r=1&

Fronstin, P., & Roebuck, C. (2014). The cost of spousal health coverage. *Employee Benefit Research Institute*, *35*(1), 2-7. Retrieved December 1, 2014 from http://www.ebri.org/pdf/notespdf/EBRI_Notes_01_Jan-14_SpslCvg-RetPlns1.pdf

Gabriel, M. H., Jones, E. B., Samy, L., & King, J. (2014). Progress and challenges: Implementation and use of health information technology among critical-access hospitals. *Health Affairs*, *33*(7), 1262–1270. doi:10.1377/hlthaff.2014.0279 PMID:25006155

Garets, D., & Davis, M. (2006). Electronic medical records vs. electronic health records: Yes, there is a difference. *HIMSS Analytics*. Retrieved December 10, 2014 from http://www.himss.org/files/HIMSSorg/content/files/WP_EMR_EHR.pdf

Hillestad, R., Bigelow, J., Bower, A., Girosi, F., Meili, R., Scoville, R., & Taylor, R. E. M. R. (2005). Can electronic medical record systems transform health care? Potential health benefits, savings, and costs. *Health Affairs*, *24*(5), 1103–1117. doi:10.1377/hlthaff.24.5.1103 PMID:16162551

Holroyd-Leduc, J., Lorenzetti, D., Straus, S. E., Sykes, L., & Quan, H. (2011). The impact of the electronic medical record on structure, process, and outcomes within primary care: A systematic review of the evidence. *Journal of the American Medical Informatics Association: JAMIA*, *18*(6), 732–737. doi:10.1136/amiajnl-2010-000019 PMID:21659445

iHealthBeat. (2011). *Texas curbs spending by $1B by deploying EHRs, telehealth in prisons*. Retrieved December 1, 2014 from http://www.ihealthbeat.org/articles/2011/8/26/texas-curbs-spending-by-1b-by-deploying-ehrs-telehealth-in-prisons

Kaiser Family Foundation. (2013). Employer Health Benefits: 2013 Summary of Findings. *The Kaiser Family Foundation and Health Research and Educational Trust*. Retrieved December 1, 2014 from http://kaiserfamilyfoundation.files.wordpress.com/2013/08/8466-employer-health-benefits-2013_summary-of-findings2.pdf

Kaushal, R., Shojania, K. G., & Bates, D. W. (2003). Effects of computerized physician order entry and clinical decision support systems on medication safety: A systematic review. *Archives of Internal Medicine*, *163*(12), 1409–1416. doi:10.1001/archinte.163.12.1409 PMID:12824090

Krupinski, E. A. (2008). Telemedicine for home health and the new patient: When do we really need to go to the hospital? *Studies in Health Technology and Informatics*, *29*(4), 614–621. PMID:18305331

Ku, L., Jones, E., Finnegan, B., Shin, P., & Rosenbaum, S. (2009). *How is the primary care safety net faring in Massachusetts? Community health centers in the midst of health reform (Issue paper no. 7878)*. Washington, DC: Kaiser Commission on Medicaid and the Uninsured.

Lettieri, E., Bartoli, L., & Masella, C. (2013). Coordinating intra-sector services in healthcare: Requirements and elements that managers should take into account. *European Management Journal*, *31*(6), 591–601. doi:10.1016/j.emj.2013.05.004

Leviss, J., Kremsdorf, R., & Mohaideen, M. (2006). The CMIO – A new leader for health systems. *Journal of the American Medical Informatics Association*, *13*(5), 573–578. doi:10.1197/jamia.M2097 PMID:16799119

Matysiewicz, J., & Smyczek, S. (2013). Relations between healthcare organizations and their patients: Three-factors models in the e-healthcare market. *Review of Business*, *33*(2), 7–25.

Mekhjian, H. S., Kumar, R. R., Kuehn, L., Bentley, T. D., Teater, P., Thomas, A., & Ahmad, A. et al. (2002). Immediate benefits realized following implementation of physician order entry at an academic medical center. *Journal of the American Medical Informatics Association*, *9*(5), 529–539. doi:10.1197/jamia.M1038 PMID:12223505

Menachemi, N., & Collum, T. (2011). Benefits and drawbacks of electronic health record systems. *Risk Management and Healthcare Policy*, *4*, 47–55. doi:10.2147/RMHP.S12985 PMID:22312227

Menon, N. M., & Kohli, R. (2013). Blunting Damocles' Sword: A longitudinal model of healthcare IT impact on malpractice insurance premium and quality of patient care. *Information Systems Research*, *24*(4), 918–932, 1164–1165. doi:10.1287/isre.2013.0484

Moukheiber, Z. (2012). *Epic systems' tough billionaire.* Retrieved December 10, 2014 from http://www.forbes.com/sites/zinamoukheiber/2012/04/18/epic-systems-tough-billionaire/

Najaftorkaman, M., Ghapanchi, A. H., Talaei-Khoei, A., & Ray, P. (2015). A taxonomy of antecedents to user adoption of health information systems: A synthesis of thirty years of research. *Journal of the Association for Information Science and Technology*, *66*(3), 576–598. doi:10.1002/asi.23181

Nussbaum, A., Tirrell, M., Wechsler, P., & Randall, T. (2010, April 5). Obamacare's cost scalpel. *Business Week*, 64-65.

O'Brien, M. S. (2006). Implementation of the EPIC Electronic Medical Record/ Physician Order-Entry System. *Journal of Healthcare Management*, *51*(5), 338–343. PMID:17039692

Pizzi, R. (2014). Nursing Informatics Adds Value as Healthcare is Transforming. *Healthcare IT News*. Retrieved December 1, 2014 from http://www.healthcareitnews.com/news/nursing-informatics-adds-value-healthcare-transforming

Razzaque, A., Eldabi, T., & Jalal-Karim, A. (2013). Physician virtual community and medical decision making: Mediating role of knowledge sharing. *Journal of Enterprise Information Management*, *26*(5), 500–515. doi:10.1108/JEIM-07-2013-0047

Romano, M. J., & Stafford, R. S. (2011). Electronic health records and clinical decision support systems: Impact on national ambulatory care quality. *National Library of Medicine. Archives of Internal Medicine*, *171*(10), 897–903. doi:10.1001/archinternmed.2010.527 PMID:21263077

Rosenbaum, S., & Margulies, R. (2011). Tax-exempt hospitals and the Patient Protection and Affordable Care Act: Implications for public health policy and practice. *National Library of Medicine. Public Health Reports*, *126*(2), 283–286. PMID:21387959

Schoen, C., Osborn, R., Squires, D., Doty, M., Rasmussen, P., Pierson, R., & Applebaum, S. (2012). A survey of primary care doctors in ten countries shows progress in use of health information technology, less in other areas. *Health Affairs*, *31*(12), 2805–2816. doi:10.1377/hlthaff.2012.0884 PMID:23154997

Somashekhar, S., & Sun, L. H. (2013). *HealthCare.gov meets deadline for fixes Obama administration says.* Retrieved December 10, 2014 from http://www.washingtonpost.com/national/health-science/healthcaregov-meets-deadline-for-fixes-white-house-says/2013/12/01/a3885612-5a13-11e3-ba82-16ed03681809_story.html

Thibodeau, P., & Gross, G. (2013). HealthCare.gov had "no chance in hell". *Computerworld*, *47*(19), 6.

Truven Health Analytics. (2014). *Disease Management Analytics*. Retrieved December 1, 2014 from http://truvenhealth.com/your-healthcare-focus/life-sciences/disease-management-analytics

U.S. Department of Health & Human Services. (2014). What is a medical home? Why is it important? *Health Resources and Services Administration (HRSA) - Health Information Technology*. Retrieved December 10, 2014 from http://www.hrsa.gov/healthit/toolbox/Childrenstoolbox/BuildingMedicalHome/whyimportant.html

U.S. Department of Health & Human Services. (2015). *Summary of the HIPAA security rule*. Retrieved April 20, 2015 from http://www.hhs.gov/ocr/privacy/hipaa/understanding/srsummary.html

Vo, A., & Bhaskar, R. (2012). Health Care Reform Requires Rethinking on the IT Strategy. *Journal of Cases on Information Technology*, *14*(2), 65–72. doi:10.4018/jcit.2012040105

Wolfstadt, J. I., Gurwitz, J. H., Field, T. S., Lee, M., Kalkar, S., Wu, W., & Rochon, P. A. (2008). The effect of computerized physician order entry with clinical decision support on the rates of adverse drug events: A systematic review. *Journal of General Internal Medicine*, *23*(4), 451–458. doi:10.1007/s11606-008-0504-5 PMID:18373144

Zai, A. H., Grant, R. W., Estey, G., Lester, W. T., Andrews, C. T., Yee, R., & Chueh, H. et al. (2008). Lessons from implementing a combined workflow-informatics system for diabetes management. *Journal of the American Medical Informatics Association*, *15*(4), 524–533. doi:10.1197/jamia.M2598 PMID:18436907

Zlabek, J. A., Wickus, J. W., & Mathiason, M. A. (2011). Early cost and safety benefits of an inpatient electronic health record. *Journal of the American Medical Informatics Association*, *18*(2), 169–172. doi:10.1136/jamia.2010.007229 PMID:21292703

ADDITIONAL READING

Agarwal, R., Sands, D. Z., Schneider, J. D., & Smaltz, D. H. (2010). Quantifying the economic impact of communication inefficiencies in U.S. hospitals. *Journal of Healthcare Management*, *55*(4), 265–282. PMID:20812527

Alpay, L., Van Der Boog, P., & Dumaij, A. (2011). An empowerment-based approach to developing innovative e-health tools for self-management. *Health Informatics Journal*, *17*(4), 247–255. doi:10.1177/1460458211420089 PMID:22193825

Ball, M. J., & Lillis, J. (2001). E-health: Transforming the physician/patient relationship. *International Journal of Medical Informatics*, *61*(1), 1–10. doi:10.1016/S1386-5056(00)00130-1 PMID:11248599

Ballantine, P. W., & Stephenson, R. J. (2011). Help me, I'm fat! Social support in online weight loss networks. *Journal of Consumer Behaviour*, *10*(5), 332–337. doi:10.1002/cb.374

Bitner, M. J. (2001). Service and technology: Opportunities and paradoxes. *Managing Service Quality*, *11*(6), 375–379. doi:10.1108/09604520110410584

Bringewatt, R. J. (2001). Making a business case for high-quality chronic illness care. *Health Affairs*, *20*(6), 59–60. doi:10.1377/hlthaff.20.6.59 PMID:11816690

Bugshan, H., Nick Hajli, M., Lin, X., Featherman, M., & Cohen, I. (2014). Social media for developing health services. *Qualitative Market Research*, *17*(3), 283–296. doi:10.1108/QMR-07-2013-0048

Chou, W. Y. S., Prestin, A., Lyons, C., & Wen, K. Y. (2013). Web 2.0 for health promotion: Reviewing the current evidence. *American Journal of Public Health*, *103*(1), 9–18. doi:10.2105/AJPH.2012.301071 PMID:23153164

Cunningham, P., Grant-Pearce, C., Green, L., Miles, I., Rigby, J., & Uyarra, E. (2005). In Sickness, in Health and in Innovation: NHS DIRECT – A Health Sector Innovation Study. Administration, 53(3), 42–65.

Ghannouchi, S. A., Mabrouk, K., & Ghannouchi, S. (2010). Proposal of data warehouse in the context of healthcare process reengineering. *Business Process Management Journal*, *16*(4), 688–712. doi:10.1108/14637151011065964

Gibbons, M. C., Fleisher, L., Slamon, R. E., Bass, S., Kandadai, V., & Beck, J. R. (2011). Exploring the potential of Web 2.0 to address health disparities. *Journal of Health Communication*, *16*(1), 77–89. doi:10.1080/10810730.2011.596916 PMID:21843097

Groselj, D. (2014). A webometric analysis of online health information: Sponsorship, platform type and link structures. *Online Information Review*, *38*(2), 209–231. doi:10.1108/OIR-01-2013-0011

Hajli, M., Bugshan, H., Lin, X., & Featherman, M. (2013). From e-learning to social learning-a health care study. *European Journal of Training and Development*, *37*(9), 851–863. doi:10.1108/EJTD-10-2012-0062

Halamka, J. D. (2014). Early experiences with big data at an academic medical center. *Health Affairs*, *33*(7), 1132–1138. doi:10.1377/hlthaff.2014.0031 PMID:25006138

Hamid, A., & Sarmad, A. (2008). Evaluation of e-health services: user's perspective criteria. *Transforming Government: People. Process and Policy*, *2*(4), 243–255.

Hardey, M. (2001). 'E-health': The internet and the transformation of patients into consumers and producers of health knowledge. *Information Communication and Society*, *4*(3), 388–405. doi:10.1080/713768551

Harjumaa, M., & Muuraiskangas, S. (2014). Building persuasiveness into information systems. *Electronic Journal of Information Systems Evaluation*, *17*(1), 23–35.

Kamel, B., Maged, N., & Wheeler, S. (2007). The emerging Web 2.0 social software: An enabling suite of sociable technologies in health and health care education1. *Health Information and Libraries Journal*, *24*(1), 2–23. doi:10.1111/j.1471-1842.2007.00701.x PMID:17331140

Liu, L., & Zhu, D. (2013). An integrated e-service model for electronic medical records. *Information Systems and eBusiness Management, 11*(1), 161-183.

Maletz, F. W. (2011). From hospital to "Healthspital": A better paradigm for health care. *The Futurist*, *45*(2), 16–19.

Neuhauser, L., & Kreps, G. L. (2003). Rethinking communication in the e-health era. *Journal of Health Psychology*, *8*(1), 7–23. doi:10.1177/1359105303008001426 PMID:22113897

Palvia, P., & Thambusamy, R. (2013). Electronic medical records application development: Perspectives of the service provider. *Journal of Information Technology Case and Application Research*, *15*(2), 11–29. doi:10.1080/15228053.2013.11082801

Phillips, A., & Thornbory, G. (2014). Apps for health professionals. *Occupational Health*, *66*(4), 27–29.

Schartinger, D., Miles, I., Saritas, O., Amanatidou, E., Giesecke, S., Heller-Schuh, B., & Schreier, G. et al. (2015). Personal health systems technologies: Critical issues in service innovation and diffusion. *Technology Innovation Management Review*, *5*(2), 46–57.

Sunyaev, A. (2013). Consumer facing health care systems. *E-Service Journal, 9*(2), 1-23, 63.

Wilson, E. V., & Lankton, N. K. (2004). Modeling patients' acceptance of provider-delivered e-health. *Journal of the American Medical Informatics Association, 11*(4), 241–248. doi:10.1197/jamia.M1475 PMID:15064290

Wilson, E. V., & Tulu, B. (2010). The rise of a health-IT academic focus. *Communications of the ACM, 53*(5), 147–150. doi:10.1145/1735223.1735259

Chapter 7
Geographic Information System Applications in Public Health:
Advancing Health Research

Sandul Yasobant
Indian Institute of Public Health Gandhinagar, India

Kranti Suresh Vora
Indian Institute of Public Health Gandhinagar, India

Ashish Upadhyay
Indian Institute of Public Health Gandhinagar, India

ABSTRACT

Geographic information systems or geographic information science is a combination of computer-mapping capabilities with additional database management/data analysis tools. GIS is widely used in various sectors such as environmental science, urban planning, agricultural applications etc. Public health is another focus area, where GIS has been used for research and practice areas such as epidemic surveillance and monitoring, among others. The journey of use of GIS in public health spans more than a century and GIS application in public health has evolved from the simple maps to the higher level geostatistical analysis and interactive WebGIS in recent times. GIS is an analytical tool which differs from conventional computer-assisted mapping and any statistical analysis programs in its ability to analyze complex data and visual presentation of spatial data. Specialized GIS techniques such as network analysis, location-allocation models, site selection, transportation models, and geostatistical analysis are well established and used in many developed

DOI: 10.4018/978-1-4666-9961-8.ch007

and developing nations. Unfortunately owing to the high cost of licensed software and specialized skills for advanced data analysis, use of these techniques is limited mainly for the research and by few experts. GIS is proved to be useful for various public health practices and research purposes including epidemiological surveys/ investigation, implementation research, program/policy decision making and dissemination of information. The advantage of using GIS is that maps provide an added dimension to data analysis, which helps in visualizing the complex patterns and relationships of public health issues, thus many unanswered questions in public health, can be understood well through use of GIS techniques. Use of GIS in public health is an application area still in its infancy. Wider use of GIS for public health practice such as program planning, implementation and monitoring in addition to building evidence base for the policy making will help reduce inequities in health and provide universal healthcare. Overall, GIS is a helpful and efficient tool especially for public health professionals working in low resource settings. In the future with inclusion of advanced GIS technology like WebGIS can help reach the goal of optimal health care services globally.

Knowing where things are, and why, is essential to rational decision making.
- Jack Dangermond, ESRI

1. INTRODUCTION

Public health is the science of ensuring and improving the health of communities through practice and research. Multidimensional public health data provides useful information to improve planning, implementation and monitoring of programs and evidence based policymaking processes; if analyzed appropriately. A number of quantitative approaches have been used for the complex analysis of these datasets but combining quantitative data with spatial data and visualization of spatial data are limited in public health research. In such circumstances Geographic information systems (GISs) or geographic information science (GIScience) is a powerful analytical tool; which differs from conventional computer-assisted mapping and any statistical analysis programs. Although computer-assisted cartographic systems emphasize map production and presentation of spatial data, they cannot analyze spatially-defined statistical data. GIS blends these different types of data to visualize, analyze, and explore geographically referenced information. Thus, a Geographic Information System can be used to address research questions or practical applications in the field of public health such as: *condition* – what is at …?; *location* – where is …?; *trend* - what has changed since…?; *pattern* – what spatial patterns exist?; and *modeling or scenario-building* – what if…?. In other words, it can be used to track the geographic location of people, places, events, actions, or impacts, to conduct spatial or statistical analysis on the variables of interest, and to create maps that display the spatial/temporal distributions and relationships of those variables (Richards, Croner, Rushton, & Brown, 1999) (Phillips et al., 2000) (Bédard & Henriques, 2002).

Recently, Geographical Information System (GIS) has emerged as an innovative and important component of research and practice in public health. GIS has proved to be useful for various research purposes including epidemiological surveys/investigation, implementation research, program/policy decision making and dissemination of information. The advantage of using GIS is that maps provide an added dimension to data analysis, which helps in visualizing the complex patterns and relationships of public health issues. Relationships among neighboring areas are explicit in maps which allows for the visualization of spatial patterns of disease or health service utilization. Some of the typical questions that can be answered by GIS are shown in Box-1. Despite the first use of GIS in the field of public health and advancement of technologies; GIS techniques has not been used extensively in this field due to difficulty in learning the technology (Sheppard, McMaster, Leitner, & Tian, 1999) (Schlundt, Mushi, Larson & Marrs, 2001) (Ferguson, Maheswaran, & Daly, 2004).

Examples of GIS scope in public health:

- Can we identify areas wherein a particular disease is prevalent?
- Can we get some geospatial clues about the possible factors that is responsible for a particular disease?
- Where to allocate additional resources for health facilities?
- What should be an ideal location of Health facility?
- Which are the areas wherein water related diseases are prevalent?
- In which area the maternal mortality rate is high?
- Which are the areas where the birth rate is high?

In short, GIS for Public Health, could be a useful decision support tool in strengthening health system in a more realistic and need based manner. So this chapter summarizes the basics of GIS for public health practitioners and its applications in public health research. Also an effort has been made to scope the extensive use of GIS to advance the public health research in future.

1.1. History of GIS

The GIS development started primarily in mid-18th century by the French geographer Charles Picquet for spatial analysis in epidemiology (GIS Lounge, 2012) and

Table 1. GIS and its evolution

Year	Type	Events	Innovators / Founders
1832	Map	Spatial analysis of mortality in Cholera epidemic in the city of Paris	Charles Picquet, France
1854	Map	Cholera outbreak map showing the cluster of cholera cases in London epidemic.	John Snow, London, UK
1963	Software Technology	Analysis of current use of land resources and ways to optimize the same in Canada	Roger Tomilnson, USA
1965	Technology	Dual Independent Map Coding (DIME) Developed for Geographic Database Files of Census	The US Bureau of Census
1971	Projects and software	General Information System for Planning (GISP) developed for Environmental Planning	UK Department of the Environment
1982	Commercial Software	ESRI Arc/Info 1.0 First Major Commercial GIS Software Designed for wider use	ESRI, USA
1985	GPS Technology	Global Positioning System more use for surveying and ground data collection for mapping	USA
1988	Digital Data Products	First public release TIGER (Topographically Integrated Geographic Encoding and Referencing) Digital Data for Census	US Bureau of Census, USA
1993	General	First Web-based interactive map viewer developed by Xerox Palo Alto Research Center (PARC)	Steve Putz, USA

John Snow who depicted a cholera outbreak in 1854 in the form of maps (John Snow Mapping, 1854). Systematic large scale use of GIS happened for the first time in Canada between 1960 to 1963 for public sector as a Canada Geographic information system (CGIS) by Roger Tomilnson to analyze inventory maps in order to identify the existing use of nations land resource and ways to optimize the same (Historica Canada, 1965). GIS has been upgraded from 19th century simple maps to the interactive web based technology of 21st century. The major evolution of GIS as a technology in general is described in Table-1.

In summarize the history of GIS; that there 'have been three distinct phases in the development of Geographic Information Systems.'

- **Phase-1. (Up to 1960's)** Initiation of the technology but the field was dominated by few individuals interested in the technology leading to limited utilization and technology development.

- **Phase-2. (1960's to Early-1980's):** GIS was used by governments in North America such as US Census bureau, Environment Protection Agency and Canadian government.
- **Phase-3. (Post 1980's):** Commercial GIS software availability led to wider use of the technology especially by the private sector. Not much use in Public health because of high cost of software and technical complexities. GIS became more interactive and simpler to use, yet public health utilization remains limited. Free GIS software developed by international development agencies such as WHO.

1.2. Historical Pathways of GIS in Public Health

The idea that location can influence health/healthcare utilization is a very old one in the health science. As far back as the time of Hippocrates (3rd century BC), physicians realized that certain diseases tended to occur in some places and not in others. In fact, different locations on Earth were thought to be associated with different physical, biological and environmental profiles of indigenous populations. Despite the realization, evidence was difficult to generate and present till about 150 years ago in 18th Century (Hall, 2000) (Meade & Earickson, 2000).

The first documented use of maps to present disease related data was in 1832 by the French geographer Charles Picquet in the city of Paris. He presented color coded maps of 48 districts of Paris depicting the percentage of deaths from cholera for every 1000 people. This was the first example of a visual representation of geographic data. In 1840, Robert Cowan used maps to show relationship between crowding and incidence of yellow fever in Glasgow-England (Lang, 2000). He recognized that in regions where there was crowding of immigrants, the frequency of disease was higher. Robert Perry used identified affected households on a map in 1843 to show typhus epidemic in Glasgow (Burrough, 1986) is another example of earlier use of maps in the public health. John Snow, an English physician is considered the father of modern epidemiology, in part because of his work in tracing the source of a cholera outbreak in Soho, London, in 1854. Original map by John Snow showing the clusters of cholera cases in the London epidemic of 1854, was drawn and lithographed by Charles Cheffins. Snow later used a dot map to illustrate the cluster of cholera cases around the pump. Snow's study was a major event in the history of public health and brought cartographic methods to the forefront of the discipline. Later on, German geographer Augustus Petermann created a series of Cholera maps of the British Isles in 1952 to show the geographical extent of the 1931–33 Cholera epidemic and discover environmental or local conditions, which might have affected the diffusion of the disease (Barrett, 2002).

These early mapping techniques proved extremely useful for elucidating the geospatial correlates of disease incidence and spread in the field of public health. The main obstacle for early physicians/medical geographers was limited technology and dearth of relevant data. Maps had to be drawn by hand, making them difficult to reproduce, and since physicians were the ones with medical data, it was they, not geographers, who first mapped disease patterns. That, however, changed at the turn of the 19th century. With advent of computers and development of information technology, now maps are created on the computer at much greater speed and accuracy. Also with availability of commercial software for industrial and research use and free application for academia and research, the used of GIS has expanded to planning and monitoring also. Access to free platforms such as Google and advanced software applications have made it possible to have dynamic and interactive GIS techniques such as Geovisualization for non-GIS public health professionals and planners. The journey of GIS from paper based hand drawn static maps to web based interactive GIS has spanned more than a century.

2. GIS: AS A TECHNOLOGY

2.1. Basics of GIS

GIS is a computerized data management system used to capture, store, manage, retrieve, analyze, and display spatial information. A GIS differs from other graphics systems in several respects. First, data are geo-referenced to the coordinates of a particular projection system. This allows precise placement of features on the earth's surface and maintains the spatial relationships between mapped features. As a result, commonly referenced data can be overlaid to determine relationships between data elements. For example; location of health service provider to the healthcare utilization of the population could be studied easily through GIS. Second, GIS software use relational database management technologies to assign a series of attributes to each spatial feature. Common feature identification keys are used to link the spatial and attribute data between tables.

The GIS components are divided in to four parts. They are Hardware, Software, Data and Human Ware etc. GIS used as to capture spatial data, data storing, processing & analysis and output production through maps. Hardware + Software + Data + Methods + User = GIS

2.1.1. GIS and Data

GIS software generally uses two types of data: Raster data (i.e., discrete cells in a rigid row by column format), such as satellite imagery or aerial photography or Vectors (points, lines and polygons) to represent features on the earth's surface. Most systems allow for full integration of both types of data. In either case, a fully functioning GIS allows the user to enter or digitize data that are georeferenced; link specific attributes to each feature using relational database management system technology; analyze relationship between various geographic features using a wide range of spatial operations and functions; and produce high-resolution images or graphics on color monitors or plotters.

a) **Raster data** is characterized by grid-cell data structure where the geographic area is divided into cells identified by row and column. The size of cells in a tessellated data structure is selected on the basis of the data accuracy and the resolution needed by the user. There is no explicit coding of geographic coordinates required since that is implicit in the layout of the cells. A raster data structure is in fact a matrix where any coordinate can be quickly calculated if the origin point is known, and the size of the grid cells is known. Since grid cells can be handled as two dimensional arrays in computer encoding many analytical operations are easy to program. This makes tessellated data structures a popular choice for many GIS software (Figure 1a).
b) **Vector data** is characterized by the use of sequential points or vertices to define a linear segment. Each vertex consists of an X coordinate and a Y coordinate. Vector lines are often referred to as arcs and consist of a string of vertices terminated by a node. A node is defined as a vertex that starts or ends an arc segment. Point features are defined by one coordinate pair, a vertex. Polygonal features are defined by a set of closed coordinate pairs. In vector representation, the storage of the vertices for each feature is important, as well as the connectivity between features, e.g. the sharing of common vertices where features connect (Figure 1b).

2.1.2. Ways to Collect GIS Based Data

2.1.2.1. Global Positioning System (GPS)

Geolocation is given two coordinates in a global address: Latitude and Longitude. Global Positioning System (GPS) is used to assign a geographic location to make

Figure 1. (a- Left) Raster data and (b-Right) Vector data

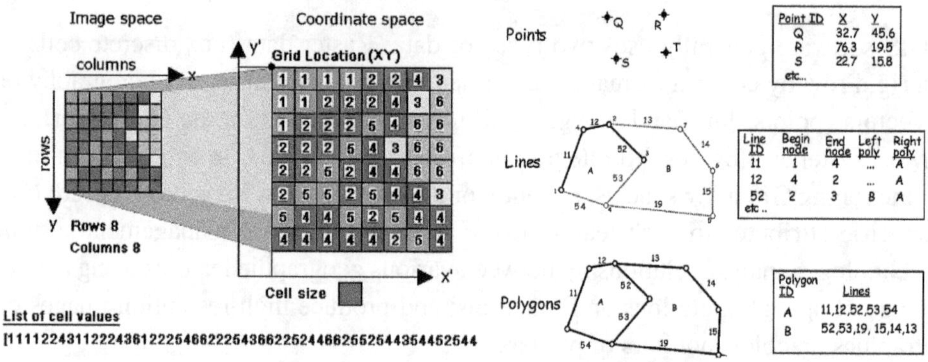

maps more accurate and effective. Positioning in three dimensions (Latitude, Longitude, and Elevation) requires at least four satellites and accuracy depends on the number of satellites and their positions (if elevation is not needed then only three satellites need be above the horizon). For example a location of health facility through GPS could be expressed as N 23o 35. 77', E 72o 57. 659' (Degree, Minute, Second) format.

2.1.2.2. Remote Sensing (RS)

Remote sensing is a method of obtaining information from distant objects without direct contact. This is possible due to the existence or the generation of force fields between the sensing device and the sensed object. Principal force field used in remote sensing is that of electromagnetic energy, as characterized by the Maxwell equations. Remote sensed imagery is integrated within a GIS. And these sensors collect data in the form of images and provide specialized capabilities for analyzing and visualizing those images.

2.2. GIS Techniques Used in Public Health

1. **Mapping and Visualization:** GIS offers tools to present spatial information at the level of individual occurrence, and to conduct predictive modeling. It determines geographical distribution and variation of diseases, and their prevalence and incidence through maps. GIS can help in generating thematic maps - ranged color maps or proportional symbol maps to denote the intensity of a disease or a vector. In comparison with tables and charts, maps developed using GIS can be extremely effective means for communicating messages clearly even to those who are not familiar with the technology. Frequently used maps in the public health research are Dot-density and Choropleth maps. Dot-density maps are the simplest way to display events. These maps use dots or other symbols

to represent the number of occurrences of a given data characteristic. Each dot or symbol used on the map represents a single entity (one dot = 1 case) or a group (one dot = 1000 cases). Choropleth maps are area maps in which polygons are shaded, colored, or patterned according to the value of a given attribute for each polygon. Choropleth maps are also called thematic maps or Shaded maps- Figure 2 (a).

2. **Overlay Analysis:** GIS can overlay different pieces of spatial and non-spatial information to combine the characteristics of several datasets into one; to find specific locations or areas that have a certain set of attribute values. In general, there are two methods for performing overlay analysis—feature overlay (overlaying points, lines, and polygons) and raster overlay. This helps in decision making and health research through multi criteria modeling (for example, in understanding the association between prevalence of certain diseases and specific geographic features)- Figure 2 (b).
3. **Buffer Analysis:** Buffer analysis is used for identifying areas with similar attributes surrounding geographic locations for specific distance. The process involves generating a buffer around existing geographic features and then identifying or selecting features based on whether they fall inside or outside the boundary of the buffer. Buffering can be done on all three types of vector data: point, line, area. The resulting buffer is a polygon file. For example, a

Figure 2a. Visualization/mapping
(MATIND Gujarat Project Data, 2015)

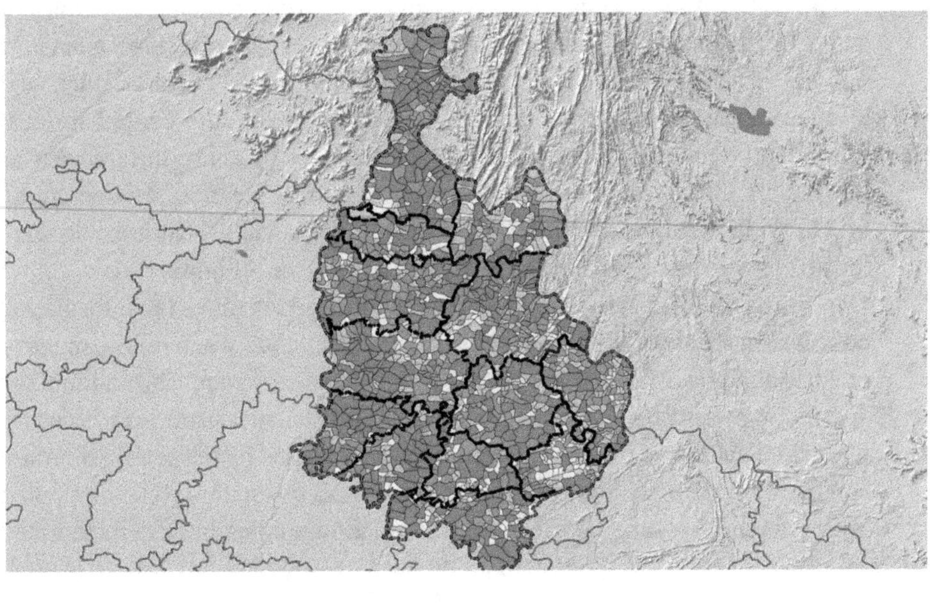

Figure 2b. Overlay analysis
(MATIND Gujarat Project Data, 2015)

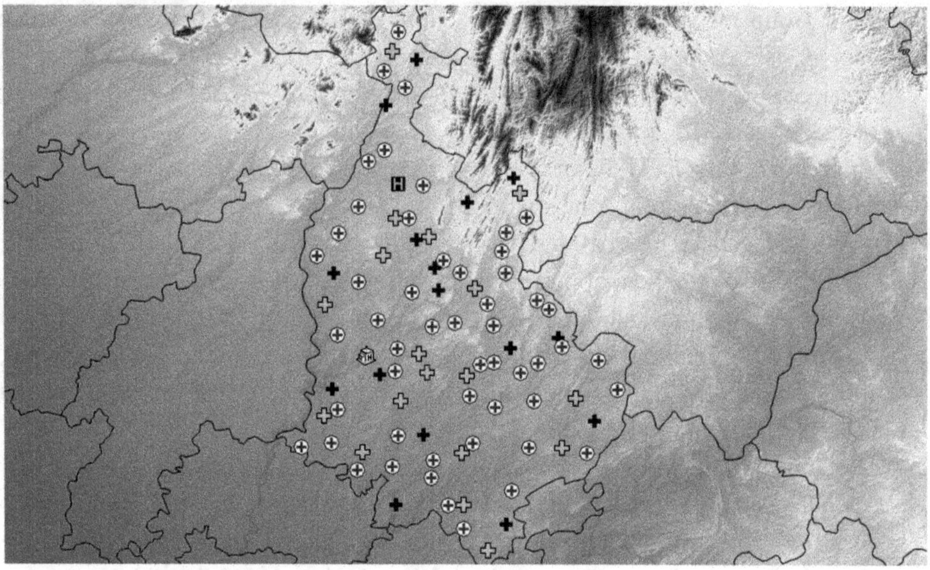

radius of 10 km around a hospital to depict its catchment area or 1 km around a health facilities coverage in village populations. The user can specify the size of the buffer and then combine this information with population access to type of health facility to determine how much population fall within the buffer- Figure 2 (c).

4. **Network Analysis:** GIS can quickly assess the geo demographic dynamics of an organization's existing service area in order to expand the service area for optimal service provision. It can identify catchment areas of health centers and also locate suitable sites for a new health facility. Health services delivered at home can be scheduled in a more efficient manner by analyzing transportation factors and street patterns, and by recommending the most efficient route. GIS Provides accurate and timely information about where health services are located and instructions and maps on how to get there- Figure 2 (d).
5. **Geo-Statistical Analysis:** of GIS uses space time index for all the information collected in the database. This is one special technique where GIS can carry out data analysis like any other quantitative analysis software while adding the spatial component. Unlike traditional analysis, geostatistical analysis account for the spatial pattern of observed frequencies as modeled by the semivariogram, and more importantly, the variance of the kriging estimator can be computed with reference to time and location. Simulation studies have demonstrated

Figure 2c. Buffer analysis
(MATIND Gujarat Project Data, 2015)

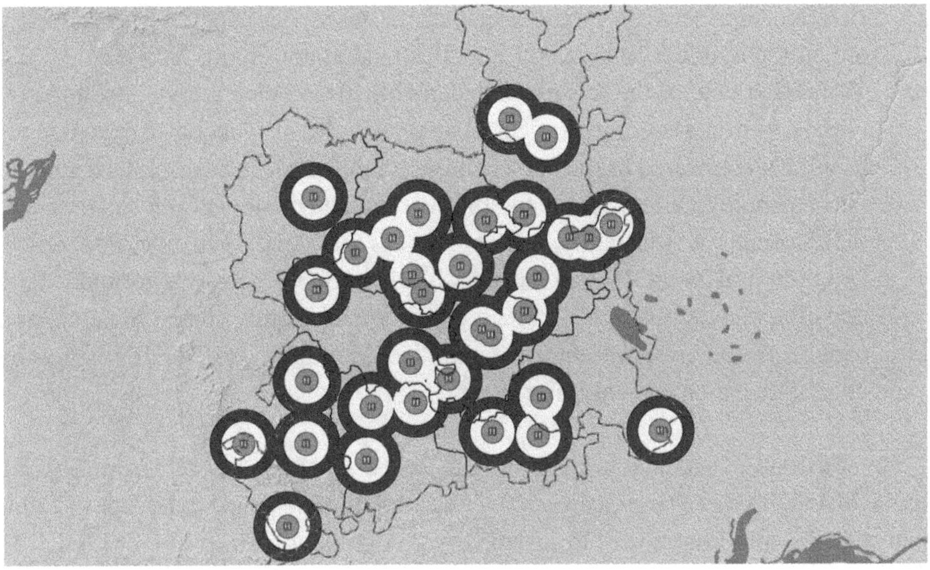

Figure 2d. Network analysis
(MATIND Gujarat Project Data, 2015)

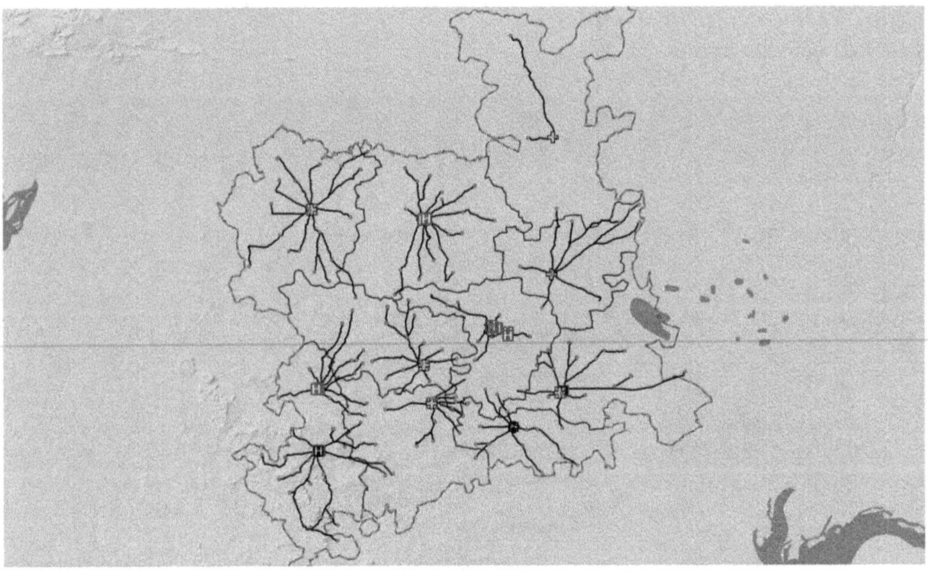

substantially improved accuracy of the risk estimated using Binomial or Poisson kriging, relative to head-banging and empirical Bayesian smoothers. Relationships between variables that vary across space (Spatial heterogeneity) are only possible to analyze through this technique- Figure 2 (e).

6. **Web GIS:** One of the recent advancements in GIS technology is web-based GIS. Health data is stored in a central server which can be accessed from various terminals connected to the server through internet or intranet. Internet based GIS technology eliminates the traditional method of flow of information, and the information is instantly available across the globe. Dynamic, interactive, and temporal WebGIS make it possible for non-GIS experts to understand and disseminate public health data which are inherently spatial in nature and cannot, as easily, be presented through the use of paper based GIS maps or by quantitative analysis only- Figure 2f.

To demonstrate GIS techniques, the authors have used MATIND data from Gujarat, India. MATIND was a large scale survey received funding from the European Community's Seventh Framework Programme under grant agreement no. 261304. The funders had no role in designing and preparation of this chapter.

Basic spatial analytic methods either investigate patterns in spatial data or seek to find relationships between such patterns and the spatial (and perhaps temporal)

Figure 2e. Geo-statistical analysis
(MATIND Gujarat Project Data, 2015)

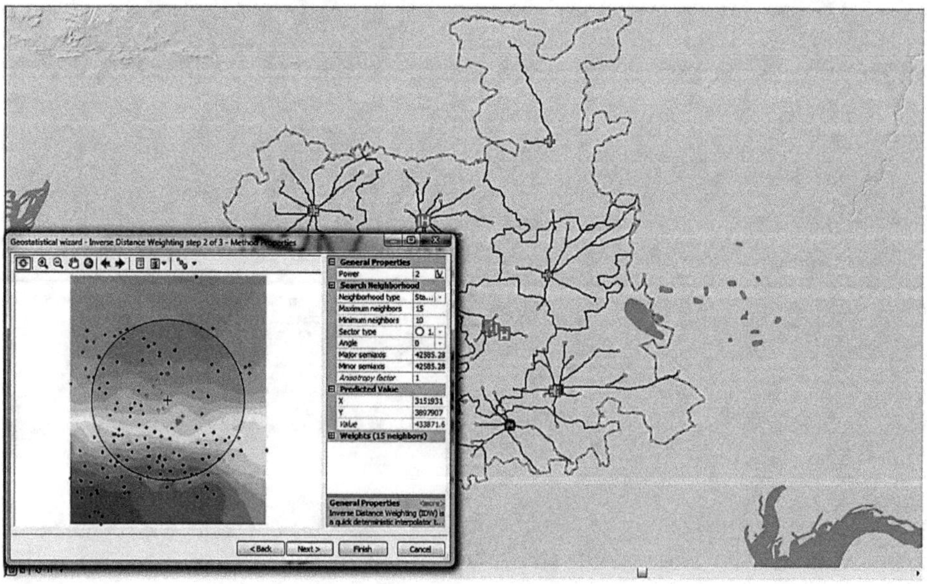

Figure 2f. WebGIS- Geovisualisaton
(MATIND Gujarat Project Data, 2015)

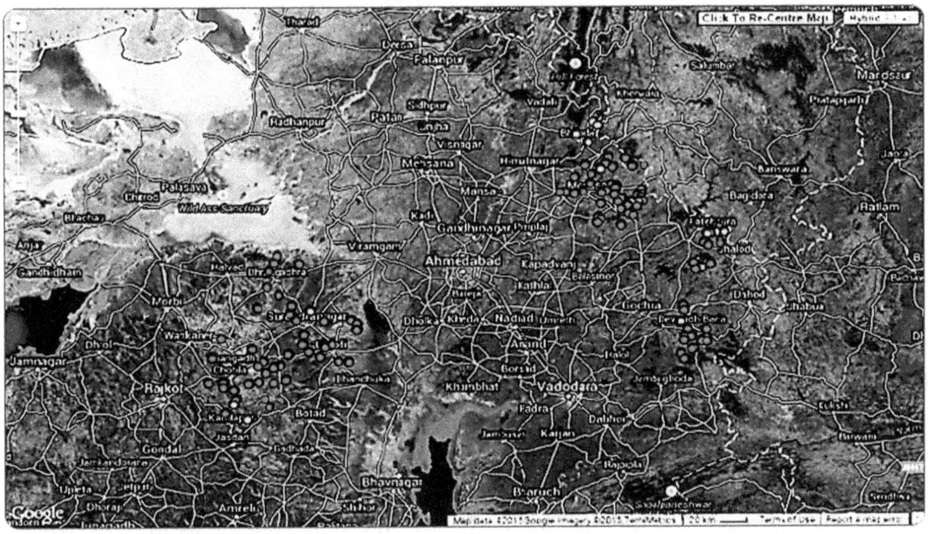

variation of other attributes, or for methods of spatial or spatio–temporal modelling. Further analysis would include network analysis, location-allocation models, site selection, and transportation models, all of which are considered to be quite well developed within many GIS. Advanced analysis by GIS is geostatistical analysis; which would include nearest neighbour methods and K-functions, Kernel and Bayesian smoothing methods, spatial autocorrelation, spatial econometric modelling, and spatial general linear models. As there are many applications available with GIS software; but it depends upon the need to decide upon which application to use. Keeping in mind the various dimensions of GIS technologies in the field of public health; Table 2 summarizes the Strength-Weakness-Opportunity-Threat (SWOT) of GIS techniques in public health.

There are also concerns or issues with use of GIS tools for public health. Most grave among those is a concern for the privacy and confidentiality of individuals. Protecting the privacy and confidentiality of those individuals is of paramount importance. Depending on the quantity and quality of data and the methodology used in analysis, a given map may be either useful or misleading (Rytkonen, 2004). For example, people expose themselves to different risk factors in different locations, and the relationship between catching a disease and the potential environmental risk factor is difficult to prove reliably. An example of this is where working-age adults may spend much of their lives outside the area where they are actually resident (Taylor, 1998). Thus, all the exposures and risks earlier in life may become

Table 2. SWOT Analysis of GIS ~ Public Health

Strength	Weakness
▪ Better insight in spatial patterns ▪ Visual presentation of data-easy to understand ▪ Multilevel modeling of complicated Data ▪ Possibility to do predictions ▪ Visualization of time series ▪ Quick	▪ Complexity of software ▪ GIS trained personnel required ▪ Cost of Software ▪ Problems with Data Sources ▪ Importance of Scales ▪ Less Qualitative research focused
Opportunity	**Threat**
▪ Internet use in Data collection ▪ Use of GPS in Data Sources ▪ Dynamics of Web based GIS Software	▪ Less Awareness of GIS opportunities ▪ Data Facilities & Skilled staff required ▪ Confidentiality of Research

associated on maps with an inaccurate geographical location and may easily lead to erroneous conclusions and etiological hypotheses without individual-level information of the exposure history. This problem is compounded when considering the exposure for diseases with a long latent period such as cancer (Poulstrup & Hansen, 2004). All these GIS techniques are only useful when there is availability of accurate relevant data; which is a major challenge in least developed countries. Therefore if public health data are not reliable; GIS cannot provide appropriate result and may sometimes mislead. Though GIS has certain advantages, these limitations are important to note.

2.3. GIS Software

There is a large range of GIS software available for use in public health; each with their own strengths and weaknesses. Some packages are open domain and can be freely downloaded from the web, but these often have limited functionality. In other hand a large number of paid licensed version software are also available and could be purchased according to the need and extend of use of professionals. Selection of software depends on the use and specific need. Table 3 provides summary of GIS software applications with sources available for Public health researchers/ practitioners.

3. GIS IN PUBLIC HEALTH RESEARCH AND PRACTICE

Great leaps of science are often made at the borders where different fields of research meet. GIS in public health is a good example of this. In many public health and epidemiology research GIS has recently emerged as an innovative and important component, sometimes even an essential tool. GIS can support public health

Table 3. GIS Software in Public Health

Name & Source of Software	Major Functions of Software
Commercial Software	
Autocad (www.autodesk.com)	Application for 2D and 3D computer-aided design (CAD) and drafting
Arcgis Desktop (www.esri.com)	Analyze, map, manage, share, and publish geographic information
Bentley System (www.bentley.com)	Design, construction and operation of infrastructure
Caliper (http://www.caliper.com)	Sophisticated, vector-based, low-end GIS desktop mapping
ERDAS Imagine (www.hexagongeospatial.com)	GIS, Remote Sensing, Photorgammetry and Image Processing
Geomedia Professional (http://www.intergraph.com/gis/products.asp)	GIS, remote sensing, and photogrammetry
Idrisi (http://www.clarklabs.org)	Functionality in the area of spatial analysis in Academia Research
MapInfo Professional (www.mapinfo.com)	Rroute analysis, 3D and statistical analysis, MapInfo MapMarker for Geocoding
Free Open Source Software	
ChildInfo (www.childinfo.org)	Simple tool for tables, graphs and maps
Crimestat III (http://www.icpsr.umich.edu/CRIMESTAT/)	Density analysis; hot spot analysis; plus a range of new modeling tools
Epi Map (http://wwwn.cdc.gov/epiinfo/)	GIS Mapping capability in Epi-Info
ESTAT(http://gis.cancer.gov/nci/spatial.html)	Exploratory Spatio-Temporal Analysis
GAM/K(http://www.ccg.leeds.ac.uk/software/gam/)	Geographic Analysis Machine / cluster hunting
GeoDa (http://geodacenter.asu.edu/software)	Exploratory spatial data analysis
GRASS (http://grass.itc.it/)	Geographic Resources Analysis Support System
HealthMapper (www.healthmap.org/en)	Analyzing epidemiological data, revealing trends, dependencies and inter-relationships
ILWIS (http://www.itc.nl/ilwis)	PC-based GIS & Remote Sensing software for image processing, spatial analysis
MapWindow GIS (www.mapwindowgis.com)	Desktop GIS Mapping Software
PostGIS (http://postgis.refractions.net/)	Geographic Object relational database software
QGIS (http://www.qgis.org/)	Visualize, analyze and publish geospatial information
SaTScan (http://www.satscan.org)	Designed for disease pattern analysis and surveillance
TNTMips (http://www.microimages.com/)	To view, create, edit, georeference, interpret, and publish any type of geospatial data
uDig (http://udig.refractions.net/)	GeoSpatial application and a platform through which developers can create new, derived applications

continued on following page

Table 3. Continued

Name & Source of Software	Major Functions of Software
ZDES(http://www.geog.leeds.ac.uk/software/zdes/)	Zone design system
Web Base Software	
Mapserver (http://mapserver.org/)	Open Source development environment for building spatially-enabled internet applications.
Open Layers (http://openlayers.org/)	OpenLayers is a pure JavaScript library for displaying map data in most modern web browsers, with no server-side dependencies
OpenSourceGIS (http://opensourcegis.org/)	Assorted open source GIS software list, including almost 250 sites and software utilities for spatial data processing

in different ways as well. First and foremost, GIS displays can help inform proper understanding and drive evidence based decisions. GIS has not only been used to measure the burden of disease and the spatial dynamics of infectious diseases (Cooke, Tanser, Barnighausen, & Newell, 2010) (Wilkinson &Tanser, 1999) and neglected tropical diseases (Simarro et al., 2010); but also been used to identify inequities in access and coverage of health services (Schuurman, Fiedler, Grzybowski, & Grund, 2006) (Schuurman, Bell, L'Heureux, & Hameed, 2009) (Tanser, 2006). In public health causality of disease is difficult to prove conclusively using GIS yet evidence for causal relationships could be strengthened through GIS related techniques. Use of GIS in public health is not new but its application in the public health area is still in its infancy. Like most new applications, there is a lot of promise, but it is important to bear in mind the limitation of the application. It is obvious that GIS has a lot to offer the health sciences (Cliff & Hagget, 1988) (Gatrell & Löytönen, 1998) hence, the broader applications of GIS in public health have been discussed below.

3.1. GIS in Public Health Services Planning:

It is evident that many questions concerning the provision of health care are related to space. People are distributed in space and they are not evenly distributed. Health problems vary in space and so do the needs of the people. Where should health care centres be situated and what services should they offer to answer efficiently to the needs of populations varying in numbers, densities, and health problems? These are problems that GIS can help resolve with their spatial analysis tools. Public health planners assess the health needs of certain populations and communities, analyze and evaluate programs and policies, and use this information to develop plans to implement public health programs and advocate for public health policies. The advantage of GIS over conventional quantitative methods is the local spatial information used to give local context to the problem and solution to match. To reach the universal health coverage it's important to look into many determinants such as social, biological, economical as well as geographical and it's the place where GIS can help planner to take decision accurately, efficiently and hastily. Thus, GIS based evaluation of health services and optimizing healthcare services have been elaborated to discuss the extent of its use.

3.1.1. Evaluation of Health Services Utilization

Geographical access is an important aspect in the planning process. GIS-based accessibility analysis is a logical method which can be applied to test the degree to which equitable access is provided. The GIS analysis is however based on the assumption of rational choice, i.e. a person will always go to their closest facility. Inputs to the analysis are supply (capacity of facilities) and demand (people seeking the service) estimates. Geography of supply is expressed through counts of the number of hospitals, their physical location and configuration and the relative size of those hospitals and numbers of services provided. The best example could be of Malawi study (Heard, Larsen, & Hozumi, 2004) where they employed to integrate health facility data from the Malawi health facilities inventory and global positioning data from the 2000 Malawi demographic and health survey. An effort to detect a plausible causal pathway was made by using distance to health services as a proxy variable for access to services. A famous report by Hanly report indicates how the proposals by the Government might affect geographical accessibility to Irish acute hospitals and modelled it within a GIS framework (Kalogirou, & Foley, 2006).

The Division of Public Health Systems, within the Public Health Practice Program Office (PHPPO), of the Centers for Disease Control and Prevention (CDC Atlanta) has addressed the geographic component for access to health services which is dependent on the individual client's location and demographic bracket, topography and travel times on route to the service and for planning purposes may be measured in the following ways.

- Geographical relationship between the location of potential clients and available services.
- Determining the market area for services by mapping the location of clients.
- Determining the proportion of eligible (or target) population that is receiving service from the facilities.
- Evaluating the relationship between client geographic access, health care use and health outcomes.
- Planning service provision at individual sites based on neighborhood demographics.

Apart from the more service-specific areas, much of the work of medical geographers and cartographers has focused on the issue of health inequalities. Quantitative measurements of health inequalities have taken a number of forms. There is a clear relationship between wealth and poverty and the different measures of health inequalities. A simple starting point for many geographers is to look at how these relationships are expressed spatially by mapping income against health indicators (Driedger et al., 2007). Another valuable example is the work of Damiani et al. (2005) who used a surface model approach to measure access to acute hospitals which in turn was weighted by a measure of choice, as expressed through levels of available beds. In this way, a normal mapped result, which identified rural and remote areas as poorly served, was considerably modified when the impact of waiting times and available beds was fed in. In the modified version, areas around the South East and South West of England showed up as under-served, an interesting example of how demand and supply affect the original models. In all cases, the ability of GIS to effectively visualize accessibility in the form of vector time maps and raster accessibility surfaces have allowed for ready analysis and interpretation as both a pointer to and a timesaving short-cut for subsequent explanatory analysis. Thus concisely saying simple evaluation of health services is incomplete without geo-spatial component of GIS; which could provide a comprehensive picture of any health program or could provide a simple potential solution of the current problem. A summary of previous studies measured accessibility using GIS have been summarized in Table 4.

Table 4. Examples of some previous studies using GIS to measure accessibility

Authors	Health Issue	Methodology	Findings
Al-Taiar *et al.* (2010)	Vaccination	Measured straight-line distances, driving distances and time.	All three measures showed strong association with vaccination of children after adjusting for socioeconomic status.
Lin *et al.* (2005)	Pain management	Measured distance between patient and facility's zip codes	Similar differences observed between revealed and potential access in both rural and urban areas.
Lou & Wang (2003)	Primary care	Two-step floating catchment area and gravity based	Two-step floating catchment area: simpler and easier to interpret, for use in improving the designation of health professional shortage areas.
Parker & Campbell (1998)	General practitioner services, accident & emergency services	Calculated network distance between patient and facility's zip codes	General practitioner services: "the majority of patients choose medical practices near their home address, many patients do not elect to receive medical services from the practice which is geographical closest to their home address."

3.1.2. Optimizing Geographic Access to Health Services:

Spatial planning of health care services concerns the identification of suitable locations for a given number of facilities in a defined territory, in such a way that the health needs have spatially dispersed population are served in an optimal way (Amer, 2007). GIS can be used in projecting the population growth in communities and ensuring that health services are going to be located in the most appropriate position and that adequate resources will exist to service projected needs. By overlaying existing health facilities on projected population growth data, planners can see where services may best be sited for future communities. Most health and social care planning systems need to plan the location of services based on number of different scenarios which can include: the location of a brand new service, the addition of a new service to existing services, the removal of a service or the multiple alteration of existing services. With the arrival of GIS and geo-computational methods working in tandem with improved spatial data, the calculation of multiple scenarios became much quicker and the arrival at optimal locations for services based on available data was easier. This new knowledge is then used to look at the location of existing services to see if they are effectively located given the modelled demand. In turn, location-allocation approaches were used to model potentially more effective locations for those services. A review paper on location allocation models for health services development in developing nation's notes that the earliest use of the model was in 1966 in Guatemala while in 1979 a study in India mentions use of such model for locating social services (Rahmana. &Smith, 2000). With use of GIS technology such as location allocation should be part of routine monitoring and a part of routine health care planning process for optimizing limited resources (Rushton. 1984) (WenHsiang, 2000).

The geographic health studies have shown extensive beneficial as of their outcomes. For example studies in New Zeeland (Rigby & Skelly, 2005) in British Columbia (Lin et al., 2002) and in Wales (Christie & Fone, 2003) used local topography and included distance as a health utilization predictors for optimizing the public health services. Some of the studies mentioned before used more robust forms of spatial modelling and moving beyond Euclidian distance to include consideration of travel distance along road networks and even more usefully, travel time. Additional sophistication was provided by studies which looked at incorporating public as well as private transport into the models (Martin et al., 2002; Lovett et al., 2002; Jordan et al., 2004). The use of multi-level modelling has also developed rapidly in the last decade with an increasing interest in the spatial aspects of health-place relationships when examined at a number of different levels in order to optimize the services.

3.2. GIS in Disease Monitoring, Control, and Surveillance

GIS has been used to produce maps of disease incidence, prevalence and mortality, morbidity at local or national levels. The information is more easily understood when visualized on a map. Besides time and person, knowledge of the spatial distribution of disease cases are essential in understanding disease transmission and determinates, as many diseases not caused directly by environmental exposure still cluster geographically (Latkin, Glass, & Duncan, 1998) (Moore & Carpenter, 1999). Studies like Lyme disease in Maryland (Glass et al., 1995), blood lead concentration (Pb-S) in Venezuela, South America would be the examples of relationship establishment and control measures planning through GIS technologies. In situations like epidemic or outbreak of any diseases; it is easier to identify the maximal affected area and control the spread of out-break. GIS should be an integral part of routine epidemic management system to ensure the quick response. Similar use of GIS for emergency preparedness or disaster management units can reduce the effect of catastrophe.

Similarly; disease surveillance system needs a technology that can provide timely information on the course of diseases and other health events. This may facilitate prompt implementation of prevention and intervention efforts, such as strengthening control action in the most affected area or initiation of epidemiological investigation. Since health related variables of interest are often spatially distributed, they require special tools for analysis and representation such as GIS technology. One of the example of disease surveillance system using GIS is Queensland Health, Australia for Dengue Fever Surveillance System; which is an automated GIS/Database system that collects, analyses and maps cases of dengue fever and vector-control work conducted in response to dengue fever outbreaks (Hart, McCulloch, 2004). Further, disease mapping has been identified as one of the tools to improve analysis and reporting within the National Notifiable Disease Surveillance System in many developed countries; which ultimately strengthens the public health system (Toms, 2004) (Spencer, 2004).

3.3. GIS in Public Health Promotion

Health promotion is the process of enabling people to increase control over, and to improve, their health. It moves beyond a focus on individual behavior towards a wide range of social and environmental interventions. In line of preventing diseases and promoting healthier life style GIS with GPS have proved its extensive capability in dual way to improve the current life style such as smoking cessation programs, diabetes education, mammography screening and cervical cancer screening as well as have been used to map activity spaces and preferred intervention sites for the distribution of targeted health promotion (Gesler et al., 2004) (CDC, 2005) (Robertson, 1998).

For example GIS has been used extensively to compare and very effectively illustrate a number of indicators of community walkability in older and newer suburbs in Georgia, USA (Frank, Engelke, Schmidt, 2003). A similar GIS-based approach to assessing community walkability has been replicated by a research group in Queensland in the PLACE 'Physical Activity in Localities and Community Environments' (Owen, 2004). In another example; GIS assisted the study of spatial relationships between food availability and dietary choices. For instance, how close does a supermarket have to be to make a difference in food choices for those who do not drive?. The classical example would be North Carolina Department of Health and Human Services are using GIS for analysis in their attempts to reach 1.3 million women at child-bearing age for their Folic Acid Project (Frank, Andresen, Schmid, 2004).

3.4. GIS in Environmental Health

Understanding the complex spatio-temporal relationships between environmental pollution and disease and identifying exposures to environmental hazards in high-risk populations are essential elements of an effective environmental and public health management program. Modern computer technologies, such as GIS, provide cost-effective tools for evaluating interventions and policies potentially affecting health outcomes. In Environmental Health, important issues are: 1. Improvements in exposure assessment. 2. Tackling the problem of the combined effect of multiple exposures. 3. Integration of experimental and epidemiologic evidence. The critical assessment of timing of exposure and its relationship to induction or promotion of disease including the human individual variation of susceptibility as well as latency periods and interaction with other factors are essential. Among the most important exploratory methods for environmental epidemiology and public health are methods for identifying clusters or clustering with respect to space and/or time (Alexander and Boyle 1996, Hjalmars, Kulldorff et al 1994, 1996and 1999, Kulldorff 1998). There has been a strong trend in modern environmental epidemiology towards the examination of individual biological factors (biomarkers, genetic epidemiology). GIS may provide tools for an integration of such aspects of case characteristics and environment including social milieu.

3.5. GIS in Healthcare Service Quality

Rapid growth of managed care, ambulatory services, telemedicine, and provider networks is fundamentally altering health care delivery with concomitant effects on the spatial organization of health services. Traditional models that describe the spatial behaviors of health care consumers and providers are not likely to fit well in the new "digital" health care landscape (Lovett et al 2014). These new spatial behaviors, which can be studied and modeled in GIS, should be prioritized for future research attention. A study from Western Indian State (Gujarat), focused on spatial assessment of a maternal healthcare service to improve the quality of services. Comprehensive Emergency Obstetric (CEmOC) services have been assessed in context of implementation of a Public Private Partnership (PPP) and resultant change in service area was observed during the year 2006-2012. The unique feature of the spatial study is inclusion of bed strength of the obstetric facilities in the GIS analysis to ensure the optimal quality of maternal services (Avoidance of overcrowding). To optimize the access to quality maternal care a further location-allocation analysis was done. The newer service centres have been decided based on the selection criteria for optimal geographic availability, to the under-served population (Vora et al. 2015). The health care industry have since long, mapped events such as sporadic epidemics of infectious diseases for epidemiological research; but now with newer GIS technology, hospitals can explore in real time (Yasobant et al 2015) and map where their patients are coming from and what are the most prevalent healthcare issues. If data collected from various sources would be triangulated through GIS/GPS, then this spatial data will enhance the ability of healthcare industry to monitor quality and research ways to improve the quality.

Historically, patient safety has been viewed as actions that minimize a patient's exposure to unnecessary risk, such as keeping patients from falling or reducing medication dosage errors while in the healthcare environment. However, the Joint Commission of Accreditation of Healthcare Organizations (JCAHO), a major quality of care organization, recently suggested that patient safety extends beyond the walls of the hospital and into the community (Davenhall WF 2003). Experts on clinical outcomes have long recognized that geography is a critical determinant in explaining differential medical outcomes. This new spatial notion of patient safety presents interesting questions as well as new opportunities for GIS experts. A healthcare organization can develop a community-based approach for patient safety beyond hospital walls. Thus, the value of using spatial and geographic intelligence to deliver quality healthcare, as well as a new analytical framework within which to think about lifelong patient safety, is tremendously important. Geography is intrinsically tied to health as well as patients receiving the highest quality care in the safest environment. Major healthcare accreditation and oversight bodies, have expressed interest in redefining the geographic aspects of patient safety and encouraging healthcare providers to consider the value of integrating internally generated healthcare information with externally available population health information including spatial information (Chae et al 2003). In conclusion, GIS is emerging as a tool to improve the quality of healthcare services and should be successfully implemented in the planning phase itself. There is a scope of innovative researches to develop GIS application for accessing and improving the quality of care in healthcare industry.

Despite the progresses in public health; there are many unanswered questions faced by public health professionals regarding causality, evaluation, policy making etc. To answer such questions, GIS can be an integral part of the tool kit; thus adding to development of an effective framework of action.

4. CONCLUDING REMARKS AND FUTURE OF GIS IN PUBLIC HEALTH

Today's public health problems are much more complex in scope than those of earlier era, and public health professionals today depend on technologies to deal with these issues. GIS can play an important role in all aspects of public health for optimal use of resources for equitable universal health.

Certainly, as the ground level situation changes very rapidly as a result of migration, extensive travelling across the globe and emergence of new diseases; hence real time data and ease of understanding the complexity are essential. As traditional GIS visualization techniques focus on the presentation of points, lines and polygons in static maps, there is an urgent need to develop more comprehensive, dynamic GIS tool. Newer techniques such as Geovisualization (a type of WebGIS) allow users to explore specific phenomena in more efficient and effective ways to uncover or clarify dimensions that may be ambiguous in traditional GIS visualizations (Yasobant et al, 2015). Thus a real time GIS in the form of "Tools for Tomorrow's Health care" could help solve many challenges in public health. Continuous monitoring of effectiveness of public health programs would be easier with inclusion of GIS in health management information system (HMIS). Same data can be used for further planning/ improvement of programs and provide evidence base for policy making.

For some health issues the impact of place is critically important. In these situations GIS can be the tool in pinpointing where public health efforts needs to be concentrated (Colantonio et al., 2011). Currently all most all the public health indicators are population based; but it's high time to add the spatial component to monitor and standardize the health indicators. Health Practitioner to population ratio is used by almost all international agency including WHO to monitor the access to universal healthcare ignoring the geographic access (McMichael, Beaglehole, 2000) (Sobal, 2001) (Huynen, Martens, Hilderink, 2005). Although GIS originally started with public health, there is a scope of wider applications and mainstreaming GIS as a public health practice and research method.

History of GIS in public health is long but applications in the field are sparse. The journey has been from the simpler maps to the higher level geostatistical analysis and interactive WebGIS. GIS has been used for public health planning and research in many countries yet there is a scope for wider and routine applications of GIS. The key benefit of deploying GIS in public health practice is that it can summarize a large amount of tabular data into visual maps that can be very insightful for the planning and evaluation of public programs, and for engaging the attention of policy makers and the non-experts in the process. By adding the "place" to the traditional person/time/place triad underlying public health epidemiology and surveillance, the use of GIS technology can help public health practitioners better appreciate how and where place matters in affecting the public's health in ways that are policy and programmatically relevant. The use of GIS technology can also help enhance the "person" component of the epidemiological triad by providing a method to add measures of socio-economic status, educational attainment, ethnicity, housing quality etc. to health data sets which often contain only very sparse person-level information such as age and gender. The use of GIS technology in public health settings can also facilitate the development of applications for the coordination of emergency response efforts and for strategic placement of health program offices and resources. Overall, GIS is a helpful and efficient tool must be used by public health professionals extensively. In near future with advancement of technology like WebGIS would contribute better to this field for optimal health of the population.

REFERENCES

Alexander, F. E., & Boyle, P. (Eds.). (1996). Methods for investigating localized clustering of disease. IARC Scientific Publications.

Amer, S. (2007). *Towards Spatial Justice in Urban Health Services Planning – A Spatial Analytic GIS based Approach Using Dares Salaam, Tanzania as a Case Study*. The Netherlands: International Institute for Geo-Information Science and Earth.

Barrett, F. A. (2002). The role of French-language contributors to the development of medical geography (1782–1933). *Social Science & Medicine*, *55*(1), 155–165. doi:10.1016/S0277-9536(01)00210-6 PMID:12137184

Bédard, Y., & Henriques, W. (2002). Modern Information Technology in Environmental Health Surveil-lance: Overview and Analysis. *Canadian Journal of Public Health*, *93*, S29–S33. PMID:12425172

Burrough, P. (1986). *Geographic Information Systems for Natural Resources Assessment*. New York: Oxford University Press.

Chae, Y. M., Kim, H. S., Tark, K. C., Park, H. J., & Ho, S. H. (2003). Analysis of healthcare quality indicator using data mining and decision support system. *Expert Systems with Applications*, *2*(24), 167–172. doi:10.1016/S0957-4174(02)00139-2

Christie, S., and Fone, D., (2003). Equity of access to tertiary hospitals in Wales: a travel time analysis. *Journal of Public Health Medicine, 25*(4), 344-350.

Cliff, A., & Haggett, P. (1988). *Atlas of disease distributions: analytic approaches to epidemiological data.* Oxford, UK: Blackwell Reference.

Colantonio, A., Moldofsky, B., Escobar, M., Vernich, L., Chipman, M., McLellan, B. (2011). Using Geographical Information Systems Mapping to Identify Areas Presenting High Risk for Traumatic Brain Injury. *Emerg Themes Epidemiol, 4*(1), 7.

Cooke, G. S., Tanser, F. C., Barnighausen, T. W., & Newell, M. L. (2010). Population uptake of antiretroviral treatment through primary care in rural South Africa. *BMC Public Health, 10*(1), 585. doi:10.1186/1471-2458-10-585 PMID:20920267

Damiani, M., Propper, C., & Dixon, J. (2005). Mapping choice in the NHS: Cross sectional study of routinely collected data. *British Medical Journal, 330*(7486), 284–288. doi:10.1136/bmj.330.7486.284 PMID:15695275

Davenhall, W. F. (2003). *Redefining Quality of Patient Care and Patient Safety using GIS.* Directions Magazine.

Division of Adult and Community Health, National Center for Chronic Disease Prevention and Health Promotion, Centers for Disease Control and Prevention. (n.d.). *Chronic Disease Prevention - The Burden of Chronic Disease and the Future of Public Health, 2005.* Retrieved from http://www.cdc.gov/nccdphp/burden_pres/

Driedger, S. M., Kothari, A., Morrison, J., Sawada, M., Crighton, E., & Graham, I. (2007). Using participatory design to develop (public) health decision support systems within GIS. *International Journal of Health Geographics, 6*(1), 53. doi:10.1186/1476-072X-6-53 PMID:18042298

Ferguson, E. C., Maheswaran, R., & Daly, M. (2004). Road-traffic pollution and asthma – using modeled exposure assessment for routine public health surveillance. *International Journal of Health Geographics, 3*(1), 24. doi:10.1186/1476-072X-3-24 PMID:15485575

Frank, L. D., Andresen, M. A., & Schmid, T. L. (2004). Obesity relationships with community design, physical activity, and time spent in cars. *American Journal of Preventive Medicine, 27*(2), 87–96. doi:10.1016/j.amepre.2004.04.011 PMID:15261894

Frank, L. D., Engelke, P. O., & Schmidt, T. L. (2003). *Health and community design. The impact of the built environment on physical activity*. Washington, DC: Island Press.

Gatrell, A. C., & Löytönen, M. (Eds.). (1998). GIS and Health. Taylor and Francis.

Gerard, R. (1984). Use of Location-Allocation Models for Improving Geographic Accessibility of Rural Services in Developing Countries. *International Regional Science Review*, *9*(3), 217–240. doi:10.1177/016001768400900303

Gesler, W. M., Hayes, M., Arcury, T., Skelly, A. H., Nash, S., & Soward, A. C. M. (2004). Use of mapping technology in health intervention research. *Nursing Outlook*, *52*(3), 142–146. doi:10.1016/j.outlook.2004.01.009 PMID:15197363

GIS Lounge. (2012). Retrieved from http://www.gislounge.com/history-of-gis/

Glass, G. E., Schwartz, B. S., Morgan, J. M. I. III, Johnson, D. T., Noy, P. M., & Israel, E. (1995). Environmental risk factors for Lyme disease identified with geographic information systems. *American Journal of Public Health*, *85*(7), 944–948. doi:10.2105/AJPH.85.7.944 PMID:7604918

Hall, W. (n.d.). *Just another Medical Geography*. Retrieved from http://healthcybermap.org/HGeo/pg1_1.htm

Hart, A., & McCulloch, B. (2004). *Dengue and Data Management. In Empowering Business For Tomorrow*. Brisbane: Spatial Sciences Institute.

Historica Canada. (1965). Retrieved from The Canada Geographic Information System (CGIS): http://www.thecanadianencyclopedia.ca/en/article/geographic-information-systems/

Hjalmars, U., Kulldorff, M., & Gustafsson, G. (1994). Risk of acute childhood leukaemia in Sweden after the Chernobyl reactor accident. *BMJ (Clinical Research Ed.)*, *309*(6948), 154–157. doi:10.1136/bmj.309.6948.154 PMID:8044093

Hjalmars, U., Kulldorff, M., Gustafsson, G., & Nagarwalla, N. (1996). Childhood leukaemia in Sweden: Using GIS and a spatial scan statistic for cluster detection. *Statistics in Medicine*, *15*(7-9), 707–715. doi:10.1002/(SICI)1097-0258(19960415)15:7/9<707::AID-SIM242>3.0.CO;2-4 PMID:9132898

Hjalmars, U., Kulldorff, M., Wahlqvist, Y., & Lannering, B. (1999). Increased incidence rates but no space-time clustering of childhood astrocytoma in Sweden, 1973-1992: A population-based study of pediatric brain tumors. *Cancer*, *85*(9), 2077–2090. doi:10.1002/(SICI)1097-0142(19990501)85:9%3C2077::AID-CNCR27%3E3.0.CO;2-4 PMID:10223251

Huynen, M. M., Martens, P., & Hilderink, H. B. (2005). The health impacts of globalization: A conceptual framework. *Globalization and Health*, *1*(1), 14. doi:10.1186/1744-8603-1-14 PMID:16078989

Jordan, H., Roderick, P., Martin, D., & Barnett, S. (2004). Distance, reality and the need for care: Access to health services in South West England. *International Journal of Health Geographics*, *3*(1), 21. doi:10.1186/1476-072X-3-21 PMID:15456514

Kalogirou, S., & Foley, R. (2006). Health, Place & Hanly: Modelling Accessibility to Hospitals in Ireland. *Irish Geography*, *39*(1), 52–68. doi:10.1080/00750770609555866

Kulldorff, M. (1998). Statistical methods for spatial epidemiology: Tests for randomness. In GIS and Health. Taylor and Francis.

Lang, L. (2000). *GIS for Health Organisations*. ESRI Press.

Latkin, C., Glass, G. E., & Duncan, T. (1998). Using geographic information systems to assess spatial patterns of drug use, selection bias and attrition among a sample of injection drug users. *Drug and Alcohol Dependence*, *50*(2), 167–175. doi:10.1016/S0376-8716(98)00025-8 PMID:9649968

Lin, G., Allen, D., & Penning, M. (2002). Examining distance effects on hospitalizations using GIS: A study of three health regions in British Columbia, Canada. *Environment & Planning A*, *34*(11), 2037–2053. doi:10.1068/a3528

Lovett, A., Haynes, R., Sünnenberg, G., & Gale, S. (2002). Car travel time and accessibility by bus to general practitioner services: A study using patient registers and GIS. *Social Science & Medicine*, *55*(1), 97–111. doi:10.1016/S0277-9536(01)00212-X PMID:12137192

Lovett, A., Poots, A. J., Clements, J. T. C., Green, S. A., Samarasundera, E., & Bell, D. (2014). Using geographical information systems and cartograms as a health service quality improvement tool. *Spatial and Spatio-temporal Epidemiology*, *10*, 67–74. doi:10.1016/j.sste.2014.05.004 PMID:25113592

Mapping the 1854 Broad Street Pump Outbreak. (2003). *John Snow and the Broad Street Pump on the Trial of an Epidemic*. Retrieved from http://www.ph.ucla.edu/epi/snow.html#YOUTH

Martin, D., Wrigley, H., Barnett, S., & Roderick, P. (2002). Increasing the sophistication of access measurement in a rural healthcare study. *Health & Place*, *8*(1), 3–13. doi:10.1016/S1353-8292(01)00031-4 PMID:11852259

McMichael, A. J., & Beaglehole, R. (2000). The changing global context of public health. *Lancet*, *356*(9228), 495–499. doi:10.1016/S0140-6736(00)02564-2 PMID:10981904

Meade, M. S., & Earickson, R. J. (2000). *Medical geography* (2nd ed.). New York: Guilford Press.

Moore, D. A., & Carpenter, T. E. (1999). Spatial analytical methods and geographical information systems: Use in health research and epidemiology [Review]. *Epidemiologic Reviews*, *21*(2), 143–161. doi:10.1093/oxfordjournals.epirev.a017993 PMID:10682254

Nathan, J. (2004). Investigating Access to Reproductive Health Services Using GIS: Proximity to Services and the Use of Modern Contraceptives in Malawi. *African Journal of Reproductive Health*, *8*(2), 164–179. doi:10.2307/3583189 PMID:15623130

Owen, N. (2004). A Spatially-Based Approach to Cancer Prevention: The *PLACE* (Physical Activity in Localities and Community Environments) Study. *4th Annual Queensland Health and Medical Scientific Meeting*. Brisbane Convention and Exhibition Centre.

Phillips, R., Kinman, E., Schnitzer, P., Lindbloom, E., & Ewigman, B. (2000). Using Geographic Information Systems to understand health care access. *Archives of Family Medicine*, *9*(10), 971–978. doi:10.1001/archfami.9.10.971 PMID:11115195

Poulstrup, A., & Hansen, H. L. (2004). Use of GIS and exposure modeling as tools in a study of cancer incidence in a population exposed to airborne dioxin. *Environmental Health Perspectives*, *112*(9), 1032–1036. doi:10.1289/ehp.6739 PMID:15198924

Rahman, S., & Smith, D. K. (2000). Use of location-allocation models in health service development planning in developing nations. *European Journal of Operational Research*, *123*(3), 437–452. doi:10.1016/S0377-2217(99)00289-1

Rigby, J. E., Skelly, C., Tate, N. J., Brabyn, L., King, R., & Borman, B. (2005). Inequalities in geographical access to healthcare services: using GIS to inform policy planning and implementation. *Proceedings of 10th International Symposium on Health Information Management Research*. SEERC.

Robertson, J. G. W., & Wier, K. R. (1998). Using geographical information systems to enhance community-based child welfare services. *Child Maltreatment*, *3*(3), 224235. doi:10.1177/1077559598003003002

Rytkonen, M. J. (2004). Not all maps are equal: GIS and spatial analysis in epidemiology. *International Journal of Circumpolar Health*, *63*(1), 9–24. doi:10.3402/ijch.v63i1.17642 PMID:15139238

Schlundt, D. G., Mushi, C., Larson, C. O., & Marrs, M. (2001). Use of innovative technologies in the evaluation of Nashville''s REACH 2010 community action plan: Reducing disparities in cardiovascular disease and diabetes in the African American community. *The Journal of Ambulatory Care Management*, *24*(3), 51–60. doi:10.1097/00004479-200107000-00009 PMID:11433556

Schuurman, N., Bell, N. J., L'Heureux, R., & Hameed, S. M. (2009). Modelling optimal location for pre-hospital helicopter emergency medical services. *BMC Emergency Medicine*, *9*(6). PMID:19426532

Schuurman, N., Fiedler, R. S., Grzybowski, S. C., & Grund, D. (2006). Defining rational hospital catchments for non-urban areas based on travel-time. *International Journal of Health Geographics*, *5*(43). PMID:17018146

Sheppard, E., McMaster, R., Leitner, H., & Tian, H. (1999). GIS-based Measures of Environmental Equity: Exploring Their Sensitivity and Significance. *Journal of Exposure Analysis and Environmental Epidemiology*, *9*(1), 18–28. doi:10.1038/sj.jea.7500023 PMID:10189624

Simarro, P. P., Cecchi, G., Paone, M., Franco, J. R., Diarra, A., Ruiz, J. A., & Jannin, J. G. et al. (2010). The Atlas of human African trypanosomiasis: A contribution to global mapping of neglected tropical diseases. *International Journal of Health Geographics*, *9*(1), 57. doi:10.1186/1476-072X-9-57 PMID:21040555

Sobal, J. (2001). Commentary: Globalization and the epidemiology of obesity. *International Journal of Epidemiology*, *30*(5), 1136–1137. doi:10.1093/ije/30.5.1136 PMID:11689535

Spencer, J. (2004). Establishment of a national surveillance system to provide early warning of disease outbreaks - Discussion Document. In Commonwealth Department of Health and Ageing. Biosecurity and Disease Control Branch, Population Health Division.

Tanser, F. (2006). Methodology for optimising location of new primary health care facilities in rural communities: A case study in KwaZulu-Natal, South Africa. *Journal of Epidemiology and Community Health*, *60*(10), 846–850. doi:10.1136/jech.2005.043265 PMID:16973529

Taylor, R. (1998). Small Area Epidemiological Analysis. In C. Kerr (Ed.), *Handbook of Public Health Methods* (pp. 627–637). Sydney: McGraw-Hill Book Company Australia Pty Ltd.

Thomas, B., Richards, C., Croner, G., Rushton, C., & Brown, K. (1999). Littleton Fowler. *Public Health Reports (Washington, D.C.)*, *114*(4), 359–373.

Toms, J. (2004). Project Summary - BSS Scoping Study Stakeholder Consultation October/November 2004. In Commonwealth Department of Health and Ageing. Population Health Division, Biosecurity and Disease Control Branch.

Vora, K. S., Yasobant, S., Patel, A., Upadhyay, A., & Mavalankar, D. V. (2015). Has Chiranjeevi Yojana changed the geographic availability of free Comprehensive Emergency Obstetric Care Services in Gujarat, India? *Global Health Action*, *8*(0). doi:10.3402/gha.v8.28977 PMID:26446287

Wen, H. W. (2000). Generalized Linear Models. Department of Statistics, Tunghai University.

Wilkinson, D., & Tanser, F. (1999). GIS/GPS to document increased access to community based treatment for tuberculosis in Africa. Geographic information system/global positioning system. *Lancet*, *354*(9176), 394–395. doi:10.1016/S0140-6736(99)01893-0 PMID:10437874

Yasobant, S., Vora, K. S., Hughes, C., Upadhyay, A., & Mavalankar, D. V. (2015). Geovisualization: A Newer GIS Technology for Implementation Research in Health. *Journal of Geographic Information System*, *7*(01), 20–28. doi:10.4236/jgis.2015.71002

Section 4
Strategy and Policy

Chapter 8
Strategies for Expanding Access and Improving the Quality of Pharmaceutical Services

Marcus Vinícius Dias-Souza
Federal University of Minas Gerais, Brazil

ABSTRACT

Pharmaceutical services are among the most accessible healthcare assistance systems worldwide, being provided generally in enterprises like Drugstores and Compounding Pharmacies. Pharmacists are highly accessible healthcare professionals considering also the availability, geographic distribution and location of pharmaceutical enterprises. However, there are several challenges for providing these services for patients with limitations such as low education, difficulties on reaching the Pharmacist, and the need for individualized monitoring (due to the complexity of therapy). Reports of low quality services are growing worldwide, and in order to expand access and improve the quality of pharmaceutical services, Pharmacists must move from being medication dispensers with focus in administrative management to a clinically-oriented practice with a humanistic view. The aim of this chapter is to make an approach on the implementation of effective strategies and ways to improve the quality of Pharmacists' work as specialized healthcare providers.

DOI: 10.4018/978-1-4666-9961-8.ch008

INTRODUCTION

If Pharmacists do not take their place in science and in professional practice, our future is condemned to be like inflammation and apoptosis. (Personal communication with Professor Flávio Figueiredo, Pharm.D, MSc).

Perception and satisfaction of patients with healthcare services are increasingly being considered important parameters to assess the quality and competence of care providers and the outcomes and impacts of their services in patients' health and in society. The World Health Organization (WHO) defines quality of care as the coverage to which the care provision achieves the most favorable outcomes when balancing risks and benefits in a given financial setting, and because of the worldwide rise in medication use in recent years, this subject has gained more attention among Pharmacists and pharmacy practice research (Schulz et al., 2001; Kheir et al., 2004; Patwardhan et al., 2014; Sakharkar et al., 2015; Shemeikka et al., 2015).

Pharmacy profession has improved to include the provision of services beyond the traditional role of medication dispensing. Pharmacists are highly accessible healthcare professionals considering also the availability, geographic distribution and location of pharmaceutical enterprises like drugstores and compounding pharmacies. Historically, the main role of pharmacy is to dispense medications and provide patients enough instructions regarding their correct use. The Pharmacist is usually the first professional addressed by a patient with minor or complex health issues, commonly due to the scarcity of physicians, or even due to financial barriers to private clinical services when public healthcare services cannot address patients' needs. Conversely, in spite of this context, differently from other health professionals, providing patient care is not an imperative activity for Pharmacists, as several technical fields of the profession (comprising both privative and non-privative activities) do not necessarily involve direct contact with patients (Hepler, 1996; Schulz et al., 2001; Kheir et al., 2004; Wiley et al., 2014; Penm et al., 2015).

The World Health Organization has pointed that more than half of the world population cannot access the medication they demand. Prices are often too high for people or health systems to afford, and therefore, spends on medicines are a major part of the total healthcare budget. Governments must control the cost of drugs through specific policies and make sure that essential medicines are not overpriced. Also, policies for pharmaceutical services must be included, given that the Pharmacists are the most appropriate professionals to provide the correct and safe use of medications, and to analyze, consider and include pharmacoeconomic and pharmacoepidemiological factors in the organization of drug dispensing (Malone et al., 2001; Murray et al., 2009; Penm et al., 2015).

In some countries, in addition to counseling patients on appropriate drug administration, dosage, side effects, storage and interactions, Pharmacists are allowed to prescribe over-the-counter and other types of medications in several countries, such as phytotherapics and homeopathic products, what can help patients to take decisions on self-treatment with medications. This helps to explain in parts why patients often seek advice in pharmacies, and frequently do not consider a physician consultation, which are also, sometimes, not accessible for patients, generally due to the scarcity of professionals. Nevertheless, there are several challenges for providing these services for patients with limitations such as low education, difficulties on reaching the Pharmacist, the need for individualized monitoring (due to the complexity of therapy), and reports of low quality services are growing worldwide. These facts have been requiring Pharmacists to rethink the way in which pharmacy practice is performed (Lewin, 2013; Sakthong et al., 2013; Sakharkar et al., 2015; Fisher et al., 2015; Malewski et al., 2015).

Pharmacy is a very dynamic profession, given that patients' and society needs regarding drug therapy are changing continually. Evidence-based pharmacy practices are the key to provide effective pharmaceutical services and to improve the quality of healthcare as a whole. In this sense, Pharmacists must move from being medication dispensers with focus in administrative and logistics management, to be patient-focused and clinically-oriented care providers, with more responsibility and commitment to improve their technical knowledge, but with a humanistic view of practice. Thus, the aim of this chapter is to discuss the implementation of effective strategies to expand the access of patients to pharmaceutical services focusing in PC, and ways to improve the quality of such services. Data regarding patients' views and satisfaction with Pharmacists' performance as a specialized healthcare provider, and Pharmacists' perception of receptiveness and evolution of patients will be also discussed in light of evidence-based practice (Straus, 2007; Sakharkar et al., 2015; Cho et al., 2015; Malewski et al., 2015).

BACKGROUND

Pharmaceutical Services: In Way of Changes

Pharmaceutical services are generally designed in agreement to medicines policies in order to ensure access, affordability, and delivery of essential medicines to the population. Usually, they comprise medication dispensing, counseling on rational use, and logistic organization of dispensing services accordingly to local epidemiologic data. Strategies for the rational use of medications are than planned to promote safe and cost-effective treatments, considering regulatory and quality standards defined by local laws. Pharmacists should, therefore, develop mechanisms for regular review or new proposals of formularies, guidelines and policies regarding drug dispensing and prescribing; therefore, developing trained human resources for this field is of paramount importance, and efforts have been made in several institutions to provide this improvement in different levels of pharmaceutical education, such as PharmBSc (Bachelor of Science in Pharmacy), PharmMS (Master of Science in Pharmacy) and PharmD (Doctor of Pharmacy) (Vijayanarayana et al., 2014).

Pharmaceutical services are among the most accessible healthcare assistance systems worldwide, being quite often provided without additional charges (beyond medication prices) by Pharmacists in enterprises like Drugstores and Compounding Pharmacies; yet, some of these services can be charged, for instance, pharmaceutical consultations, the time spent in blood pressure measurements or preparation of healing bandages. The published experience on the traditional way that pharmaceutical services are established and offered to the population has shown that they have historically been working relatively well for patients in conditions such as: a) common and controlled acute or chronic diseases, b) use of not many medications (like two or three formulations), c) simple therapeutic schemes, and d) adequate education level to understand pharmaceutical advising on rational use of medications (Straus, 2007; Citrome, 2011; Fisher et al., 2015; Gabr & Shams, 2015).

However, what can Pharmacists do to patients with limitations such as low literacy, difficulties on reaching the Pharmacist, or unusual needs like individualized care and monitoring for complex diseases and/or drug therapies?

The answer is neither simple nor easy, and varied barriers can be mentioned. However, these difficulties can be overcome with adequate strategic planning, training and management. In this chapter, I will present different strategies for improving and expanding pharmaceutical services which have provided encouraging results that strongly indicates their effectiveness in providing pharmaceutical services with equity, justice, and addressing patients' needs.

PHARMACEUTICAL CARE

Overview of the Implementation Process

Since the 1990s, Pharmaceutical Care (PC) has been described as an important service and element of pharmacy practice and healthcare, in which Pharmacists are responsible for the quality. Because of the extension of this subject, the approach of this chapter is limited to demonstrate how PC can influence pharmaceutical services to become more accessible and with a broader coverage of patients.

PC is a pharmaceutical service designed to achieve definitive therapeutics outcomes through preventing or solving drug related problems, and is generally defined as a direct provision of drug related care by the Pharmacist through health education, in order to improve patients' quality of life when using medication. It represents a shift of practice in pharmacy from being drug product-oriented to a patient-oriented view (Hepler & Strand, 1990; Penna, 1990; Cipolle et al., 2004; Dias-Souza & Barros, 2012c). As described by Hepler (1996), PC services comprise:

1. Recognition and correct identification of clinical conditions requiring safe and efficient drug therapy;
2. Prescribing for definite outcomes;
3. Dispensing and patient counseling, involving the patient or family/caregiver in all decisions;
4. Monitoring and management of outcomes;
5. Documentation of all actions.

PC activities also include medication dispensing, providing education on drug use through patient counseling, drug use monitoring, preparation of formulations for parenteral nutrition, monitoring adverse drug reactions, development of drug use guidelines, and cooperation with the healthcare team; these are offered in a mutually beneficial exchange way, in which the patient asks and consents to be supported by the Pharmacist regarding pharmacotherapeutics needs, and the Pharmacist accepts the responsibility to provide drug therapy support with competence and commitment. The Pharmacist provides this service for one patient each time, but groups can also be reached by PC services, in consultations that vary in time and frequency according to the patient's needs (Dias-Souza & Barros, 2012a; Alturkia et al., 2013; Cheng et al., 2015).

The steps of pharmaceutical consultations include (but are not limited to):

1. Collection and organization of patient-specific information (such as demographic data, body mass index and blood pressure);
2. Identification of health problems;
3. Analysis of all the medication being used, in order to identify potential drug-related problems (DRP) like dosage form, therapeutic schemes, administration, and drug-drug and drug-food interactions;
4. Patient counseling on pharmacological and non-pharmacological management of the disease;
5. Monitoring of the desired outcomes through clinical investigations.

These steps will be discussed in the following paragraphs.

In PC services, the Pharmacist work in concert with the patient and other healthcare professionals to promote health, prevent diseases, and to assess, monitor, and when necessary, modify medication use in order to assure that drug therapy regimens are adequate, safe and therefore, effective. PC services should optimize quality of life regarding drug therapy, and achieve positive and definitive clinical outcomes within realistic financial expenditures (Malone et al., 2001; Wait, 2005; Straus, 2007).

The implementation of PC depends essentially on data collection and documentation systems that register patients' information, such as demographic data and clinical history, communications with other professionals like nutritionists, physician in charge, dentist, and also for scientific research purposes, like the study of medication use profile. Moreover, specific equipments are needed to assess drug therapy adherence and effectiveness, and also patient education materials, as described in the previous section. Interactions between the Pharmacist in charge and the patient (and the family and/or caregivers, when necessary) should occur to assure efficient mutual communication and cooperation, and that the decision making process on drug therapy is shared by the Pharmacist and the patient. The Pharmacist uses technical knowledge and skills to optimize drug therapy and the patient agrees to supply personal information and actively participate in the process of PC (Pispati, 2003; Cohen et al., 2009; Schmelz et al., 2010).

Nevertheless, varied barriers have been described for the implementation and success of PC services (Schulz et al., 2001; Lada and Delgado, 2007; Maher et al., 2011; Kaufmann et al., 2015; Kuhmmer et al., 2015; Pauwels et al., 2015; Srivastava & McGuire, 2015), and some of them will be briefly presented:

- **Access to Effective Drug Information Resources:** Some professionals have scarce training in searching for evidence-based data in articles, for example. This can be overcome with specific training in articles search platforms;
- **Access to Full Patient Information:** This happens especially when the Pharmacist is dealing with the caregiver and not directly with the patient, or when the patient has some type of limitation that affects this parameter;
- **PC Courses in Graduate and Undergraduate Curricula:** Many pharmacy faculties still do not give attention to social activities of Pharmacists;
- **Comprehensive Understanding to Care Concepts:** PC is still often regarded as pharmaceutical assistance and vice-versa;
- **Continuity of Quality Improvement:** The lack of interest and motivation for quality improvement is very common when the Pharmacist is not properly valued;
- **Counseling Guideline or Plan for Effective Patient Counseling:** This is a critical point in PC: although patients have different needs, all steps in PC

must be standardized when possible, to guarantee that care will be delivered to all patients in a similar way;

- Disparity of cultures and believes, often affecting the use of medication;
- **Poor Documentation of the Provided Care:** For an effective follow-up, all actions must be registered and properly saved;
- **Fear of Change to New Profession and Poor Education in Communication Skill:** The lack of training in these is the most critical issue regarding human resources in PC. However, it is possible that trainings with strategies like the simulated patient may help to improve this ability;
- Education in skills needed to deal with technology;
- Financial capital to start the service;
- Improper utilization of registration formularies;
- Inadequate private counseling area;
- **Lack of Insurance Assistance:** Most insurance services world-wide do not cover pharmaceutical services at all;
- **Legislation Barriers:** In some countries, pharmacy clinical practice is still poorly regulated, what may cause doubts when implementing PC;
- **Pharmacy Location:** Sometimes, the location makes it difficult for patients to reach the Pharmacist;
- **Professional Resistance to Interactions with the Pharmacist:** Often, some prescribing or care professionals do not interact with the Pharmacist. A good alternative is to try a personal contact and provide scientific literature as an ice breaker;
- **Patient Interest:** Not all patients will be interested in PC. When the patient is adult and in his own, there is not much to do but to show the advantages of PC. When the patients demands family or caregiver support, it is important that the Pharmacist clearly shows how much the service can help the improvement of quality of life, promote financial savings and adequations on the use of medication;
- **Patient Literacy and Socioeconomic Status:** This is also critical for the patient that demands instructions. Memorizing is not always possible because of the load of information. However, some alternatives will be shown further in this chapter;
- **Profession Fees to Reward Care Services:** PC services are charged in some countries. Although it is a fair practice, not all patients with real need of PC services can afford them;
- **Software for Medication Assessment Support:** To avoid handwritten formularies, softwares for registration of the activities are necessary;
- Space and layout within the pharmacy;
- Trained Staff.

Pharmacists must collect subjective and objective information regarding the patient's general health status, past medical history, medication use history, social habits history (like alcohol use, smoking), diet, physical activities routine history, history of the current clinical condition, financial and insurance status, when necessary. To perform this, Pharmacists should ask patients for access to medical prescriptions, charts and reports, and should create health/physical assessment instruments. Some validated instruments have been published elsewhere, and often, adaptations are not required. Furthermore, interviews with family members or the caregiver are important, mainly for pediatric or senior patients. Other healthcare providers including physicians, nurses, and mid-level practitioners should also be contacted when necessary. All this information will form the basis for decisions on the development and modification of therapeutic schemes. Therefore, patient data must be updated, accurate, complete, organized and recorded with operational standard procedures, to assure that they are readily retrievable and recorded confidentially (Stewart et al., 1995; Hepler, 1996; Cipolle et al., 1998; Isetts et al., 2003; Dias-Souza et al., 2012a; Holtzman et al., 2015; Kaló et al., 2015).

Pharmaceutical consultations have professional limitations such as providing diagnosis; however, the experience of patients in pharmaceutical consultations generates opinions and views for both patients and Pharmacists, which are important tolls to evaluate and optimize the quality of services and to assess the need for new services. To perform PC services, Pharmacists must have characteristics like being a caregiver, communicator, decision-maker, teacher, researcher, leader, and manager, in order to offer individualized care to patients (Hepler, 1996; Cipolle et al., 1998). Conversely, the experience reported in the literature describes lack of training in such abilities during academic life (Sakharkar et al., 2015).

All the information is then evaluated and a drug therapy plan is developed with the patient. Based on a thorough understanding of the clinical picture of the patient and the treatment options available and affordable, the Pharmacist plans an outcomes-oriented drug therapy plan. For this, the Pharmacist considers not only clinical aspects of the disease, but also psychological and social consequences, including the complexity of therapy and alternatives to improve patient adherence (Hepler & Strand, 1990; Cipolle et al., 2004; Weiss et al., 2015).

Regarding medication use, the patient should be instructed about side effects, important negative or positive interactions with food and other medication, and eventually, of other therapeutic options and non-pharmacological complementary alternatives. The therapeutic therapy plan must be documented in the patient's pharmacy record and communicated to the patient's other healthcare providers when necessary. The therapeutic plan must be completely explained to the patient, including the responsibilities shared with the Pharmacist. Information should be provided to the patient at a level that the patient will understand; thus, appropriate language should be used, avoiding, for example, detailing drug mechanism of action. At the end of the consultation, the patient must know how to take the medication, why it is being administered, for how long it will last, risks and benefits of the use and what other health-related behaviors can increase quality of life (Seybert et al., 2008; Dias-Souza & Barros, 2012b; Dias-Souza & Barros, 2012c; Ross et al., 2015).

A short guide on how to start a PC consultation will be described as follows, and will be summarized in Figure 1:

Data Collection

An initial interview should be conducted with the patient/family/caregiver for establishing a professional working relationship and to open the patient's record, with confidentiality and privacy. In this first interview, all patient's needs concerning

Figure 1. PC consultation flow summary. Modified from Hepler (1996)

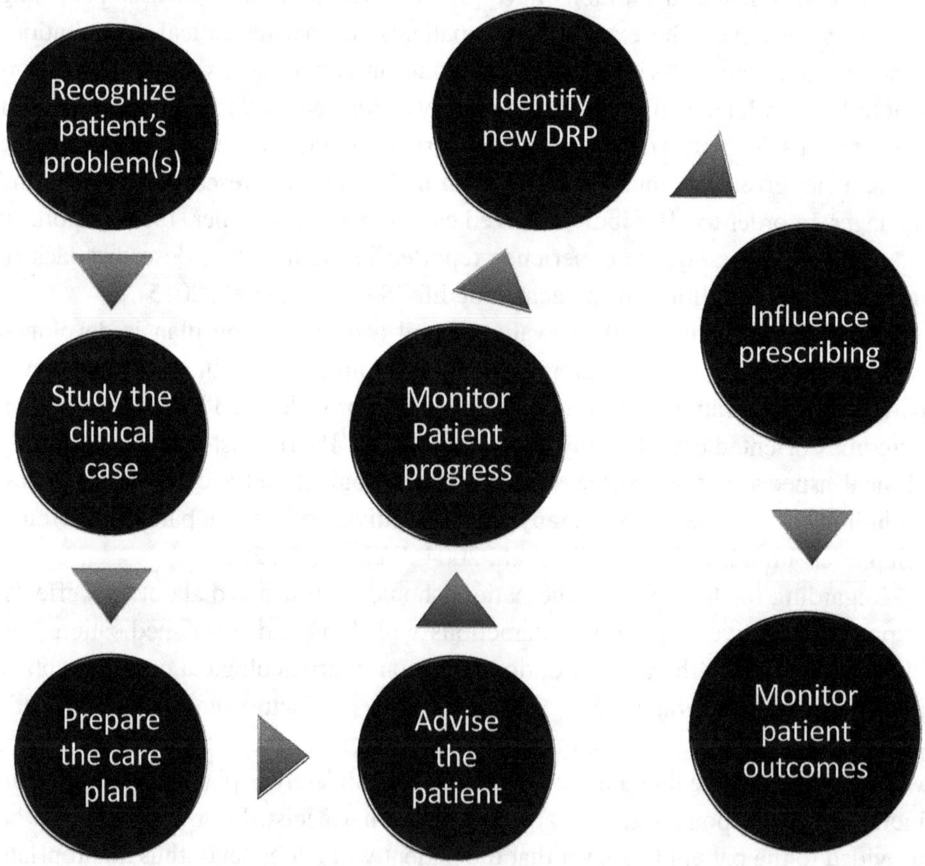

drug therapy should be met, therefore, sufficient time (often 30 to 60 minutes) is spent to assure that questions and answers are provided without embarrassment or hurry. The interviewee should be comfortable with the questions, and for scientific and professional protection of both Pharmacist and patient, a consenting form approved by an Ethics committee should be signed by them (Penna, 1990; Kroenke, 2001; Cadogan & Ryder, 2015).

Standard procedures should be used to systematically record patient-specific subjective information, including health and activity status, past medical history, medication history, social history (including economic situation), family history, and history of present illness. Patients' perceptions, thoughts, beliefs and feelings of the diseases should be included on the formulary. When necessary, physical assessment techniques like blood-pressure monitoring, capillary measurements of lipids and sugars, should be appropriately performed to obtain patient-specific objective information (Toubro et al., 1999; Schwartz et al., 2008; Sancar et al., 2011; Safaeian et al., 2015).

The Pharmacist must guarantee that patients' records are properly organized, kept updated, and with all important points discussed in all consultations.

Evaluation of the Information Obtained at the Interview

After the patient left the consultation office, the Pharmacist begins an evaluation of the subjective and objective information gathered from the patient and 1) investigates what drug-related problems are happening or can happen in the current clinical picture; 2) analyses opportunities for optimizing the safety, effectiveness, and financial aspects of the drug therapy; 3) discuss the conclusions with the patient in the second consultation. The discussions with the patient, as necessary and appropriate, should guarantee an appropriate understanding of the clinical picture, treatment strategies and administration schemes, and what will be necessary to do for an effective management (Hepler, 1996; Cipolle et al., 1998; Cipolle et al., 2004; Cheng et al., 2013; Al-Quteimat & Amer, 2014).

Preparation of the Care Plan

This preparation happens during step b. The Pharmacist identifies, evaluates and then chooses the most appropriate actions to improve and/or assure the safety, effectiveness, and/or cost-effectiveness of current or planned drug therapy, and to minimize the existing or potential drug-related problems. The care plan is prepared according to the desired outcome. The plan may include work with the patient as well as with other health professionals to provide therapy protocol adjustments or to modify prescribed drug therapy, implement clinical monitoring, recommend alterations on diet, add non-prescription medications or non-pharmacological treatments, or recommend a visit to a specific professional (Spencer et al., 2005; Montgomery et al., 2008; Petrillo et al., 2011; Vijayanarayana et al., 2014).

For each identified problem, the Pharmacist should consider each of the patient's needs and determine the desirable and mutually agreed outcome and incorporate these to the care plan. The plan may include specific disease state and drug therapy endpoints and monitoring endpoints. The Pharmacist reviews the plan and desirable outcomes with the patient and with other healthcare professionals when it is necessary (Odedina & Segal, 1996; Campbell & Saulie, 1998).

Implementing the Care Plan

The Pharmacist take the steps necessary to implement the plan, which include contacting other health professionals when necessary for any modifications on drug therapy, counseling the patient and/or the caregiver about the correct use of the medication and all problems associated to the incorrect use, coordinate the acquisition of medications and related supplies and begin the clinical monitoring. The Pharmacist should maximize patients' understanding and involvement in the care plan, guaranteeing that the parameters for drug therapy monitoring like blood pressure, molecular markers, blood glucose and cholesterol testing, are made and understood by the patient, family and the caregiver (Moore, 1998; Spitzer et al., 2001; Diez-Quevedo et al., 2001; Ojasalo, 2001).

The patient should be instructed on how to properly use all medications and related products when necessary. Information should be provided to the patient in an easy way to understand. All this information must be registered in the pharmacy record, as well as the steps taken to implement the plan including the appropriate baseline monitoring parameters (Knapp et al., 2004; Spencer et al., 2005; Austin et al., 2006, Nkansah et al., 2008).

Monitoring Outcomes and Modifying the Care Plan

The Pharmacist should review subjective and objective monitoring parameters in order to determine if the desired outcomes will be achieved as outlined in the drug therapy plan. If any problems are detected, the Pharmacist must make the required modifications with the patient, family and caregiver. As progress towards outcomes is achieved, the Pharmacist should provide positive reinforcement and update the care plan. The Pharmacist uses appropriate professional judgment to assess the need to notify other healthcare professionals involved in the patient's case about the registered evolutions (Classen et al. 2002; Brown et al., 2003; Cranor & Christensen, 2003; Malone et al., 2003; Osterberg & Blaschke, 2005; Scuffham et al., 2008; Fiz et al., 2011)

Establishing evidence-based practice is important for effective, updated and relevant PC services. Furthermore, the implementation of PC is relevant to patients because not only drug therapy will be optimized, but complex pharmacological regimens prescribed may be restructured or simplified by the Pharmacist in order to make it more understandable to the patient. This becomes even more important when we consider that a single patient may visit more than one physician in a given clinical condition and get different prescriptions, and the communication among them about drug prescription is often insufficient. Additionally, medication costs often consume a significant proportion of patients' and public health financial resources, what makes PC services economically relevant. Different pharmacoeconomics analysis described that significant financial savings could be achieved by patients, institutions and health insurances through PC services (Isetts et al., 2003; Kiel & McCord, 2005; Morello et al., 2006; Nkansah et al., 2008; Dias-Souza & Barros, 2012b; Lewin, 2013).

Different methodologies of PC have been used worldwide, and the most explored (and published) will be presented briefly:

A. **PWDT (Pharmacists Workup of Drug Therapy):** In this method, patients are assessed by a single Pharmacist for the all drugs used for any health problems that the patient might be affected by, and the DRP are analyzed for each formulation used. Therefore, if the patient has migraine and diabetes, the same Pharmacist is responsible for optimizing the drug therapy of both diseases (Isetts et al., 2003; Kiel & McCord, 2005).
B. **TOM (Therapeutic Outcomes Monitoring):** In this method, patients are assessed by more than one Pharmacist for the drugs used for each health problem that the patient might be affected by, and the DRP are analyzed for each formulation used. Therefore, if the patient has asthma and arthritis, a specialist Clinical Pharmacist in asthma and another, specialist in arthritis, shall be visited (Dias-Souza & Barros, 2012b; Dias-Souza & Barros, 2012c)
C. **Dáder:** This method was developed by a Spanish group of PC headed by Maria José Fáus-Dáder, and has similarities with PWDT in its organization and coverage of diseases, but DRP are analyzed in a different way. This method is widely used also in Latin America (Amariles et al., 2012).

Other methodologies for PC services include FARM (Findings, Assessment, Resolution and Monitoring), DOT (Direct Observed Treatment), and SOAP (Subject, Objective, Assessment, Planning) (Amariles et al., 2012).

Providing Written Information in PC

A critical point regarding PC is that most of the counseling offered by Pharmacists to patients is provided orally, and hardly ever the patient or the Pharmacists take notes of the information in a standardized and validated way. As a result, patients may misunderstand or forget important details like drug onset of action and side effects, leading to poor compliance problems and negative results. Doubts regarding the need for therapy may arise and complex therapeutic schemes, usually difficult to be managed by patients without professional support, also contributes to poor compliance. The use of written and/or pictorial aids and other educational approaches is still scarce in pharmacy practice, and here, I would like to encourage the reader to explore this resource to improve the access of patients to pharmaceutical services. In this sense, previous works of our group provided evidence of the relevance of written information for patient counseling and education on drug administration (Worley-Louis et al., 2003; Worley et al., 2007; Seybert et al., 2008; Dias-Souza & Andrade, 2010; Dias-Souza & Barros, 2012c, Khan et al., 2013).

A clinical case of chronic pain in an elderly patient had drawn our attention at first: because of the use of several medications, the patient had difficulties in administrating them correctly, and several interactions were detected in the first pharmaceutical consultation. We reorganized the therapeutic scheme and provided handwritten information in a simple and accessible language such that the elderly patient could easily understand. As the clinical monitoring followed, the evolution of the patient was positive and pain was finally under pharmacological control. We recommended physical therapy sections for the patient, and advised for a clinical-functional assessment by a Physiotherapist (Dias-Souza & Andrade, 2010).

Nevertheless, all this was directed for a single patient. How to deal with several people that simultaneously demand specific written information like this patient? And how to do this for so many possible medications – isolated or combined – in compounding pharmacies or drugstores? A possible answer comes in a study developed by our group. The development of drug use instructional cards (DUIC) for different pharmacological groups and its use in compounding pharmacies was described in 2012 for the first time (Dias-Souza & Barros, 2012c).

The DUICs were developed due to a rising demand of basic advising on the correct use of medications on the pharmaceutical setting where the work was developed (a Brazilian compounding pharmacy located at the state of Minas Gerais). Using patients' complaint formularies (PCF) – a document that the good manufacturing practices (GMP) laws from the National Sanitation Regulatory Agency (ANVISA, an agency equivalent to the FDA in the U.S.A.) obligate compounding pharmacies to have in order to register any complaints from patients or clients – we have explored the most frequent drug-related problems to delineate how the DUICs should be designed. The parameters we considered were:

1. Drug-drug interactions
2. Drug-food interactions
3. Correct way and time of administration
4. Storing the dosage form
5. Experienced side effects and potential toxicity

After analyzing these data, we performed an extensive literature review for collecting technical information for correct drug using, regarding:

1. Most common drugs and indication;
2. Pharmacokinetics and metabolism;
3. Drug-drug interactions (obtained at the drug interaction checker in Medscape website);
4. Drug-food interactions;
5. Basic Nutritional Support;
6. Best time of administration;
7. Pregnancy, lactation and fertility impairment warnings;
8. Contraindications;
9. Common Clinical Adverse Reactions.

DUICs were then developed for the following groups:

1. Antihistamines;
2. Antimicrobials;
3. Anti-hypertensives;
4. Anti-lipemics;
5. Proton pump inhibitors
6. Non Steroidal Anti-inflammatory Drugs (NSAID);
7. Psychotropic drugs

After, the design was created and adjusted for the size of the document, such that it could be attached to the medication that was dispensed through the delivery service or at the counter. DUICs samples (in Portuguese) are shown in Figure 2.

We showed through our data that the DUICs not only were effective in counseling patients in a standardized way, but also improved telepharmacy services: the basic instructions provided in the DUICs could be assimilated by non-Pharmacists attendants, and some basic information about drug use could be rapidly provided

Figure 2. DUIC samples (available only in Portuguese) developed by Dias-Souza & Barros (2012c): a) antihistamine drugs; b) NSAID; c) antilipemic drugs; d) antimicrobials. DUICs are still being distributed for patients that are costumers of the compounding pharmacy where the study was conducted

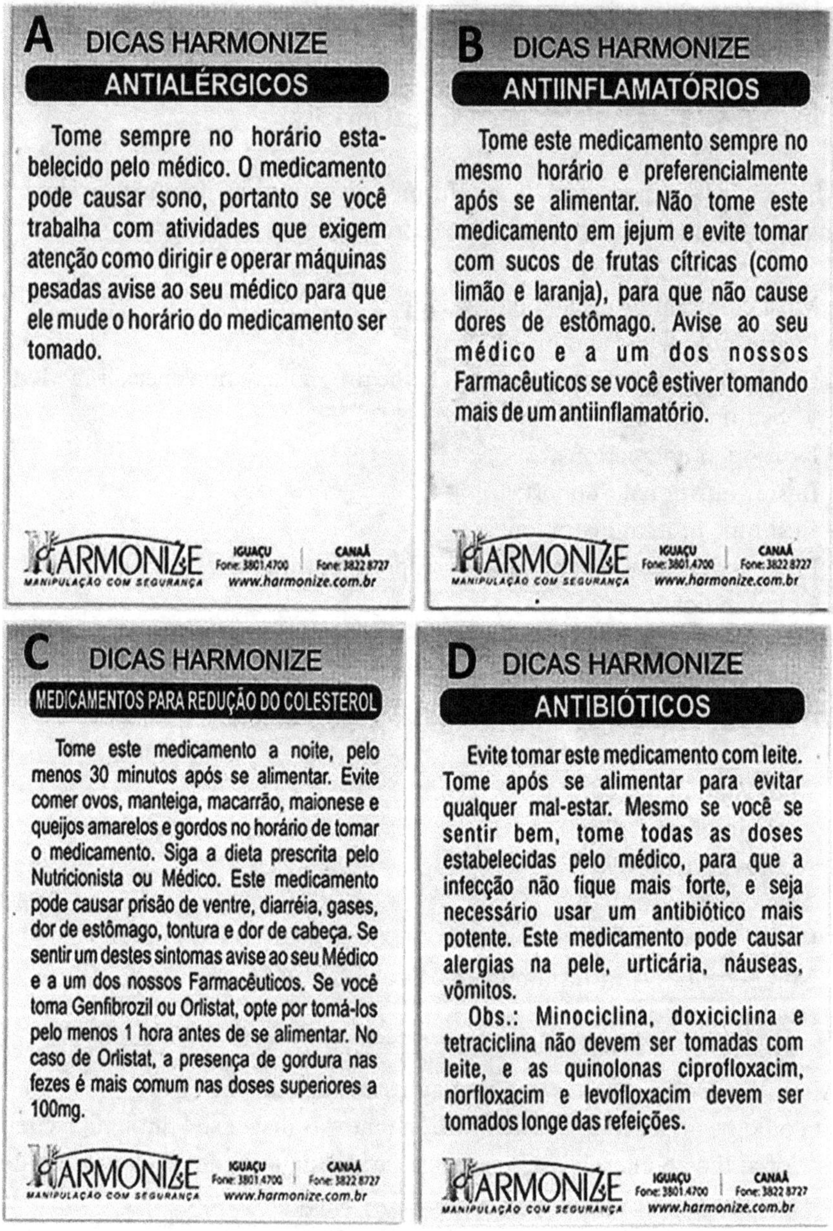

A DICAS HARMONIZE

ANTIALÉRGICOS

Tome sempre no horário estabelecido pelo médico. O medicamento pode causar sono, portanto se você trabalha com atividades que exigem atenção como dirigir e operar máquinas pesadas avise ao seu médico para que ele mude o horário do medicamento ser tomado.

HARMONIZE MANIPULAÇÃO COM SEGURANÇA — IGUAÇU Fone: 3801.4700 | CANAÃ Fone: 3822.8727 — www.harmonize.com.br

B DICAS HARMONIZE

ANTIINFLAMATÓRIOS

Tome este medicamento sempre no mesmo horário e preferencialmente após se alimentar. Não tome este medicamento em jejum e evite tomar com sucos de frutas cítricas (como limão e laranja), para que não cause dores de estômago. Avise ao seu médico e a um dos nossos Farmacêuticos se você estiver tomando mais de um antiinflamatório.

HARMONIZE MANIPULAÇÃO COM SEGURANÇA — IGUAÇU Fone: 3801.4700 | CANAÃ Fone: 3822.8727 — www.harmonize.com.br

C DICAS HARMONIZE

MEDICAMENTOS PARA REDUÇÃO DO COLESTEROL

Tome este medicamento a noite, pelo menos 30 minutos após se alimentar. Evite comer ovos, manteiga, macarrão, maionese e queijos amarelos e gordos no horário de tomar o medicamento. Siga a dieta prescrita pelo Nutricionista ou Médico. Este medicamento pode causar prisão de ventre, diarréia, gases, dor de estômago, tontura e dor de cabeça. Se sentir um destes sintomas avise ao seu Médico e a um dos nossos Farmacêuticos. Se você toma Genfibrozil ou Orlistat, opte por tomá-los pelo menos 1 hora antes de se alimentar. No caso de Orlistat, a presença de gordura nas fezes é mais comum nas doses superiores a 100mg.

HARMONIZE MANIPULAÇÃO COM SEGURANÇA — IGUAÇU Fone: 3801.4700 | CANAÃ Fone: 3822.8727 — www.harmonize.com.br

D DICAS HARMONIZE

ANTIBIÓTICOS

Evite tomar este medicamento com leite. Tome após se alimentar para evitar qualquer mal-estar. Mesmo se você se sentir bem, tome todas as doses estabelecidas pelo médico, para que a infecção não fique mais forte, e seja necessário usar um antibiótico mais potente. Este medicamento pode causar alergias na pele, urticária, náuseas, vômitos.

Obs.: Minociclina, doxiciclina e tetraciclina não devem ser tomadas com leite, e as quinolonas ciprofloxacim, norfloxacim e levofloxacim devem ser tomados longe das refeições.

HARMONIZE MANIPULAÇÃO COM SEGURANÇA — IGUAÇU Fone: 3801.4700 | CANAÃ Fone: 3822.8727 — www.harmonize.com.br

for patients. Although the DUICs were planned (and are still being used) for compounded medication, the same instructional material can be adapted for industrialized medication, for which, information commonly found on package inserts has been described as poorly designed by professionals and not completely understood by patients. Also, patients often describe that written information on prescription drug labels are confusing or incomplete.

To overcome these problems, Kripalani et al. (2007) developed illustrated medication schedules for helping low-literacy patients to administrate medications correctly. The development of the cards design began by raising the needs of the patients through surveying local Pharmacists by telephone and posted emails on national pharmacy list servers, asking about the use of medication aids, visuals, or other patient education tools. Physicians with expertise in medication adherence, patient education, and literacy helped to draft the cards, using pictures to illustrate instructions to follow drug therapy schedules. A multidisciplinary team of healthcare providers then reviewed the content and format of the design draft. Twelve patients of different age and educational attainment reviewed sample pill cards to provide input into the types of pictures used, the size of the text and overall document, and the desired content. The instrument could maximize comprehension across levels of health literacy, providing only the most essential medication instructions like name, purpose, appearance, and time of administration. Patients with inadequate or marginal literacy skills, less than high school education, or cognitive impairment were most likely to refer to the card on a regular basis initially and after 3 months. Patients found it easy to understand and helpful for remembering important medication information, such as the name, purpose, or time of administration.

Kassardjian et al. (2008) validated a Pictorial Representation of Illness and Self Measure (PRISM) as a measure of suffering in patients with chronic non-cancer pain. Patients were recruited from 2 hospital pain clinics, and the majority of them were middle-aged women, in whom chronic pain is more prevalent and also more treated with medication. For that task, patients were shown a letter size white paper with a fixed yellow circle glued in the bottom left-hand corner of the piece of paper. Then, they were asked to imagine that the paper represented his/her life and that the yellow disk represented his/her concept of self. They were given a red paper disk representing their pain and asked to glue it in a location related to the "self" disk, reflecting the impact of pain into their lives. The same request was made regarding work, family, spouse/partner and recreation. Patients glued the disks onto the page in whatever order they wanted. Blind patients also completed the task, indicating that it also behaved as a tactile tool. Eight main parameters were assessed: Physical functioning, role-physical, bodily pain, general health, vitality, social functioning, role-emotional, and mental health. Higher scores in a scale of 0–100 indicated better health-related quality of life. Different situations were identified using this PRISM system: Patients reported that their close relatives were a negative influence to the treatment because they were overly controlling, or did not believe in the state of disability due to pain. Patients with high scores felt controlled by partners or family members, or emotionally distant from them. It was also reported by group of patients that their partner and family have either very little influence over their lives, or a significant negative influence. Patients found PRISM thought-provoking, and it was described by the authors as a quick, simple, and manageable tool for patients with chronic pain to complete.

A randomized blind trial comparing picture-based versus prose-based information pamphlets was conducted by Thompson et al. (2010). The authors compared memory, comprehension, and preference for medication information presented in a prose-based medication information pamphlet versus a pictorial-based information pamphlet. Specific information regarding methotrexate was used in this study. A total of 100 participants aged 18–65 years of age, who had not completed high school, could read English, and had no prior knowledge about methotrexate were included. The (better) effects of pamphlet type were assessed using immediate free recall, cued recall and comprehension. In the end, each participant was shown a card displaying both the picture and prose-based pamphlets and asked to decide which pamphlet they felt to be most visually appealing, which they would rather receive, which looked more useful, and which was easier to read. According to the statistical analysis, no differences were detected between picture and prose pamphlets in free recall, cued recall, and comprehension either immediately or after a 1-week interval, and the pictorial pamphlet was preferred over the prose-based pamphlet.

Mohan et al. (2013) conducted research with focus groups and interviews with Latino patients with diabetes at two safety net clinics in the USA to understand medication taking practices and perceptions of illustrated medication instructions. They explored PictureRx™, a software platform that generates illustrated, patient-centered medication lists in a daily medication schedule. The following essential information for patients is included: name, dose, frequency, purpose, and special instructions when needed. The design of PictureRx cards (Fig 3) was evidence-based, drawing on research and best practices for the creation of patient education materials with illustrations for medication instructions and other health-related information. Patients reported confidence in being able to take medications and expressed preference for illustrated medication instructions, which could overcome patients' difficulties on administrating the medication.

Pictorial representations of clinical scenarios for asthmatic patients and of commonly used inhalers devices were developed by Roberts et al. (2010). Initial images were developed, designed and reviewed in consultation with medical and nursing respiratory members of staff before testing it with patients. A computerized software package was developed for the preparation of personalized asthma action

Figure 3. Adapted schematic sample of how the charts for drug information are disposed on the works developed by Kripalani et al. (2007) and Mohan et al (2013)

Drug Name	Use	How to take	Morning	Afternoon	Night
Sinvastatin 10 mg	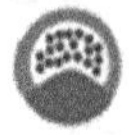 Lipid metabolism	1 tablet at night	X	X	✓
Atenolol 100 mg	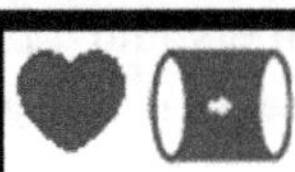 Blood pressure	1 tablet at morning	✓	X	X

plans during a consultation: the health professional should select the options according to the patient's needs. Following a series of sequential screens, the professional identifies appropriate images and scenarios to build a plan. In the end, a pictorial action plan is generated, which should be printed and provided to the patient. The software package automatically checks dosages used, and maximizes inhaled therapy. When the patient uses peak flow for self-monitoring, the program calculates the personalized action levels based upon the reported best peak flow. Users can print out a picture only plan, a words only version or a plan containing pictures and words. According to the authors, the pictorial care plans are quickly prepared to be printed for the patient to take away in several formats, and the data can be stored in the patient's record.

A recent work evaluated the efficacy of a pictorial medication sheet to improve adherence in patients with heart failure and cognitive impairment (Hawkins & Firek, 2014). A total of 36 patients were enrolled. Four study visits spread over approximately four months were performed. At visit one, subjects were asked to bring in all of their regularly prescribed medication for a direct count of administered tablets. After 30 days, in visit two, another tablet count was performed, and adherence was estimated. The subject then received a customized pictorial medication sheet with brief instruction on how to use the pictorial medication sheet that represented their actual prescribed medication regimen. Subjects were asked to use the new sheet in place of any prior medication instruction sheet they may have been using. The medication sheet included of images of the subject's current medications printed in full color and dose range, arranged in columns for morning, noon, and evening administrations. Descriptions of the medication name, indication and dose were also included. Authors reported that although medication adherence was poor, statistically significant improvements (described in tablets counting) were detected after the interventions.

Nevertheless, written information must be used properly, and should be used regardless of problems not related to the patient. A negative example in this sense was described. Hamrosi et al. (2013) examined and compared the use and provision of written medicine information in Australia, focusing in Consumer Medicine Information (CMI) - available for medicines as package inserts, computer prints, or leaflets - by Pharmacists and consumers. The reasons surrounding readership and provision of the CMI and comparisons on its use by both consumers and pharmacists were also investigated. A total of 1000 consumers and 1100 Pharmacists were interviewed by postal or telephone surveys. The authors found that 66% of consumers usually read the CMI looking for information regarding side effects and clinical use of the medication. Reasons mentioned for not reading the CMI comprised previous experience with the medications, enough information was provided verbally from the Pharmacist, and also that the document was too long or contained too much information. Interestingly, the disparity detected by the authors amongst the types of written medicine received by patients and provided by pharmacists is strongly suggestive of incomplete/inadequate (or both) provision of pharmaceutical services. Almost 90% of pharmacists reported providing package inserts, but 88% of consumers reported receiving them when provided with written medicine information. Personalized computer-generated CMI was provided by 99% of pharmacists, but only 37% of consumers reported receiving it. Around 40% of pharmacists and 25% of GPs (n = 45) also reported providing loose leaflets/brochures yet only 7% (n = 47) of consumers reported receipt.

Telepharmacy Services

In this section, I would like to introduce the need and the context of telepharmacy services, a powerful tool for expanding pharmaceutical services when used correctly. According to the World Health Organization (WHO, 2010), telemedicine is defined as the delivery of healthcare services, where distance is a critical factor using information and communication technologies for the exchange of information for diagnosis, treatment and prevention of diseases, research and for the continuing education of healthcare providers, all in the interests of advancing the health of individuals and their communities. Telepharmacy, following the example of telemedicine, offers pharmaceutical services at a distance, i.e., with the Pharmacist and patient communicating through telephone, videoconferencing systems such as Skype®, or any online communication system such as WhatsApp® and social networks. Online chat services available at the website of the pharmacy are also a good alternative.

And why this is important? Telepharmacy technologies can improve patient access to pharmaceutical services beyond remote medication dispensing, including PC. This sort of communication is especially important when the patient cannot reach the Pharmacist due to several possible limitations like mobility issues (the patient does not have access to a vehicle), or if the patient is affected by a disease that impairs the patient to meet the Pharmacist (Garrelts et al., 2010).

Nevertheless, to use this sort of service, a Pharmacist must work exclusively on it, and must have trained people on using the system for technical support or as workmates, to make the service work in a normal flow. In this service, patients can be advised about any aspects of the medication. Also, as some are not comfortable on going to the pharmacy for several reasons (embarrassment on talking to the Pharmacist face-to-face about the health problem, embarrassment on talking about it in public), the service may make the patient more comfortable on talking to the Pharmacist through typing or by phone.

Bynum et al. (2001) assessed the effect of telepharmacy counseling and using interactive compressed video, on how to use the asthma inhaler and patient satisfaction among adolescents with asthma. The telepharmacy service provided accessible education regarding asthma inhaler techniques for adolescents.

Moser et al. (2004) found 4136 documents using the search term "telemedicine" in MEDLINE from 1964 to 2003. They reported significant correlations between publications per million inhabitants and GDP per capita. Fatehi and Wootton (2012) examined the occurrence of the terms "telemedicine", "telehealth", and "e-health" in the Scopus database and a total of 11.642 documents were found in 2012. They found that "telemedicine" was the most common term with 8.028 documents.

Stubbings et al. (2005) described a telepharmacy call center service that was developed at a multidisciplinary health service through collaboration among the health professionals and the health plan to care for patients with medication-related questions. Pharmacists work close to physicians, nurses, and service associates of the call center. The team answered approximately 1.200 calls daily, regarding their transition into the health insurance plan and drug therapy questions. The service improved the quality and cost-effectiveness of drug therapy regimens and significant cost savings were registered.

The group of Lam et al. (2009) reported telepharmacy-related services and outcomes in western Washington State (USA) from 2007 to 2008. Five network clinics without in-house pharmacies were remotely connected to a central pharmacy to provide telepharmacy services, and automated drug dispensing system (ADDS) units, webcams, and electronic medical charts were used to provide remote medication order processing/dispensing, patient counseling, refill authorizations, and medication assistance referral services. Patient demographics, numbers of dispensed medications, patient consultations, and refill authorizations were registered, and service referrals, Pharmacist feedback and workflow changes as well. Antimicrobial drugs were the most frequently dispensed medication, and Pharmacists described webcam-enabled interviews as an excellent method for better privacy and longer counseling.

Garrelts et al. (2010) implemented a telepharmacy service at five hospitals from a Catholic, nonprofit, integrated delivery network health system. Telepharmacy services were provided by a team of Pharmacists employed by the health system. Using a virtual private network or terminal server, Pharmacists directly accessed hospital servers and information systems to conduct their work. The time spent in routine orders of medication reduced significantly after telepharmacy services were implemented. The number of clinical interventions documented increased and annual savings reached 1 million dollars.

Sankaranarayanan et al. (2014) documented remote Pharmacist interventions for patients at eight rural hospitals in the Midwestern United States during prospective prescription order review/entry from 2008 to 2011. Remote Pharmacists' interventions were divided in three broader-level definitions: (a) interventions in interactions and potential interactions, contraindications, adverse effects, drug product selection, drug regimen and recommendations, (b) patient medication management regarding therapy review and action, and (c) health system-centered medication use process, regarding medication prescribing, transcribing and documenting, administering, and monitoring clinical results. Frequencies of intervention levels were compared by year, hospital, remote Pharmacist, and hospital pharmacy status. Frequency of interventions significantly increased each year, and differed significantly across the hospitals, suggesting that patients' needs were addressed particularly.

Service Quality Perspectives

The quality of healthcare services, included the ones provided by Pharmacists, is a topic of intense discussion. The aim of this section is to briefly present important aspects of the services that should be focused such that patients' perspectives are built on positive experiences.

As mentioned, Pharmacists are key professionals to improve medication compliance among users, given their availability of contact with patients, specific knowledge and skills. The burden of several diseases can be reduced through improving medication compliance, and the implementation of clinical pharmaceutical services has positive impacts on patient care, satisfaction and perspectives on these services. Patients' perceived quality of interaction with the Pharmacist, service facilities and outcomes have a significant effect on a patient's choice to use the medication or not (Khan et al., 2013; Al-Quteimat et al., 2014; Fisher et al., 2015).

Managing quality is clearly not a simple task, given that not only technical and regulatory points of clinical services are involved, but values, knowledge and behavior of the Pharmacists regarding patient care are included. Although there is some agreement on how Pharmacists can manage patients' therapy-related needs, there is less agreement on whether the pharmacists are able to meet those needs. Services are generally designed to be broad enough to meet several clinical needs of patients - such as the so called cognitive services (characterized by direct interaction between patient and pharmacist, making use of the pharmacist's knowledge), however, due to the exposed reasons, patients' perspectives of the services are variable. Also, standards to evaluate services vary among patients, once previous experiences are the starting point. All this data, however, is essential for understanding patients' interaction, satisfaction and trust in the Pharmacist (Cho et al., 2015; Malewski et al., 2015; Gabr & Shams, 2015).

Understanding the intricate communication between these features helps us to improve the quality of services. Clinical effectiveness, safety, positive outcomes, patient experiences (self-rated health), proximity, availability and access are the main items to build patients perspectives of the services. However, the pressures for the development of adequate and efficient services can sometimes present divergent logics considering the economic aspects of an enterprise. This technical difficulty should be overcome and negotiated in a way that economic needs of productivity are in line with professional and patients' values regarding high quality health services. This is not a simple endeavor, but in a middle-term perspective, these actions support the growth of the enterprise, as more people tend to look for the service after patients spread the word about the experiences with the service (Dias-Souza & Barros, 2012a; Kaufmann et al., 2015; Kuhmmer et al., 2015).

When patients are engaged in the development of services, it is more likely that they will use these services more frequently (whenever it is necessary) and will be more compliant to recommended treatment plans, leading to the expected health outcomes. The existence of high quality patient-centered services based on reliable and safe patient-Pharmacists relationships, the convenience and ease of access to services and the responsiveness to their therapeutic needs - and when adequate, the quick and safe provision of medication supply, are elements of paramount importance for patients' compliance and development of positive perspectives. These are also important requirements of the patient and caregivers as clients of the pharmaceutical enterprise, especially if the clinical services are charged. Young, highly educated consumers and recently diagnosed patients tend to consider these items with even more importance (Ross et al., 2015; Safaeian et al., 2015).

CONCLUSION

Strategies on expanding and improving pharmaceutical services have been presented in opportunities that are still poorly explored in daily practice: the provision of written information for patients and telepharmacy services. Written information may help patients to remember and reinforce how medication should be correctly taken, and in case of low literacy, alternatives of pictorial support were discussed. Telepharmacy services may help patients and health professionals to quickly reach the Pharmacist and solve drug-related problems, especially when there mobility issues. The implementation of these services in PC context is not a simple endeavor; however, to overcome the technical difficulties, the Pharmacist must work together with patients, families and caregivers, generating solid services, and along with other health professionals. This team work is the key for improving and expanding pharmaceutical services.

ACKNOWLEDGMENT

The author is thankful to GPqFAR (*Integrated Pharmacology and Drug Interactions Research group*) scientists and students, for the outstanding work developed so far. MVDS is head of GPqFAR and is currently at the Federal University of Minas Gerais, Brazil; his research is supported by grants from Fundação de Amparo à Pesquisa do Estado de Minas Gerais (FAPEMIG).

REFERENCES

Abdel-Tawab, R., James, D. H., Fichtinger, A., Clatworthy, J., Horne, R., & Davies, G. (2011). Development and validation of the Medication-Related Consultation Framework (MRCF). *Patient Education and Counseling*, *83*(3), 451–457. doi:10.1016/j.pec.2011.05.005 PMID:21621944

Al-Quteimat, O. M., & Amer, A. M. (2014). Evidence-based pharmaceutical care: The next chapter in pharmacy practice. *Saudi Pharmaceutical Journal*. doi:10.1016/j.jsps.2014.07.010

Alturkia, M., & Khanb, T. M. (2013). A study investigating the level of satisfaction with the health services provided by the Pharmacist at ENT hospital, Eastern Region Alahsah, Kingdom of Saudi Arabia. *Saudi Pharmaceutical Journal*, *21*(3), 255–260. doi:10.1016/j.jsps.2012.09.001 PMID:23960841

Amariles, P., Sabater-Hernández, D., García-Jiménez, E., Rodríguez-Chamorro, M. Á., Prats-Más, R., Marín-Magán, F., & Faus, M. J. et al. (2012). Effectiveness of Dader Method for pharmaceutical care on control of blood pressure and total cholesterol in outpatients with cardiovascular disease or cardiovascular risk: EMDADER-CV randomized controlled trial. *Journal of Managed Care Pharmacy*, *18*(4), 311–323. doi:10.18553/jmcp.2012.18.4.311 PMID:22548691

Austin, Z., Gregory, P. A., & Martin, J. C. (2006). Characterizing the professional relationships of community Pharmacists. *Research in Social & Administrative Pharmacy*, *2*(4), 533–546. doi:10.1016/j.sapharm.2006.02.007 PMID:17161810

Cadogan, C. A., & Ryder, S. A. (2015). Community Pharmacists' role in benzodiazepine supply in Ireland: A questionnaire of Pharmacists' views and experiences. *International Journal of Pharmacy Practice*, *23*(6), 415–422. doi:10.1111/ijpp.12182 PMID:25756294

Campbell, R. K., & Saulie, B. A. (1998). Providing pharmaceutical care in a physician office. *Journal of the American Pharmacists Association*, *38*, 495–499. PMID:9707960

Cheng, Y., Raisch, D. W., Borrego, M. E., & Gupchup, G. V. (2013). Economic, clinical, and humanistic outcomes (ECHOs) of pharmaceutical care services for minority patients: A literature review. *Research in Social & Administrative Pharmacy*, *9*(3), 311–329. doi:10.1016/j.sapharm.2012.05.004 PMID:22835704

Cheng, Y., Raisch, D. W., Borrego, M. E., & Gupchup, G. V. (2015). Development of Patient-Reported Outcomes Measure of Pharmaceutical Therapy for Quality of Life (PROMPT-QoL): A novel instrument for medication management. *Research in Social & Administrative Pharmacy*, *11*(3), 315–338. doi:10.1016/j.sapharm.2014.10.002 PMID:25453539

Cho, M. H., Yoo, K. B., Lee, H. I., Lee, K.-S., Kwon, J. A., Han, K.-T., & Park, E.-C. et al. (2015). The effect of new drug pricing systems and new reimbursement guidelines on pharmaceutical expenditures and prescribing behavior among hypertensive patients in Korea. *Health Policy (Amsterdam)*, *119*(5), 604–611. doi:10.1016/j.healthpol.2015.01.002 PMID:25630635

Chumney, E. C., & Robinson, L. C. (2006). The effects of Pharmacist interventions on patients with polypharmacy. *Pharmacy Practice*, *4*, 103–109. PMID:25247007

Cipolle, R. J., Strand, L. M., & Morley, P. C. (1998). *Pharmaceutical Care Practice*. New York: McGraw-Hill.

Cipolle, R. J., Strand, L. M., & Morley, P. C. (2004). *Pharmaceutical Care Practice: the Clinicians Guide*. New York: McGraw-Hill.

Citrome, L. (2011). Evidence-based medicine: It's not just about the evidence. *International Journal of Clinical Practice*, *65*(6), 633–635. doi:10.1111/j.1742-1241.2011.02669.x PMID:21564431

Classen, D. C. M., Lloyd, R. C. P., Provost, L. P., Griffin, F. A. R., & Resar, R. M. (2008). Development and Evaluation of the Institute for Healthcare Improvement Global Trigger Tool. *Journal of Patient Safety*, *4*(3), 169–177. doi:10.1097/PTS.0b013e318183a475

Cohen, V., Jellinek, S. P., Hatch, A., & Motov, S. (2009). Effect of clinical Pharmacists on care in the emergency department: A systematic review. *American Journal of Health-System Pharmacy*, *66*(15), 1353–1361. doi:10.2146/ajhp080304 PMID:19635771

Cranor, C. W., & Christensen, D. B. (2003). The Asheville Project: Short-term outcomes of a community pharmacy diabetes care program. *Journal of the American Pharmacists Association*, *43*(2), 149–159. doi:10.1331/108658003321480696 PMID:23945854

Dias-Souza, M. V., & Barros, G. C. (2012). Development of Drug Use Instructional Cards for Compounded Formulations as a Complementary Patient Education Tool. *Brazilian Journal of Hosptal Pharmacy and Health Services*, *3*, 6–9.

Dias-Souza, M. V., & Barros, G. C. (2012a). Pharmaceutical Care and Clinical Monitoring of the Allergic Patient: A Case Report. *Brazilian Journal of Hospital Pharmacy and Health Services*, *3*, 338–341.

Dias-Souza, M. V., & Barros, P. H. (2012b). For a Paperless Pharmaceutical Practice: Development and Implementation of FEEDPHARMA System. *Brazilian Journal of Hospital Pharmacy and Health Services*, *3*, 20–22.

Diez-Quevedo, C., Rangil, T., Sanchez-Planell, L., Kroenke, K., & Spitzer, R. L. (2001). Validation and utility of the patient health questionnaire in diagnosing mental disorders in 1003 general hospital Spanish inpatients. *Psychosomatic Medicine*, *63*(4), 679–686. doi:10.1097/00006842-200107000-00021 PMID:11485122

Dowse, R., Ramela, T., & Browne, S. H. (2011). An illustrated leaflet containing antiretroviral information targeted for low-literate readers: Development and evaluation. *Patient Education and Counseling*, *85*(3), 508–515. doi:10.1016/j.pec.2011.01.013 PMID:21306856

Fakhran, S., Alhilali, L., Kale, H., & Kanal, E. (2015). Assessment of rates of acute adverse reactions to gadobenate dimeglumine: Review of more than 130,000 administrations in 7.5 years. *AJR. American Journal of Roentgenology*, *204*(4), 703–706. doi:10.2214/AJR.14.13430 PMID:25794059

Fisher, J. A., Cottingham, M. D., & Kalbaugh, C. A. (2015). Peering into the pharmaceutical "pipeline": Investigational drugs, clinical trials, and industry priorities. *Social Science & Medicine*, *131*, 322–330. doi:10.1016/j.socscimed.2014.08.023 PMID:25159693

Fiz, J., Duran, M., Capella, D., Carbonell, J., & Farre, M. (2011). *Cannabis* Use in Patients with Fibromyalgia: Effect on Symptoms Relief and Health-Related Quality of Life. *PLoS ONE*, *6*(4), e18440. doi:10.1371/journal.pone.0018440 PMID:21533029

Gabr, W. M., & Shams, M. E. E. (2015). Adherence to medication among outpatient adolescents with epilepsy. *Saudi Pharmaceutical Journal*, *23*(1), 33–40. doi:10.1016/j.jsps.2014.05.003 PMID:25685041

Garrett, D. G., & Bluml, B. M. (2005). Patient self-management program for diabetes: First-year clinical, humanistic, and economic outcomes. *Journal of the American Pharmacists Association*, *45*(2), 130–137. doi:10.1331/1544345053623492 PMID:15868754

Gourley, G. A., Portner, T. S., Gourley, D. R., Rigolosi, E. L., Holt, J. M., & Solomon, D. K. (1998). Humanistic outcomes in the hypertension and COPD arms of a multicenter outcomes study. *Journal of the American Pharmacists Association*, *38*, 586–597. PMID:9782692

Gourley, G. K., Gourley, D. R., Rigolosi, E., Reed, P., Solomon, D. K., & Washington, E. (2001). Development and validation of the pharmaceutical care satisfaction questionnaire. *The American Journal of Managed Care*, *7*, 461–466. PMID:11388126

Hamrosi, K. K., Raynor, D. K., & Aslani, P. (2014). Pharmacist, general practitioner and consumer use of written medicine information in Australia: Are they on the same page? *Research in Social & Administrative Pharmacy*, *10*(4), 656–668. doi:10.1016/j.sapharm.2013.10.002 PMID:24239213

Hawkins, L. A., & Firek, C. J. (2014). Testing a novel pictorial medication sheet to improve adherence in veterans with heart failure and cognitive impairment. *Heart & Lung: The Journal of Acute and Critical Care*, *43*(6), 486–493. doi:10.1016/j.hrtlng.2014.05.003 PMID:24928185

Hepler, C. D. (1996). Pharmaceutical Care. *Pharmacy World & Science*, *18*(6), 233–236. doi:10.1007/BF00735965 PMID:9010887

Hepler, C. D., & Strand, L. M. (1990). Opportunities and responsibilities in pharmaceutical care. *American Journal of Hospital Pharmacy*, *47*, 533–543. PMID:2316538

Holtzman, C. W., Brady, K. A., & Yehia, B. R. (2015). Retention in Care and Medication Adherence: Current Challenges to Antiretroviral Therapy Success. *Drugs*, *75*(5), 445–454. doi:10.1007/s40265-015-0373-2 PMID:25792300

Isetts, B. J., Brown, L. M., Schondelmeyer, S. W., & Lenarz, L. A. (2003). Quality Assessment of a Collaborative Approach for Decreasing Drug-Related Morbidity and Achieving Therapeutic Goals. *Archives of Internal Medicine*, *163*(15), 1813–1820. doi:10.1001/archinte.163.15.1813 PMID:12912717

Kaló, Z., Holtorf, A. P., Alfonso-Cristancho, R., Shen, J., Ágh, T., Inotai, A., & Brixner, D. (2015). Need for multicriteria evaluation of generic drug policies. *Value in Health*, *18*(2), 346–351. doi:10.1016/j.jval.2014.12.012 PMID:25773570

Kassardjian, C. D., Gardner-Nix, J., Dupak, K., Barbati, J., & Lam-McCullock, J. (2008). Validating PRISM (Pictorial Representation of Illness and Self Measure) as a Measure of Suffering in Chronic Non-Cancer Pain Patients. *The Journal of Pain*, *9*(12), 1135–1143. doi:10.1016/j.jpain.2008.06.016 PMID:18755635

Kaufmann, C. P., Stämpfli, D., Hersberger, K. E., & Lampert, M. L. (2015). Determination of risk factors for drug-related problems: A multidisciplinary triangulation process. *BMJ Open*, *5*(3), e006376. doi:10.1136/bmjopen-2014-006376 PMID:25795686

Khan, M. U., Khan, A. N., Ahmed, F. R., Feroz, Z., Rizvi, S. A., Shah, S., & Adil, Z. et al. (2013). Patients' opinion of Pharmacists and their roles in healthcare system in Pakistan. *Journal of Young Pharmacists*, *5*(3), 90–94. doi:10.1016/j.jyp.2013.08.001 PMID:24396248

Kheir, N. M., van Mil, J. W. F., Shaw, J. P., & Sheridan, J. L. (2004). Health-related quality of life measurement in pharmaceutical care - Targeting an outcome that matters. *Pharmacy World & Science*, *26*(3), 125–128. doi:10.1023/B:PHAR.0000026811.37414.4f PMID:15230357

Kiel, P. J., & McCord, A. D. (2005). Pharmacist impact on clinical outcomes in a diabetes disease management program via collaborative practice. *The Annals of Pharmacotherapy*, *39*(11), 1828–1832. doi:10.1345/aph.1G356 PMID:16219894

Kitano, H. (2004). Biological robustness. *Nature Reviews. Genetics*, *5*(11), 826–837. doi:10.1038/nrg1471 PMID:15520792

Kitano, H. (2007). Innovation: A robustness-based approach to systems-oriented drug design. *Nature Reviews. Drug Discovery*, *4*(3), 202–210. doi:10.1038/nrd2195 PMID:17318209

Knapp, K. K., Okamoto, M. P., & Black, B. L. (2005). ASHP survey of ambulatory care pharmacy practice in health systems – 2004. *American Journal of Health-Systems Pharmacists*, *62*, 274–284. PMID:15719585

Kripalani, S., Robertson, R., Love-Ghaffari, M., Henderson, L. E., Praska, J., Strawder, A., & Jacobson, T. A. et al. (2007). Development of an illustrated medication schedule as a low-literacy patient education tool. *Patient Education and Counseling*, *66*(3), 368–377. doi:10.1016/j.pec.2007.01.020 PMID:17344015

Kroenke, K., Spitzer, R. L., & Williams, J. B. (2001). The PHQ-9: Validity of a brief depression severity measure. *Journal of General Internal Medicine*, *16*(9), 606–613. doi:10.1046/j.1525-1497.2001.016009606.x PMID:11556941

Kuhmmer, R., Lima, K. M., Ribeiro, R. A., Hammes, L. S., Bastos, G., & Cotta de Souza, M. et al. (2015). Effectiveness of pharmaceutical care at discharge in the emergency department: Study protocol of a randomized controlled trial. *Trials*, *16*(1), 579. doi:10.1186/s13063-015-0579-3 PMID:25888343

Lada, P., & Delgado, G. (2007). Documentation of Pharmacists' interventions in an emergency department and associated cost avoidance. *American Journal of Health-System Pharmacy*, *64*(1), 63–68. doi:10.2146/ajhp050213 PMID:17189582

Lewin, B. (2013). Patient satisfaction with physician responses during interactions prompted by pharmaceutical advertisements. *The Social Science Journal*, *50*(4), 491–500. doi:10.1016/j.soscij.2013.03.002

Maher, A. R., Maglione, M., Bagley, S., Suttorp, M., Hu, J.-H., Ewing, B., & Shekelle, P. G. et al. (2011). Efficacy and comparative effectiveness of atypical antipsychotic medications for off-label uses in adults: A systematic review and metaanalysis. *Journal of the American Medical Association*, *306*(12), 1359–1369. doi:10.1001/jama.2011.1360 PMID:21954480

Malewski, D. F., Ream, A., & Gaither, C. A. (2015). Patient satisfaction with community pharmacy: Comparing urban and suburban chain-pharmacy populations. *Research in Social & Administrative Pharmacy*, *11*(1), 121–128. doi:10.1016/j.sapharm.2014.05.001 PMID:24933533

Malone, D. C., Carter, B. L., Billups, S. E., Valuck, R. J., Barnette, D. J., Sintek, C. D., & Amato, M. G. et al. (2001). Can clinical Pharmacists affect SF-36 scores in veterans at high risk for medication-related problems? *Journal of Medical Care*, *39*(2), 113–122. doi:10.1097/00005650-200102000-00002 PMID:11176549

Malone, M., & Alger-Mayer, S. A. (2003). Pharmacist intervention enhances adherence to Orlistat therapy. *The Annals of Pharmacotherapy*, *37*(11), 1598–1602. doi:10.1345/aph.1D183 PMID:14565841

Montgomery, A. T., Kalvemark-Sporrong, S., Tully, M. P., & Kettis-Lindblad, A. (2008). Follow-up of patients receiving a pharmaceutical care service in Sweden. *Journal of Clinical Pharmacy and Therapeutics*, *33*(6), 653–662. doi:10.1111/j.1365-2710.2008.00965.x PMID:19138243

Moore, T. J., Psaty, B. M., & Furberg, C. D. (1998). Time to act on drug safety. *Journal of the American Medical Association*, *27919*(19), 1571–1573. doi:10.1001/jama.279.19.1571 PMID:9605903

Morello, C. M., Zadvorny, E. B., Cording, M. A., Suemoto, R. T., Skog, J., & Harari, A. (2006). Development and clinical outcomes of Pharmacist-managed diabetes care clinics. *American Journal of Health-System Pharmacy*, *63*(14), 1325–1231. doi:10.2146/ajhp050430 PMID:16809752

Murray, R. L., Bauld, L., Hackshaw, L. E., & McNeill, A. (2009). Improving access to smoking cessation services for disadvantaged groups: A systematic review. *Journal of Public Health*, *31*(2), 258–277. doi:10.1093/pubmed/fdp008 PMID:19208688

Nkansah, N. T., Brewer, J. M., Connors, R., & Shermock, K. M. (2008). Clinical outcomes of patients with diabetes mellitus receiving medication management by Pharmacists in an urban private physician practice. *American Journal of Health-System Pharmacy*, *65*(2), 145–149. doi:10.2146/ajhp070012 PMID:18192260

Norman, G. R., Sloan, J. A., & Wyrwich, K. W. (2003). Interpretation of changes in health-related quality of life: The remarkable universality of half a standard deviation. *Medical Care*, *41*(5), 582–592. doi:10.1097/01.MLR.0000062554.74615.4C PMID:12719681

Odedina, F. T., & Segal, R. (1996). Behavioural pharmaceutical care scale for measuring Pharmacists' activities. *American Journal of Health-System Pharmacy*, *53*, 855–865. PMID:8728382

Ojasalo, J. (2001). Managing customers expectations in professional services. *Managing Service Quality*, *11*(3), 200–212. doi:10.1108/09604520110391379

Osterberg, L., & Blaschke, T. (2005). Adherence to medication. *The New England Journal of Medicine, 353*(5), 487–497. doi:10.1056/NEJMra050100 PMID:16079372

Patwardhan, P. D., Amin, M. E., & Chewning, B. A. (2014). Intervention research to enhance community Pharmacists' cognitive services: A systematic review. *Research in Social & Administrative Pharmacy, 10*(3), 475–493. doi:10.1016/j.sapharm.2013.07.005 PMID:24071523

Pauwels, K., Simoens, S., Casteels, M., & Huys, I. (2015). Insights into European drug shortages: A survey of hospital Pharmacists. *PLoS ONE, 10*(3), e0119322. doi:10.1371/journal.pone.0119322 PMID:25775406

Penm, J., Chaar, B., Rose, G., & Moles, R. (2015). Pharmacists' influences on prescribing: Validating a clinical pharmacy services survey in the Western Pacific Region. *Research in Social & Administrative Pharmacy, 11*(1), 63–73. doi:10.1016/j.sapharm.2014.04.001 PMID:25042568

Penna, R. P. (1990). Pharmaceutical Care: Pharmacists mission for the 1990s. *American Journal of Hospital Pharmacy, 47*, 543–549. PMID:2316539

Petrillo, J., van Nooten, F., Jones, P., & Rutten-van Mölken, M. (2011). Utility estimation in chronic obstructive pulmonary disease: A preference for change? *PharmacoEconomics, 29*(11), 917–932. doi:10.2165/11589280-000000000-00000 PMID:21988291

Pispati, P. K. (2003). Evidence-based practice in rheumatology. *APLAR Journal of Rheumatology, 6*(1), 44–49. doi:10.1046/j.0219-0494.2003.00026.x

Roberts, N. J., Evans, G., Blenkhorn, P., & Partridge, M. R. (2010). Development of an electronic pictorial asthma action plan and its use in primary care. *Patient Education and Counseling, 80*(1), 141–146. doi:10.1016/j.pec.2009.09.040 PMID:19879092

Ross, E. L., Heizer, J., Mixon, M. A., Jorgensen, J., Valdez, C. A., Czaja, A. S., & Reiter, P. D. (2015). Development of recommendations for dosing of commonly prescribed medications in critically ill obese children. *American Journal of Health-System Pharmacy, 72*(7), 542–556. doi:10.2146/ajhp140280 PMID:25788508

Safaeian, L., Mahdanian, A. R., Salami, S., Pakmehr, F., & Mansourian, M. (2015). Seasonality and Physician-related Factors Associated with Antibiotic Prescribing: A Cross-sectional Study in Isfahan, Iran. *International Journal of Preventive Medicine, 6*(1), 1. doi:10.4103/2008-7802.151431 PMID:25789136

Sakharkar, P., Bounthavong, M., Hirsch, J. D., Morello, C. M., Chen, T. C., & Law, A. V. (2015). Development and validation of PSPSQ 2.0 measuring patient satisfaction with Pharmacist services. *Research in Social & Administrative Pharmacy, 11*(4), 487–498. doi:10.1016/j.sapharm.2014.10.006 PMID:25481330

Sakthong, P., Suksanga, P., Sakulbumrungsil, R., & Winit-Watjana, W. (2013). Economic, clinical, and humanistic outcomes (ECHOs) of pharmaceutical care services for minority patients: A literature review. *Research in Social & Administrative Pharmacy, 9*(3), 311–329. doi:10.1016/j.sapharm.2012.05.004 PMID:22835704

Sancar, M., Yalcin, B., & Mutlu, B. (2011). Determination of geriatric patients' drug profile and identify their pharmaceutical care requirements by determining potential risk factors. *European Geriatric Medicine, 2*(5), 280–283. doi:10.1016/j.eurger.2011.07.011

Sankaranarayanan, J., Murante, L. J., & Moffett, L. M. (2014). A retrospective evaluation of remote Pharmacist interventions in a telepharmacy service model using a conceptual framework. *Telemedicine and E-Health Journal, 20*(10), 893–901. doi:10.1089/tmj.2013.0362 PMID:24611489

Schmelz, A. N., Nixon, B., McDaniel, A., Hudmon, K. S., & Zillich, A. J. (2010). Evaluation of an online tobacco cessation course for health professions students. *American Journal of Pharmaceutical Education, 74*(2), 36. doi:10.5688/aj740236 PMID:20414451

Schulz, M., Verheyen, F., Muhlig, S., Müller, J. M., Mühlbauer, K., Knop-Schneickert, E., & Bergmann, K.-C. et al. (2001). Pharmaceutical care services for asthma patients: A controlled intervention study. *Journal of Clinical Pharmacology, 41*(6), 668–676. doi:10.1177/00912700122010438 PMID:11402636

Schwartz, S. M., Bansal, V. P., Hale, C., Rossi, M., & Engle, J. P. (2008). Compliance, behavior change and weight loss with Orlistat in an overthe- counter setting. *Obesity (Silver Spring, Md.), 16*(3), 623–629. doi:10.1038/oby.2007.96 PMID:18239553

Scuffham, P. A., Yelland, M. J., Nikles, J., Pietrzak, E., & Wilkinson, D. (2008). Are N-of-1 Trials an Economically Viable Option to Improve Access to Selected High Cost Medications? The Australian Experience. *International Society for Pharmacoeconomics and Outcomes Research, 11*(1), 97–109. doi:10.1111/j.1524-4733.2007.00218.x PMID:18237364

Seybert, A. L., Kobulinsky, L. R., & McKaveneya, T. P. (2008). Human patient simulation in a pharmacotherapy course. *American Journal of Pharmaceutical Education, 72*(2), 37. doi:10.5688/aj720237 PMID:18483603

Shemeikka, T., Bastholm-Rahmner, P., Elinder, C. G., Vég, A., Törnqvist, E., Cornelius, B., & Korkmaz, S. (2015). A health record integrated clinical decision support system to support prescriptions of pharmaceutical drugs in patients with reduced renal function: Design, development and proof of concept. *International Journal of Medical Informatics*, *84*(6), 387–395. doi:10.1016/j.ijmedinf.2015.02.005 PMID:25765963

Smythe, M. A., Shah, P. P., Spiteri, T. L., Lucarotti, R. L., & Begle, R. L. (1998). Pharmaceutical care in medical progressive care patients. *The Annals of Pharmacotherapy*, *32*(3), 294–299. doi:10.1345/aph.17068 PMID:9533058

Sokka, T., & Pincus, T. (2001). Markers for work disability in rheumatoid arthritis. *The Journal of Rheumatology*, *28*, 1718–1722. PMID:11469487

Spencer, M., Briggs, A. H., Grossman, R. F., & Rance, L. (2005). Development of an economic model to assess the cost effectiveness of treatment interventions for chronic obstructive pulmonary disease. *PharmacoEconomics*, *23*(6), 619–637. doi:10.2165/00019053-200523060-00008 PMID:15960557

Srivastava, D., & McGuire, A. (2015). Patient access to healthcare and medicines across low-income countries. *Social Science & Medicine*, *133*, 21–27. doi:10.1016/j.socscimed.2015.03.021 PMID:25829195

Stewart, M., Brown, J. B., & Weston, W. W. (1995). *Patient-centered Medicine: Transforming the Clinical Method*. California, USA: SAGE Publications Inc.

Straus, S. E. (2002). Individualizing treatment decisions. The likelihood of being helped or harmed. *Evaluation & the Health Professions*, *25*(2), 210–224. doi:10.1177/016327870202500206 PMID:12026754

Streiner, D. L., & Norman, G. R. (1995). *Health measurement scales: a practical guide to their development and use* (2nd ed.). Oxford, UK: Oxford University Press.

Thompson, A. E., Goldszmidt, M. A., Schwartz, A. J., & Bashook, P. G. (2010). A randomized trial of pictorial versus prose-based medication information pamphlets. *Patient Education and Counseling*, *78*(3), 389–393. doi:10.1016/j.pec.2010.01.010 PMID:20153597

Toubro, S., Dahlager, L., Hermansen, L., Herborg, H., & Astrup, A. (1999). Weight loss maintenance at one year follow-up after initial 12 weeks course in fat reduction on Danish pharmacies. *Ugeskrift for Laeger*, *161*, 5308–5313. PMID:10536516

Vijayanarayana, K., Sekhar, M. S., Surulivelrajan, M., Rajesh, R., Suhaj, A., Kumar, S. P., & Sreedharan, N. et al. (2014). Bridging pharmaceutical education. *Currents in Pharmacy Teaching and Learning*, *6*(5), 745–747. doi:10.1016/j.cptl.2014.05.017

Vinks, T. H., de Koning, F. H., de Lange, T. M., & Egberts, T. C. (2006). Identification of potential drug-related problems in the elderly: The role of the community Pharmacist. *Pharmacy World & Science*, *28*(1), 33–38. doi:10.1007/s11096-005-4213-4 PMID:16703267

Wait, S. (2005). Cost sharing for medications: To what end? *Evidence-Based Healthcare & Public Health*, *9*(3), 261–262. doi:10.1016/j.ehbc.2005.03.033

Weiss, M. C., Grey, E., Harris, M., & Rodham, K. (2015). Dispensing doctor practices and community pharmacies: Exploring the quality of pharmaceutical services. *Primary Health Care Research and Development*, *17*, 1–14. PMID:25777160

WHO document in TELEMEDICINE: Opportunities and developments in Member States, 2010. (n.d.). Available at: http://www.who.int/goe/publications/goe_telemedicine_2010.pdf

Wiley, M. T., Jin, C., Hristidis, V., & Esterling, K. M. (2014). Pharmaceutical drugs chatter on Online Social Networks. *Journal of Biomedical Informatics*, *49*, 245–254. doi:10.1016/j.jbi.2014.03.006 PMID:24637141

Worley, M. M., Schommer, J. C., Brown, L. M., Hadsall, R. S., Ranelli, P. L., Stratton, T. P., & Uden, D. L. (2007). Pharmacists' and patients' roles in the Pharmacist–patient relationship: Are Pharmacists and patients reading from the same relationship script? *Research in Social & Administrative Pharmacy*, *3*(1), 47–69. doi:10.1016/j.sapharm.2006.03.003 PMID:17350557

Worley-Louis, M. M., Schommer, J. C., & Finnegan, J. R. (2003). Construct-identification and measure development for investigating Pharmacist–patient relationships. *Patient Education and Counseling*, *51*(3), 229–238. doi:10.1016/S0738-3991(02)00222-7 PMID:14630379

KEY TERMS AND DEFINITIONS

Drug-Related Problems: Any problem on drug therapy, such as side effects, high cost, allergies, poor adhesion to therapy, etc.

Pharmaceutical Care: A model of pharmacy practice in which the Pharmacist takes the responsibility of the pharmacological treatment of a patient and optimizes it, preventing drug-related problems.

Pharmaceutical Consultations: An ambulatorial service provided by the Pharmacist to conduct clinical interviews and assessment; however, no clinical diagnosis of diseases is made.

Pharmaceutical Counseling: A pharmaceutical service to provide patients the most relevant information on the best way of drug use.

Pharmaceutical Enterprise: Any place where a Pharmacist works with medication or subjects related to medication, like manufacturing industries, compounding pharmacies or drugstores.

Pharmaceutical Services: Activities developed by the Pharmacist for the well-being of a patient, considering (or not) drug use.

Phytotherapics: Plant-based natural products.

Side Effects: Adverse reactions due to incorrect or even correct use of medications.

Chapter 9
Hospital Units Merging Reasons for Conflicts in the Human Resources

Athanasia Stamatopoulou
Piraeus University of Applied Sciences, Greece

Eleni Stamatopoulou
Ministry of Health, Greece

Denis Yannacopoulos
Piraeus University of Applied Sciences, Greece

ABSTRACT

The necessity for the control of expenses of health and the reduction of cost, led the Ministry of Health and the government of Greece to the decision-making for fusions of hospitals units of health following the new tendency of health's policy that prevails also in other countries. The research purpose was to appoint the positive and negative results from the fusions of hospitals. Any changes in the health care system aim at the reduction of expenses, however, they constitute the most frequent causes of conflicts among employees. The Hospital is characterized as a natural space for the growth of conflicts. Despite the oppositions that are recorded as for the positive and negative results, it appears finally that through the fusions, resources have been saved, management systems have been improved but in the same time, conflicts in the labour place between the individuals and the teams recruiting hospitals have been aggravated.

DOI: 10.4018/978-1-4666-9961-8.ch009

INTRODUCTION

The human resources in the health sector is an essential chapter not only its quantitative but also qualitative composition. Although more and more modern technology permeates the health sector, health remains relatively an intensive labor. According to the World Health Organization (WHO) more than 60% of health expenditure is devoted to human resources. So issues that are related to the management and development of human resources in the health sector are of major importance (Liaropoulos, 2007).

The health system is primarily a set of human relations and especially interdependencies. These relationships are hardly disturbed and even harder solutions are "positive sum", where everybody benefits from possible changes. Health services have multi- professional structure and require corporation of an appropriate number of different professionals in order to have a satisfactory result that corresponds to quantitative and qualitative criteria (Liaropoulos, 2010).

It is obvious that in hospitals, which are complex organisms, there is a need for interdisciplinary cooperation, in order to achieve clinical goals related to the sick, and the other objectives related to management issues. The need for interdisciplinary cooperation increases the degree of interaction between health professionals and it is a fact that the more increasing the interactions are, the greater the possibility of a conflict. The maintance of harmonious labor relations and the interdisciplinary cooperation are considered a necessity for health professionals, along with the performance of their duties (Stathopoulou, 2006).

Many groups interact and engage in conflicts during the provision of health care. The conflict is associated with human emotions, such as feelings of neglect and underestimation and indifference. The anger grows inside the person, which can be transformed into rage, and behaviors such as melancholy, or even violence might appear (Papadopoulou, 2009).

Feelings and attitudes that are developed impede the smooth execution of work and as a result the productivity is reduced and errors or omissions are made (Swansburg & Swansburg, 2003).

In a constantly changing society and with the current global economic crisis, which also hit Greece in recent years, the need for state intervention in the economy for the rational allocation of resources was obligatory, including the health sector, as well. Empirical studies record dramatic changes in the epidemiological map of the country, causing an increase in demand for health services and as a result increase the expenses of health care (Stiglitz, 2010; Adamakidou and Kalokairinou-Anagnostopoulou, 2009; Selgelid, 2007).

In times of crisis, when resources are limited there is a need for changes in consequent adverse situations, accompanied by stress, confrontations and conflicts

(Likert & Likert, 1976). Conflicts within organizations are inevitable and arise because of rapid and unpredictable pace of upcoming changes, new technological developments, competition for scarce resources, differences in cultures and beliefs, as well as different human personality types (Brown, 1983). Factors such as the size and the complexity of the organization, the increased interdependence and the rapid social and technological change influence the cause of conflicts in a high degree (Bateman & Snell, 2004).

The right to health is a basic human right enshrined in the Constitution of the World Health Organization and most UN treaties and more recently by the Treaty (Roth, 2004) establishing a European Constitution (Article II-95 of the Charter the European Union's Fundamental Rights) (European Union, 2004) which recognizes the right of every person to have medical care, and states that this right must be recognized through the laws of each Member State of the European Union, as a prerequisite to support the health system.

The establishment of the National Health System (NHS) in Greece under Law.1397 / 83 (Government Gazette 143A / 1983) came as an urgent need for the establishment of a modern health system responsive to the real needs and aspirations of the Greek population, ranking the country according to the World Health Organization in 2000 to 14th place in developed countries health (WHO, 2000).

The need to control health care costs and to reduce costs, as far as 10% of gross national product (GNP) is binded, led the NHS to decide for hospitals merging. Bed mergers and the rational allocation of human and material resources, following the new trend of health policy prevailing in other European Union countries, in order to increase efficiency, evaluates the hospitals and public health system as a whole, maintaines the equal access to health services as an important social criterion (Tsavalias et al., 2012).

The Hospital mergers in Europe are implemented as part of an overall reform of the health services. Aimed at the improvement of efficiency and effectiveness to the enhancement of the quality of health services and the rationalization of the distribution to health services in hospitals that is often regarded as a means of improving the provision of health services (Rotter et al., 2012).

According to a publication in the European Journal of Health Economics is reported that hospitals in Portugal have restructured with wide mergers, after convictions were made between institutions, policymakers in the larger hospitals that argue to the reduction of the average cost (Azevedo & Mateus, 2013). Incentives for integrating clinical wards and hospitals are the reduction of costs and the increase of productivity (Tsavalias et al., 2012).

In a multivaried analysis carried out by the Department of Health Management and Health Economics Institute Health and Society, School of Medicine University of Oslo, it is argued that the merger of hospitals is held for their best performance. It is reported that mergers are complicated and difficult processes which consistently lead to variable results. Changes may occur in the health of workers, resulting in long-term absence from the hospital. (Kjekshus et al., 2014).

Despite the contradictions recorded as to the positive and negative results, it seems finally that through mergers resources are saved and there is an increase of efficiency. On the contrary the conflicts are being increased among staff of health units as these mergers have the exact opposite effects (Tsavalias et al., 2012).

LITERATURE REVIEW

Conceptual Approach to Conflict

The term conflict can be attributed to multiple meanings. A conflict is defined as the result of a disagreement, incompatibility or mistrust within the people (with themselves) or even among groups and organizations (Rahim & Magner, 1995). It is considered a race condition in which one side tries to prevent the other to achieve its goals. A particularly important problem that an organization may face due to conflicts internally, is the non-recognition of compatible objectives. In other words, the contrasting sides of the conflict have different values and goals, which negatively affect the cooperation between them and the subsequent effectiveness of the organization (Wilmot & Hocker, 2001).

Generally, the term of the conflict suggests a collapse of the established decision-making mechanisms, resulting in the person or group to face difficulty in selecting of an alternative energy. Therefore, conflicts arise when an individual or a group face a problem in making decisions (Alper et al., 1998).

According to Robbins, three kinds of views characterize the cause of conflict in the collision theory. The traditional view, which the conflict is mallfunctional and is a result of poor communication, mistrust and maladministration in labor relations. In this regard the conflict is bad and directors or consultants must identify the causes and deal with them, by bringing stability and harmony. The next theory is that of human relations, which claims that the presence of conflict in groups is natural. That means that the conflict can be an advantage for one of the groups at time, which is why organizations must learn to coexist with it. The third approach proposes to encourage the conflict as a means of introducing changes and establishing of new structures and conditions for this change (Robbins, 1993).

Based on the last two concepts, conflict is a natural and inevitable phenomenon for an organization, except from the negative consequences, can bring positive results for an organization, such as to enable individuals to greater efford, be a driving force for positive changes in the organization or constitute development experience (Hellriegel & Slocum, 2010).

It is evident that the conflicts have both positive and negative effects. Positive effects include new ideas, the creation of innovation and changes, making better decisions, increase of participation, the potential increase in productivity, as well as the strengthening of relations, when they are solved positively by both sides. The negative effects include waste of energy, reduction of job satisfaction, reduction of productivity, making biased decisions and the creation of irresponsible behavior (Jameson, 1999).

The management of conflict within the organization is not necessarily refered to as a strategy of avoidance, reduction or elimination of the conflict. Instead it is regarding the strategic planning of effective strategies, which are primarily aim to minimize non-functional elements (malfunctional conflict) of this conflict with the parallel strengthening of its operating elements (functional conflict) (Menon et al., 1996).

As non-functional elements of the conflict are meant the negative reactions that hinder effectivness and are characterized by a low degree of emotional intelligence (Polychroniou, 2008a). Contrary to operating elements are referred to all these that help the organization to achieve its objectives and to improve performance, by keeping the conflict in middle levels. The maintance of operational conflict in middle levels strengthens communication, encourages the interaction among the individuals or groups and it is also associated with high levels of efficiency (Polychroniou, 2008a).

However, it is the duty of managers of an organization, to distinguish each time the functionality of a conflict, as well as the intensity that is desirable in order for the company to reap the highest benefits. A specific type of conflict may be desirable at a minimum level, but it can become uncontrollable after a particular point. An excellent level of conflict is that does not create stagnation, stimulates creativity and relieves tension, so as to increase productivity and create conditions for change without the creation of phenomena of disorganization and detuning or dissatisfaction and trends for withdrawal of emploees (Hellriegel & Slocum, 2010).

The way in which the manager will handle the conflict and will use it as a benefit of the organization is cosnidered a major issue for the smooth proccess.

Conflict Types

Conflicts can be formulated according to their origins. Based on this, they are divided into two broad categories: a) the conflicts that occur in the same individual and b) the conflicts that occur among individuals / groups / organizations.

From an organizational point of view conflicts could be categorized as:

- Hierarchical conflicts, these are among different hierarchical levels, eg between the Board and General Manager.
- Functional conflicts, among different functions or departments of the organization, e.g. between sales departments and production departments
- Conflicts of stems (Jehn, 1997).

The conflicts between individuals and groups are concidered a common and daily phenomenon in the workplace. Typically their symptoms are wariness, hesitation, aggression, indifference, anxiety and distress. The individuals and the groups that have different values, experiences, knowledge, skills, attitudes, responsibilities, needs and goals are obliged to coexist and to cooperate in an organizational environment, which is characterized by uncertainty and complexity in terms of structures, procedures, techniques, rules, and, concequently, conflicts are considered a natural consequence of this situation (Schermerhorn et al., 2007).

Then the conflicts within the person and conflicts between individuals / groups / organizations are analyzed in detail.

Conflicts in person: They are related to two opposite views that the individual can have. A person's value system can be opposite to the values of the organization. The individuals who are involved in situations in which their values come in conflict with their expectations, or when their morallity differs radically from the values that have been adopted by the organization and they may experience internal conflicts, which can get dangerous dimensions (Smither, 1994).

Conflicts of individuals / groups / organizations:

The conflict of the people is a product of organizational roles which are undertaken by individuals in an organization. Those individuals that fulfil their occupational role are involved in coflictions with themselves, because they compete in order to obtain limited organizational resourses (Alper et al., 1998).

The conflict of groups has to do with two reasons: a) the groups compete for the acquisition of limited resources and b) there are many different ways to manage the effective functioning of the parts of an organism.

The conflict of organizations is caused due to the attempt of increasing share in market (Schermerhorn et al., 2007).

Conflicts in the Workplace

Rapid developments, which cause changes in the working environment affect the way of resolving objective conflicts, show as to consider a basic goal of senior management. One of the factors, among others, which can contribute significantly to the proper functioning of an organization and particularly the hospital, except from teamwork among employees is the correct and continuous communication management with all employees, since it has proven that it can contribute effectively and efficiently to the constructive resolution of a conflict (Pavlakis et al., 2011).

It is a fact that the hospital can be described as a natural place for the development of conflict, especially when it is 'threatened' by industrial changes such as mergers of clinics etc. and as it is staffed by people of various professional groups, with different experiences, knowledge, attitudes, behaviors and perceptions and they are "obliged" through teamwork, to interact, contribute to the achievement of the organization's objectives (Tenglilimoglu & Kisa, 2005).

The uncertainty and the lack of resources in the health care environment create conditions of anxiety leading to increased conflict. A study of Whetten & Cameron (1991) found that the increase of the ethnocentric behavior makes workers have lower expectations, and, as a consequence, to reduce their participation in the decision-making process.

The conversation for changes in organizational structures can lead to uncertainty about the impact of the predictable changes to which people are involved. Any change to an existing role is thought to reduce its importance and also create conflict (Shortell, 1990).

The conflict may be characterized as hierarchical (among individuals or groups in a vertical relationship) or horizontal (among individuals or groups, on the same level), temporary or long term, and procedural (disagreement on the means) or and result-oriented (a disagreement on the ends or the results are obtained) (Shortell, 1990).

Types of Conflict in the Area of Health

The conflicts are considered a common phenomenon in the area of nursing and generally in the field of health and their solution often requires a considerable part of time of the Head of the Department. Usually managers / leaders do not suppress nor deny the conflict, but they see it as an opportunity and they do not feel threatened but they accept it as a challenge (Bennis, 1976).

Conflicts are created in cases where there is a discrepancy of views and values and also an incompatiblity in needs and in objectives. In complicated organizations, such as hospitals, the need for decentralization of decision-making and interdisciplinary collaboration increases the degree of interaction between health professionals so as to achieve clinical and administrative objectives. Thomas et al (2003) characterized conflicts as a phenomenon that leads to negative results. As interactions increase, the possibility for conflicts is multiplied.

According to Stathopoulou (2006) the concept of conflict refers to an expression of disagreement. Depending on the level at which the conflict occurs, the conflicts in the health sector are divided into: a) horizontal conflicts between individuals or departments that have similar power with the organization and b) Vertical conflicts between employees and management.

Another distinction of the conflict can be occurred by the members that are involved in, such as: a) Internal conflicts: these are psychological conflicts that occur within the same person and are related to incentives, beliefs and choices, b) interpersonal conflicts are between two or more people, c) the conflicts within a group which is related to the distribution of roles inside the group and the structure of relationships and d) the conflicts between groups which are associated with and resource allocation issues and delimitation of the area control of each group (Swansburg & Swansburg, 2003).

Finally the conflicts are classified into cold and hot. The hot conflicts operate efficiently and increase the creativity of the group while the cold inhibit communication and are not usually perceived (Swansburg & Swansburg, 2003).

Ways of Expressing of Conflicts in Hospital

Although there are common features in the ways of expresing a conflict in all organization, their occurrence in hospitals presents some peculiarities that are associated to with the nature of work and the structure of hospitals. Initially a smoldering dispute, which gradually takes the form of explicit contrast. A period of disagreement follows, which it depends on the mood, the position and the interests of the parts that are involved and it can stop or peak to an open conflict with disastrous consequences for the coherence and effectiveness of teams. Besides the direct confrontation between the parts, the conflict can be expressed and in other ways, such as: unacceptable behavior, negative body language (Gerardi, 2004), conflicts, denial, withdrawal (Porter, 1996), uncontrollable and aggressive competition (Constantino & Merchant, 1996), sabotage, frustration, apathy, decreased productivity (Constantino & Merchant, 1996; Gerardi, 2004).

Hospital Mergers

Since 1983, which is considered an important year for the development of the NHS, till nowdays it could be argued that the lack of adequate financial resources, retractions in health policy, the reactions of the insurance funds, inefficiencies in public administration and the absence of serious monitoring mechanisms and feedback were some of the reasons why the health system has faced crisis so soon. Undermining or canceling the fundamental principles of equality, universality and effectiveness which were inspired by Law1397/1983, caused discontent among users of health services in Greece, according to a report by the Organization for Economic Cooperation and Development OECD that was published in 2010 (European Commission, 2010).

The change in the epidemiological profile of Greece has to do with an aging population that creates needs that were not so intense as they were 50 years ago. It is taken for granted that the political factor has created a very expensive and particularly ineffective heritage, the change of population and of transporting data and also the current economic situation in combination with the low efficiency of hospitals resulted in the need of hospitals to reduce costs in the health, the proper management of beds, the reduction of the duration of hospitalization and the rational allocation of human resources, which are some of the issues that are significant for the Greek Health System (Athanassopoulos et al., 1999).

Despite the fact that the modern hospital sector in Europe shows decreasing in the number of hospitals and beds, according to data (OECD) in Greece, there has been an increase in general hospitals and acute inpatient beds in recent years (Tsavalias et al., 2012).

The heterogeneity is observed between the Regional Health Authorities of the Greek Territory related to the number of hospitals and health centers, the number of clinics and beds per department and as well as the different perceptions of the respective boards of directors on management issues in the areas of health which, differ from European standards, in consequence, there are major problems with the efficiency of hospitals, because effectiviness is the main means of the control and rational allocation of human and financial resources (Boutsioli, 2011).

In international literature, however, there are not several studies before and after hopitals mergers through which the assessment of efficiency could be done correctly. Even so, Greece is heading for the restructuring of the health system with hospitals mergers, parts and beds by saving resourses according to the cost-benefit analysis. It is considered to be necessary that in many countries the reduction in the number of hospital beds is accompanied by an increase in their occupancy rates, while the occupancy rate of therapeutic beds came at 76% on average across OECD countries in 2009 (Alexopoulou, 2013).

Additionally CEO of the Massachusetts General Hospital, the executive vice president of the University of Pennsylvania, the CEO, the vice president for health sciences and dean of the medical school, the College of Physicians and Surgeons of the University "Columbia", and senior Vice President and CEO of Alexandria Children's Hospital argue that the Merger supports an important strategy for leaders of academic medical centers who seek to develop the health system for their institutions. The factors of success for the implementing of mergers of university hospitals are after all their personal experience, which includes effective leadership in the fields of creativity and confidence, managing uncertainty, ensuring the stability of the medical staff and bridging cultural differences between organizations. The importance of success plays an important role in the evaluation of management, organizational and individual dynamics when large university hospitals are merged. (Their et al., 2014).

The University "Carnegie Mellon" of the United Kingdom, argues that mergers between private hospitals often produce little benefit. Despite this fact, the UK government has pursued an active policy of mergers in hospitals, arguing that consolidation will bring improvements for patients, if it is taken for granted that mergers reduce the field of competition among hospitals. (Gaynor et al., 2011).

In a recent published study that was conducted in America it is argued that for autonomous hospitals, the merger may be the only option to remain viable in the emerging new system of the country's healthcare. (Grauman & Tam, 2012). A disadvantage of mergers in hospitals is the result of the attitude which is held by the boards of the individual hospitals. Proposed to target boards to adopt new business dogmas regarding the risk, pricing, competition, regulation, innovation, and resource management. (Cain, 1982).

In the Netherlands it is argued that the Compulsory health insurance disconnects economic and consumer side of the healthcare markets. The concept of control of hospital mergers is not apparent. Patients do not visit the merging hospitals and they are still affected by changes in prices through their premiums. (Katona & Canoy, 2013).

In Florida and Texas it is argued that the benefits of mergers of hospitals may increase competition through access. (Singer et al., 2012). It is certainly investigated in another study how much the merger of hospitals in Florida and Texas favors officers, which would lead to higher prices by a merger in relation to other competitive hospitals. (Garmon, 2013).

The Possible Causes of Conflicts in the Hospital

It is widely known that any change in a healthcare system and especially when it comes to implementing mergers departments and clinical hospitals, as in this case to reduce expenditure in accordance with the cost-effective, are considered to be the most common causes of collisions between the employees. Usually the changes that would take place are not always welcome, although they are considered necessary for the organization, as they create anxiety, insecurity and reactions from employees (Sullivan & Decker, 1988). Despite all the insecurities, the manager should be able to solve problems, to manage the conflicts that will be created with proper communication, which if they are not treated in time, they can even disorientate the operation of the entire Organization (Forte, 1997; Stathopoulou, 2006).

Many, of course, are the factors that are considered causes of conflict within the Hospital. Different goals, competition, poor communication and misunderstanding of information, disagreement on performance standards and disagreements with the organizational structure being some of them (Montana & Charnov, 2002).

Some of the causes of conflict listed in the expretion event of discrepancy, due to issues such as: a) the validity and enforcement (Richardson, 1991) b) working conditions-increased levels of stress, c) denial of responsibility, d) overlapping roles and responsibilities because of the problematic definition of tasks, e) the different levels of education (Jameson, 1999), f) the defiant attitude to leadership, discrimination (Singleton et al., 1998) and i) the complicated working environment (Bourandas, 2002).

The following Table 1 shows the sources of conflict and related issues that are the focus.

Consequences of Conflicts

Conflicts can have both negative and positive effects in an organization. Most people initially have the impression that the conflict is bad or malfunctional. This occurs because the conflict shows that something is not right or that there is a problem that needs to be solved and therefore, the conflict seems to have disastrous consequences. When a collision occurs, its consequences often lead to further conflict and, thereby, a vicious cycle feedback of conflict is created (Cherrington, 1989).

The negative consequences that are possible to exist, including the procedures or upcoming changes associated with the devastating conflict and are as follows:

- The appearance of cases of inappropriate behaviors from health professionals (Stathopoulou, 2006).
- The division of labor relations and the creation of tension, when it is accumulated that can lead to new conflicts in the future (Gerardi, 2004).
- The increase of stress of health professionals (Stathopoulou, 2006).

Table 1. Sources of conflict

Personal Differences Perceptions and Expectations
Informative Insufficiency Misinformation & Deception
Incompatibility role Goals and Objectives
Environmental Stress Rarity of Resources & Uncertainty
Source: Whetten and Cameron (1991)

- The reduction in the efficiency of employees, since collaboration and teamwork, which are needed to achieve common goals, are hit (Davis & Newstrom, 1989).
- The decrease in the morale of employees (Stathopoulou, 2006).
- The emotional loading of those who are involved (frustration, anger, disappointment) and the escalation of the conflict (Lewicki et al., 2004).
- The reduced and poor communication between/of the dissidents.
- The form of communication, which probably exists between those who are involved, is part of an effort to overcome, to reduce or to reverse the side of a view from another or even to emphasize previous arguments of its own side (Lewicki et al., 2004).
- Rigid commitments. The two sides are stable and firm in their positions even more stuck to their positions, by accepting challenges from the other side. They do not recede because of fear of losing their prestige or being ridiculed (Stathopoulou, 2006).
- High cost. The conflicts that are difficult, complicated, unresolved, last longer or become more and more intense, they produce great cost both for employees and for the organization (Davis & Newstrom, 1989). This cost includes probably expenditure for jury, loss of wages, reduced productivity, physical and emotional injuries (Ury et al., 1993). The loss of time and energy is taken for granted when the stressful situation of conflict is personified and becomes obsession for who are involved in. It is also rational that the negotiation process is more time-consuming than a simple administrative decision. It has been estimated that a head consumes 20% of the time for conflict management and this, by itself, represents a significant loss of time (Torrington et al, 2009).

The positive effects of conflict include:

- The avoidance of stagnation and apathy. The agitation, which may be caused by the conflict, makes individuals be active, participate in procedures and stop them from being inerted (Papadopoulou, 2009).
- The contribution to organizational change and to adaptation (Zavlanos, 2002).
- The increase in the productivity of employees and the improvement of performance of the organization (Zavlanos, 2002).
- The emergence of problems that need to be faced (which probably were not obvious) and the dialogue which arises from the situational awareness so as to find solutions (Davis & Newstrom, 1989).

- The increase in creativity and the introduction of innovation in the organization, that has as a consequence the organizational development (Zavlanos, 2002).
- The personal development and maturation of those who are involved in the conflict management process. The better self-awareness and a deeper understanding of others is promoted, through the process of "fermentation" (Stathopoulou, 2006).
- The stimulation of employees by in participating in the decision-making processes. The people who are involved in when the conflict is resolved, feel more committed to the outcome if they are involved in solving it (Davis & Newstrom, 1989).

Conflicts between Doctors and Nurses

According to the results of the study of Casanova et al (2007) professional respect is necessary for successful communication. The conflicts between doctors and nurses are the result of a different way of working, in which nurses focus on teamwork while the doctors attribute to themselves a dominant role in providing care. Consequently, a negative climate is created that easily triggers negative behaviors, thereby affects communication.

Schmidt & Svarstad argued that teamwork through effective communication in the field of hospital improves clinical outcomes, increases patient satisfaction and contributes to the reduction of the costs in human and material resources (Schmidt & Svarstad, 2002).

Vazirani et al (2005) report that the dominating pattern of behavior of the doctor to nurse affects negatively the communication between them. This fact is attributed to the different working philosophy, responsibility and education. The majority of doctors are informed by nurses for the condition of the patient. Also, as Reader et al (2007) argue effective communication in the hospital, especially in the Intensive Care Unit ensures effective cooperation and subsequent treatment efficacy.

According to the results of the study of Puntillo & Mc Adam physicians were more optimistic in the information of patients and less clear, precise and realistic in prognosis of the disease. They were using constantly medical terminology, they were removing early from the patient and they were avoiding family, and as a result there were not having good communication between doctors-nurses-patients. At the same time, they were allowing nurses to explain the details, but they often ignored their views.

The health care system requires from nurses to communicate successfully and be effective both in providing care, reveling information and also relate with physicians (Puntillo & Mc Adam, 2006).

Today, the communication of physicians with nurses plays an important role in providing care in which modern nurse coordinates the activities of all members of the interdisciplinary team and informs them adequately. In conclusion, effective communication and the conflicts which are caused among health professionals is prerequisite for the safe management of patients. The final outcome is determined by the abilities of each manager and the application of appropriate crisis-handling methods by the Agency.

Management of the Conflicts

The management of a conflict starts with the decision whether and when someone will intervene to resolve it. This happens when disagreements are insignificant especially when they appear between two people and it is better to settle between the two parts that are involved in. If it is allowed to the two sides to resolve their own disagreement, this may be an experience of development and improvement of their skills for resolving disputes in the future. But when the disagreement can lead to significant negative effects, then the head must immediately intervene. Sometimes the intervention can be deliberately postponed, so as to leave the dispute to escalate, because the increase in the intensity can motivate participants to seek an acceptable decision. Also, the entrust to the two sides of a common task in a conflict can help and especcially a task that is not directly related to the dispute and can help one side understand the other (Stathopoulou, 2006).

The conflict management is a process that necessitates time and energy. The management of health organizations should be interested and be committed to resolve any dispute, by showing willingness to listen to the positions of all parts, so as to find common solutions. Conflicts in the business area usually involve disputes over real facts, for procedures or rules for values and objectives or formal and informal cultures. The overlapping responsibilities, poor communication among departments of an organization, the declared and undeclared ambitions, lack of teamwork, inadequate leadership, the system of remuneration and penalties may be responsible for the polarization of people or groups (Papanis & Rondos, 2005).

In surveys that are conducted in the Greek business reality has shown that conflicts are more common when job satisfaction is low, the incentives to work are utilitarian, the culture of the company is hierarchical and education is of lower importance. In the light of an external threat such as the merger of an organization, the understanding of the kind of conflict helps to the awareness of its degree complexity, in flexibility, which is needed to vent, to the type of communication to be developed for the smoothness of differences and to the deep investigation of the causes. (Papanis & Rondos, 2005).

Additionally the National Health Policy should identify the real targets on how to avoid conflict over hospital management systems, to have legislative competence to validate the expectations that the senior management (governmental and non) have. Consequenclty the Ministries of Health, Education, Labour and Finance will be coordinated through intensive training programs for managers, Physicians Public Health staff, general practitioners, Epidemiological studies, Structure of society so as to be viable to the fulfilment of changes without this burdening patients and the effectiveness of the organization (Koutis, 2011).

Conflict Management Strategies

There are different ways for a conflict to be dealt with. However, there are three main categories of conflict management strategies which are: a) the Win-Lose Strategy, b) the Win-Win strategy and c) Lose-Lose Strategy (Runde & Flanagan, 2007).

In addition, the individual strategies for dealing with conflicts are:

- **The Method of My Way:** In this method a situation which is difficult to be maintained is created. In this case the one side uses its power against another to force it to agree with her. This method belongs to the category of Win-Lose, which means, that they will definitely find a solution to the problem but it is not the best. This method is only necessary in emergency situations in which the leader must take a decision immediately (Janssen & Van de Vliert, 1996).
- **The Method Your Way:** For the application of this method the two sides that have been clashed must be followed. One of its basic features is the degradation of the differences from both sides resulting in compromise (Jameson, 1999).
- **The Method Half Way:** This method aims to compromise the two sides so that there is neither loser nor winner at the end of the conflict. All the concerned issues that differentiate the two sides must meet in the middle in order to reach a compromise. The disadvantage that the compromise has is that is not considered a solution of Win-Win strategy but a proposal Lose-Lose. Both sides think that they gave many or that they took few without giving special attention to the result (Runde & Flanagan, 2007).
- **The Method Our Way:** It is considered one of the most successful methods. It offers long-term solutions to the problems and belongs to the category of Win-Win strategy. The reason why it is not used as often as it should, is that it takes much time and effort. This method is ideal but in real conditions it cannot often be applied. This happens because of time and delvation of the real causes that led to conflict (Runde & Flanagan, 2007).

It is mentioned that there is not more appropriate way of negotiating a collision. All management styles are useful and effective, according to the circumstances by assuming and understanding of the impact of the conflict and the costs will have on the organization (Jameson, 1999).

However, avoidance of dealing with a conflict represses anger or indignation and consistently results in greater. Being aggressive may be useful to end an offensive behavior or to end of a relationship. Therefore it is important for someone to understand what his or her personal style is and to recognize his or her limitations (Wilmot & Hocker, 2001).

Strategies for Conflict Resolution

Depending on the degree of claimance and emphasis on collaboration, some conflict resolution strategies are distinguished in accordance with the model conflict model. (Thomas, 1992). This model has already been used in previous research in the hospital and is internationally considered as a study tool of how to resolve conflicts (Valentine, 2001). According to this model, five types of conflict resolution techniques are distinguished (Hendel et al., 2005):

- **Avoidance:** The individuals who are involved in a conflict avoid to face the problem that leads to conflict. People that take part in the conflict remain neutral, ignore friction and they do not take any kind of action. This strategy is suitable for situations in which the subject of the conflict is trivial or the expected benefit from the resolution of the conflict is not commensurate with the costs and does not outweigh the effort that must be done. Also, if one of those who are involved in is stronger than the other or if the necessary amount of time to deal with the problem does not exist.
- **Accommodation-Retreat:** When this strategy is followed, one side retreats to satisfy the other. This strategy is usually applied in cases in which the maintenance of good relations is considered more important than the issue of conflict and the retreat is presented as a good act. It is a way of self-sacrifice which is not assertive and does not conduce to cooperation.
- **Compromise:** Both sides sacrifice something in order to reach agreement, and both find solutions that satisfy some of the needs of people. It is about an appropriate strategy when it is necessary to provide a temporary solution in a short time, when both sides are equal, or when there is strong interest of each person who gets involved in a different aspect of the problem.
- **Competition:** One side tries to satisfy its aspirations on the other. A person uses the power and authority which are conferred on from his or her position to force others to accept a specific solution. It can be used when one side has

the knowledge and ability to take a right decision by itself and in emergency situations when a quick decision is required. It is usual between those who are involved in and there is a current-head relation.The strategy of competition, although it provides short-term benefits in the long run may prove detrimental to cooperation and labor relations, because during the implementation of the strategy emotions are generated.

- **Collaboration:** The two sides work together so as to find a solution that it would be satisfactory to both sides. Both try to reach mutual benefits while satisfying their needs. This process takes a lot of time and energy, so it is preferable to be used in important issues that deserve the payment of all this effort (Hendel et al., 2005).

Conflict Resolution and Emotional Intelligence

The conflict permeates most organizations. The Management and generally the Manager can handle those who are involved with proper management, organization and emotional intelligence. The researchers argue that the conflict management is signigicant to the effectiveness of the organization (Lemieux - Charles, 1994).

Resolving the conflict is more feasible when it is tried in the bud. As the treatment delays and as more people get involved in, the dynamics of access turns into knot and the flow of information and misinformation becomes chaotic (Papanis, 2011).

According to Daniel Goleman (1997) emotional intelligence is "the ability to recognize their own feelings and those of others and can effectively handle his emotions and interpersonal relationships." It is true that emotion can be an important source of information and a valuable tool in the proccess of prevention and resolution of conflicts. The shift to emotional intelligence about organizational problems during the last few years is due to the implementation of the work model in groups and secondly to globalization (Goleman, 1998).

According to the results of a major investigation into American companies for the skills considered essential for success, 85% of superiority and success of individuals in the higher hierarchy levels is due to their emotional abilities. The high EQ of a leader contributes to the formulation of a more fertile working environment, where employees work for the achievement of goals, giving their best. (Goleman, 1995).

For a manager, the Emotional Intelligence is concidered a skill which can increase personal effectiveness both in personal and in professional level. Developing communication relationships and trust with colleagues and subordinates, the leader improves his social image, while he or she collects emotional information that will help him or her during the decision making process.

Benefits of the Conflicts in the Workplace

Despite the fact that the conflict is a word that generally has a negative meaning, this is not correct. Conflicts can be very useful for the generation of new ideas, stimulation of creativity and also to be able to bring people closer (Ritsema Van Eck & Huguenin, 1993).

An organization without conflicts is characterized without any change and with few incentives for employees. An optimal amount of conflict will generate creativity, resolution of problems in the atmosphere, a strong team spirit, motivation and therefore changes. When conflicts become abundant, the organization will show a loss of energy, reduction of productivity, increased anxiety and, finally, disintegration. So, we must realize that conflict can be helpful and that are inevitable when people work together, but also they can destroy an organization. According to Williams (1998), benefits can be achieved only if the dealing of the employees "Top Manamement" before or after the process of merging is done in such a way so as to obtain their loyalty, in order to optimize the quality of providing health services (Williams, 1998).

An excess of conflicts is an indicator of the failure of leadership. Therefore, the dynamic of conflicts should be understood by knowing their handling in a way so as to become fertile (Schijndel van Strack & Burchardi, 2007).

CONCLUSION

Conflicts are a natural and an inevitable phenomenon, particularly in health services. It is impossible to be eliminated, but according to modern principles of management science, this is not desirable. The management of conflicts is primarily an administrative process, which is an important aspect of organizational activity.

The current wave of mergers is mainly a reaction to a competitive environment, which gives more emphasis on control of cost. The development of managing care has come under considerable pressure on healthcare providers. The success in organizing the merger requires focusing on two crucial elements: a) the clarity of the objectives of the merger and b) how the process itself will be managed and will be communicated to the employees.

The success of this project requires sophisticated management as it should be carefully supported from a considered policy management personnel preventing in that way the nascent labor conflict.

For the proper function of the hospital and the parts that were going to merge, the manager is required to enhance the interconnection of personnel departments by providing proper guidance and information as well as to contribute to the improvement of communication with the holding of regular meetings among the directors, the heads of departments and their subordinates.

The Mergers will be right to act only when there are convincinctive arguments when the potential benefits outweigh the costs of making the change on important providing human services.

Mergers may be the result of either the needs to reduce operating costs or to revise the organizational structure of the NHS in light of new management models imposed both by the evolution of technology and by demographic changes. In any case it must be ensured the improvement of the efficiency and quality of services provided through the therapy of bad situations and the forecasting emergency situations. To do this it requires:

- Manager selection with experience in the management of hospitals, with specific qualifications required by the responsibilities of the position (management staff from different disciplines and incentives, patient handling etc.) with a developed emotional intelligence to normalize extreme situations resulting from the increased stress of the medical and nursing staff.
- Use of business models concerning time optimization, operating costs and forecasting changes
- Management of conflicts exacerbate the forced movement of staff at best and layoffs at worst in the case of mergers
- Development of accompanying outpatient services to meet needs arising from the reduction of beds (home care etc.)
- Rationalisation of operating costs and primarily the supplies.

Considering that the concept of total quality mainly refers to the satisfaction of both the provider and recipient of services, we consider it essential to develop and implement barometers of satisfaction that will be updated periodically through repeated measurements with emphasis on mapping of pre- and post-merger situation.

There must be found ways to obtain information on the benefits of merging organizations in NHS about how the process of the merger must be managed. The evidence elements can then be used by the leaders of this change, both for national policy makers and for local councils and organizations.

REFERENCES

Adamakidou, T., & Kalokairinou-Anagnostopoulou, A. (2009). The methods of financing of hospital and primary health care in Greece. *Nosileutiki*, *48*(1), 37–49.

Alper, S., Tjosvold, D., & Law, K. S. (1998). Interdependence and controversy in-group decision-making: Antecedents to effective self-managing teams. *Organizational Behavior and Human Decision Processes*, *74*(1), 33–52. doi:10.1006/obhd.1998.2748 PMID:9719650

Athanassopoulos, A. D., Gounaris, C., & Sissouras, A. (1999). A descriptive assessment of the production and cost efficiency of general hospitals in Greece. *Health Care Management (Philadelphia, Pa.)*, *2*(2), 97–106. doi:10.1023/A:1019023408924 PMID:10916606

Azevedo, H., & Mateus, C. (2013). Cost effects of hospital mergers in Portugal. *The European Journal of Health Economics*, *15*(9), 999–1010. doi:10.1007/s10198-013-0552-6 PMID:24379130

Bateman, T., & Snell, S. (2004). *Management The new Competitive landscape* (6th ed.). New York: McGraw- Hill/ Irwin.

Bennis, W. (1976). *The Unconscious Conspiracy: Why leaders can't lead.* New York: Amacon.

Bourandas, D. (2002). *Management: Background and Current Practices.* Athens: Publications Benou. [in Geek]

Boutsioli, Z. (2011). A promising Health Care Reform in Greece. *International Journal of Healthcare Delivery Reform Initiatives*, *3*(2), 23–27. doi:10.4018/jhdri.2011040102

Brown, L. D. (1983). *Managing conflict at Organizational Interfaces.* Massachusetts: Addition-Wesley.

Cain, D. M. (1982). Is the decision to merge really a question of access to capital? *Trustee*, *35*(7), 30–32, 34–35. PMID:10256858

Casanova, J., Day, K., Dorpat, D., Hendricks, B., & Wiesman Theis, L. S. (2007). Nurse-physician work relations and role expectations. *The Journal of Nursing Administration*, *37*(2), 68–70. doi:10.1097/00005110-200702000-00007 PMID:17273025

Cherrington, D. (1989). *Organizational Behavior.* Simon & Schuster Inc.

Constantino, C. A., & Merchant, C. S. (1996). *Designing Conflict Management Systems: A Guide to Creating Productive and Healthy.* San Francisco: Publiser Jossey- Bass.

Davis, K., & Newstrom, J. (1989). *Human Behavior at work. Organizational Behavior at work* (5th ed.). USA: McGraw-Hill.

European Commission. (2010). Patient safety and quality of health care. Brussels, Belgium: Author.

European Union. (2004). *Official Journal of the European Union 47(C 310/01): 1480*. Retrieved from http://eurhttp://lex.europa.eu/LexUriServ/LexUriServ.do?uri=OJ:C:2004:310:FULL:EN:PDF

Forte, P. S. (1997). The High Cost of Conflict. *Nursing Economics*, *15*(3), 119–123. PMID:9305111

Garmon, C. (2013). Employer-provided health insurance and hospital mergers. *Health Economics, Policy, and Law*, *8*(3), 365–384. doi:10.1017/S1744133112000357 PMID:23347566

Gaynor, M., Laudicella, M., & Propper, C. (2011). *Can governments do it better? Merger mania and hospital outcomes in the English NHS*. National Bureau of Economic Research, Working Paper No. 17608.

Gerardi, D. (2004). Using mediation techniques to manage conflict and create healthy work environments. *AACN Clinical Issues*, *15*(2), 182–195. doi:10.1097/00044067-200404000-00003 PMID:15461035

Goleman, D. (1995). *Emotional intelligence*. New York: Bantam Books.

Goleman, D. (1997). *Emotional Intelligence*. Athens, Greece: Editions Ellinika Grammata. (in Greek)

Goleman, D. (1998). *Working with emotional intelligence*. London: Bloomsbury.

Grauman, D. M., & Tam, M. P. (2012). The urge to merge. *Healthcare Financial Management*, *66*(11), 76–82, 84, 86. PMID:23173365

Greek Gazette, Law 1397/1983. National Health System. Gazette 143A / 1983.

Hellriegel, D., & Slocum, W. J. Jr. (2010). *Organizational Behavior* (10th ed.). USA: South-Western Cengage Learning.

Hendel, T., Fish, M., & Galon, V. (2005). Leadership style and choice of strategy in conflict management among Israeli nurse managers in general hospitals. *Journal of Nursing Management*, *13*(2), 137–146. doi:10.1111/j.1365-2934.2004.00525.x PMID:15720483

Jameson, J. K. (1999). Toward a comprehensive model for the assessment and management of intraorganizational conflict: Developing the framework. *The International Journal of Conflict Management*, *10*(3), 268–294. doi:10.1108/eb022827

Janssen, O., & Van de Vliert, E. (1996). Concern For the Other's Goals: Key to (DE-) Escalation of Conflict. *The International Journal of Conflict Management*, *7*(2), 99–120. doi:10.1108/eb022777

Jehn, K. A. (1997). A Qualitative Analysis of Conflict Types and Dimensions in Organizational Groups. *Administrative Science Quarterly*, *42*(3), 530–557. doi:10.2307/2393737

Katona, K., & Canoy, M. (2013). Welfare standards in hospital mergers. *The European Journal of Health Economics*, *14*(4), 573–586. doi:10.1007/s10198-012-0403-x PMID:22688439

Kjekshus, L.E., Bernstrom, V.H., Dahl, E., & Lorentzen, T. (2014). The effect of hospital mergers on long-term sickness absence among hospital employees: a fixed effects multivariate regression analysis using panel data. *BMC Health Serv Res*, *3*(14), 50. doi:.10.1186/1472-6963-14-50

Koutis, X. (2011). *Notes to the Postgraduate Studies Program "Applied Public Health"*. Athens, Greece: National School of Public Health. (in Greek)

Lemieux-Charles, L. (1994). Physicians in health care management: 10 Managing conflict through negotiation. *Health Care Management. Canadian Medical Association Journal*, *151*(8), 1129–1132. PMID:7922944

Lewicki, R., Saunders, D., & Minton, J. (2004). The nature of the negotiations. Athens Publications Kritiki. (In Greek)

Liaropoulos, L. (2007). *Organization of Health Services and Health Systems*. Athens, Greece: Publication Bita. (In Greek)

Liaropoulos, L. (2010). *International Health Systems. Organization of Health Services and Health Systems*. Athens, Greece: Publication Bita. (In Greek)

Likert, R., & Likert, J. G. (1976). *New ways of managing conflict*. New York: McGraw-Hill.

Menon, A., Bharadwaj, G. S., & Howell, R. (1996). The quality and effectiveness of marketing strategy: Effects of functional and dysfunctional conflict in intraorganizational relationships. *Journal of the Academy of Marketing Science*, *24*(4), 299–313. doi:10.1177/0092070396244002

Montana, P., & Charnov, B. (2002). *Management: Management classical theory, organizations structures Management staff and dynamic working groups*. Athens, Greece: Publication Klidarithmos. (in Greek)

Papadopoulou, D. (2009). Violence in the workplace nurses. *Nosileutiki*, *48*(4), 379–387.

Papanis, E. (2011). *Online counseling and Communication*. Athens, Greece: Publications Kyriakidis. (in Greek)

Papanis, E., & Rondos, K. (2005). *Psychology-Sociology of Labour and Human Resource Management*. Athens, Greece: Publications Sideri. (in Greek)

Pavlakis, A., Kateilidou, D., Theodorou, M., Galanis, P., Sourtzi, P., & Siskou, O. (2011). Conflict management in public hospitals: The Cyprus case. *International Nursing Review*, *58*(2), 242–248. doi:10.1111/j.1466-7657.2011.00880.x PMID:21554299

Polychroniou, P. (2008a). Styles of Handling Conflict in Greek Organizations: The impact of Transformation Leadership and Emotional Intelligence. *International Journal of Organizational Behavior*, *13*(1), 52–67.

Porter, L. (1996). Conflict. *Seminars in Perioperative Nursing*, *5*(3), 119–126. PMID:8718405

Puntillo, K. A., & Mc Adam, J. L. (2006). Communication between physicians and nurses as a target for improving end-of-life care in the intensive care unit: Challenges and opportunities for moving forward. *Critical Care Medicine*, *34*(11Suppl), 332–340. doi:10.1097/01.CCM.0000237047.31376.28 PMID:17057595

Rahim, A., & Magner, R. (1995). Confirmatory factor analysis of the styles of handling interpersonal conflict: First- Order factor model and its invariance across groups. *The Journal of Applied Psychology*, *80*(1), 122–132. doi:10.1037/0021-9010.80.1.122 PMID:7706190

Reader, T. W., Flin, R., Mearns, K., & Cuthbertson, B. H. (2007). Interdisciplinary communication in the intensive care unit. *British Journal of Anaesthesia*, *98*(3), 347–352. doi:10.1093/bja/ael372 PMID:17272386

Richardson, J. M. (1991). Management of conflict in organizations. *Physician Executive*, *17*(1), 39–42. PMID:10110137

Ritsema Van Eck, J.R., & Huguenin, P. (1993). *Conflicthantering en onderhandelen; een praktische inleiding*. Houten/Diegem: Bohn Stafleu van Loghum.

Robbins, S. P. (1993). *Organizational Behavior* (1st ed.). New York: Prentice Hall International.

Roth, K. (2004). Defending Economic, Social and Cultural Rights: Practical Issues Faced by an International Human Rights Organization. *Human Rights Quarterly, 26*(1), 63–73. doi:10.1353/hrq.2004.0010

Rotter, T., Popa, D., Riley, B., Ellermann, T., Ryll, U., Burazeri, G., & Brand, H. et al. (2012). Methods for the evaluation of hospital cooperation activities (Systematic review protocol). *Syst Rev, 1*(1), 11. doi:10.1186/2046-4053-1-11 PMID:22587989

Runde, C. E., & Flanagan, T. A. (2007). *Becoming a Conflict Competent Leader: How You and Your Organization Can Manage Conflict Effectively*. Jossey-Bass.

Schermerhorn, J. R., Hunt, J. G., & Osborn, R. (2007). *Organizational Behavior* (10th ed.). Hoboken, NJ: Wiley.

Schijndel van Strack, J. M. R., & Burchardi, H. (2007). Bench-to-bedside review: Leadership and conflict management in the intensive care unit. *Critical Care (London, England), 11*(6), 1–7. PMID:18086322

Schmidt, I. K., & Svarstad, B. L. (2002). Nurse-physician communication and quality of drug use in Swedish nursing homes. *Social Science & Medicine, 54*(12), 1767–1777. doi:10.1016/S0277-9536(01)00146-0 PMID:12113434

Selgelid, M. J. (2007). The importance of "throwing money at" the problem of global health. *Ind J Med Ethics, 4*, 73–75. PMID:18630228

Shortell, S. M. (1990). *Effective Hospital-Physician Relationships, Hospital Administration United States*. Ann Arbor, MI: Administration Press Prespectives.

Singer, T., Heifetz, B., & Morrissey, T.S. (2012). The benefits of mergers. Hospital mergers can increase competition through access to capital and economies of scale. *Trustee, 65*(10), 1-43.

Singleton, C., Weeks, S., & Flatt, S. (1998). Bully tactics. How can trust bosses combat bullying? *Nursing Standard, 12*(31), 21. PMID:9653231

Smither, R. D. (1994). *The Psychology of Work and Human Performance* (2nd ed.). New York: Harper Collins College Publishers.

Stathopoulou, Ch. (2006). Resolving conflicts in a hospital environment. *Nosileutiki, 45*(1), 50–58.

Stiglitz, J. E. (2010). A new capitalist order. In J. E. Stiglitz (Ed.), *Freefall: America, free markets, and the sinking of the world economy* (1st ed.). New York: W.W. Norton & Co.

Sullivan, E. J., & Decker, P. J. (1988). *Effective Management in Nursing* (2nd ed.). Addition Wesley.

Swansburg, R. C., & Swansburg, R. J. (2003). *Introductory Management and Leadership for Clinical Nurses* (2nd ed.). Athens, Greece: Publication Iatrikes Lagos Dimitrios. (in Greek)

Tenglilimoglu, D., & Kisa, A. (2005). Conflict management in public university hospitals in Turkey: A pilot study. *Health Care Management (Philadelphia, Pa.)*, *24*(1), 55–60. PMID:15825820

Their, S. O., Kelley, W. N., Pardes, H., Knight, A. W., & Wietecha, M. (2014). Success factors in merging teaching hospitals. *Academic Medicine*, *89*(2), 219–223. doi:10.1097/ACM.0000000000000094 PMID:24362373

Thomas, E., Sexton, J., & Helmreich, R. (2003). Discrepant attitudes about teamwork among critical care nurses and physicians. *Critical Care Medicine*, *31*(3), 956–959. doi:10.1097/01.CCM.0000056183.89175.76 PMID:12627011

Thomas, K. W. (1992). Conflict and Conflict Management: Reflections and Update. *Journal of Organizational Behavior*, *13*(3), 265–274. doi:10.1002/job.4030130307

Torrington, D., Hall, L., Taylor, S., & Atkinson, C. (2009). *Fundamentals of Human Resourse Management Managing People at Work* (1st ed.). Edinburgh, UK: Prentice Hall.

Tsavalias, K., Siskou, O., & Liaropoulos, L. (2012). Hospital Mergers in Europe Lessons and prospects for Greece. *Arxia Ellinikis Iatrikis*, *29*(2), 233–239.

Ury, W., Brett, J., & Goldberg, S. (1993). *Getting disputes resolved. Designing systems to cut the costs of conflict. The program of Negotiation at Harvard Law School, Cambridge* (2nd ed.). Jossey- Bass.

Valentine, P. E. (2001). A gender perspective on conflict management strategies of nurses. *Journal of Nursing Scholarship*, *33*(1), 69–74. doi:10.1111/j.1547-5069.2001.00069.x PMID:11253585

Vazirani, S., Hays, R. D., Shapiro, M. F., & Cowan, M. (2005). Effect of a multidisciplinary intervention on communication and collaboration among physicians and nurses. *American Journal of Critical Care*, *14*(1), 71–77. PMID:15608112

Whetten, D. A., & Cameron, K. S. (1991). *Developing Management Skills* (2nd ed.). New York: Harper Collins.

Williams, A. (1998). Trust mergers. Turning threates into opportunities. *The Health Service Journal*, *108*(5604), 30–31. PMID:10180008

Wilmot, W., & Hocker, G. L. (2001). *Interpersonal Conflict* (6th ed.). New York: McGraw-Hill Higher Edukation.

World Health Organization (WHO). (2000). *The world health report 2000, Health systems Improving performance*. Geneva: WHO.

Zavlanos, M. (2002). *Organizational behavior*. Athens, Greece: Publication Stamouli. (in Greek)

KEY TERMS AND DEFINITIONS

Conflict: The conflict is a disagreement between two or more individuals or between individuals and groups or between groups, which begins when one individual or group perceives that the other side seeks to prevent or block the aspirations and interests.

Contact: Transmition of messages from one person to another or from one group to another, in order to accept and understand them. An interpersonal relationship in which you send and receive messages through symbols and gestures. The messages may be specific information, opinions, feelings.

Cooperation: For someone working jointly with another or others, (the development of mutual relations between individuals and groups that are designed to achieve common objectives) These people use information together, work together in teams and managing projects.

Emotional Intelligence: It is the ability to control your desires, to regulate moods of others, feeling isolated from thought to fall into each other's position and to hope.

Empathy: The ability to recognize the feelings of others and behave accordingly.

Group: Number of people in a particular place and time develop relations between them and experiencing common emotional experiences, realizing that they are a total that pursues specific goals.

Social Skills: The ability to communicate with other people and to provoke any reactions wanted.

Chapter 10
Towards European Modern Societies with Health Systems That Are Able to Add More Years to Life, But Also to Add More Life to Years

Androutsou Lorena
University of Thessaly, Greece

Androutsou Foulvia
University of Crete, Greece

ABSTRACT

The political context in Europe is changing including health. Among the priorities in seeking to influence the future of healthcare is a renewed attachment to health for all, health in all policies and a better coordination between social and health policy. Health issues are by definition international, and Europe has a duty to extend solidarity to the wider world population, in strategy and in delivery. Ensuring equitable access to high-quality healthcare constitutes a key challenge for health systems throughout Europe. The chapter will emphasise the importance of European public health policies. The chapter will offer a real opportunity to address public health areas and values such as right to access to healthcare into the detailed mechanisms of European policy. The chapter will form a tool for health leaders, to enrich their knowledge in the public health spectrum from a European perspective, to support, promote and improve healthcare access at a national level.

DOI: 10.4018/978-1-4666-9961-8.ch010

INTRODUCTION

The political context in Europe is changing including health. Health systems in EU Member States are varied, reflecting different societal choices. However, despite organisational and financial differences, they are built on common values, as recognised by the Council of Health Ministers in 2006 (Council Conclusions, 2006/C 146/01): universality, access to good quality care, equity and solidarity. The sustainability of national health systems is a core concern of the European Member States, the European Commission, and the World Health Organisation (WHO). The aim of the chapter is to offer insights for the health inequalities policies in the EU as a whole by presenting the most recent picture and trends across time.

BACKGROUND

Among the priorities in seeking to influence the future of healthcare, is a renewed attachment to health for all, health in all policies and a better coordination between social and health policy. High performing health systems are critical to address key health challenges faced by Member States in the European region, such as changes in disease burden and population dynamics, in governance and funding mechanisms, and in technology and clinical management practice (WHO, 2012). As outlined in the WHO report a set of key challenges facing health systems in the European region are:

- Ageing and the rising burden of (multiple) chronic conditions
- Unequal distribution of health across the region
- Financial crisis raises concerns of affordability and sustainability
- Access to technological advances and medicines
- Fragmentation, commercialisation and hospital-centric systems (WHO, 2012).

Health issues are by definition international, and Europe has a duty to extend solidarity to the wider world population, in strategy and in delivery.

WHO defined health systems as comprising 'all public and private organisations, institutions and resources mandated to improve, maintain and restore health. Health systems encompass both personal and population services, as well as activities to influence the policies and actions to address the social, environmental and economic determinants of health' (WHO, 2008a).

The WHO acknowledges that due attention must be given to all levels of care as well as the integration and coordination of functions and care mechanisms to meet the challenges of an ageing population, with increasing expectations of service quality and safety and with the ability to access these services nationally and through cross border care (WHO, 2012).

The importance and implications of the 1977 World Health Assembly resolution " Health for All" and the 1978 Declaration Systems development placed special emphasis on primary health care and stressed family health services. The mix of various sources of financing of Health care systems, which determined the policy and nature of Health Systems, has a great impact on the equity and accessibility.

The Lisbon Strategy in 2000 set out to make the EU: "the most competitive and dynamic knowledge-based economy in the world capable of sustainable economic growth with more and better jobs and greater social cohesion" through economic, social, and environmental renewal and sustainability. It stressed the importance of poverty reduction and elimination of social exclusion in the EU, (The Lisbon Special European Council, 2000).

One of the first Commission Communications to address health inequalities was "The health status of the European Union: Narrowing the health gap", published in 2003. This report highlighted areas of action for Member States, and at EU level, to narrow health inequalities, (European Commission, 2003).

In 2007, the European Commission developed this agenda in the white paper "Together for Health: A Strategic Approach for the EU 2008-2013", Commission of the European Communities (2007). This indicated that reducing inequalities in health must be a core value of future EU level activities on health and tasked the Commission with developing actions to take this forward. The European Council underlined this commitment in the Presidency Conclusion of 2008 which stressed the importance both of "closing the gap in health and in life expectancy between and within Member States and of preventative activities in the field of major chronic non-communicable diseases", (Council of the European Union, 2008).

The 'Council conclusions (2011); towards modern, responsive and sustainable health systems' under the Hungarian Presidency further emphasise innovative approaches and models of health care focusing on effective investment with the overall aim of "moving away from hospital centred systems towards integrated care systems" (Council of the European Union, 2011) moreover the Council conclusions (2013) on the "Reflection process on modern, responsive and sustainable health systems", took under consideration the progress achieved in the reflection process, in terms of including health in other policies in the frame of the implementation of the Europe 2020 Strategy, identification of themes for possible closer cooperation among Member States, exchange of best practices and progress towards more coordinated EU-level cooperation in order to support Member States, where appropriate, in their efforts to ensure that their health systems meet future challenges; and welcome the on-going work on the reflection process on the five defined objectives:

- Enhancing the adequate representation of health in the framework of the Europe 2020 Strategy and in the process of the European Semester;
- Defining success factors for the effective use of Structural Funds for health investments;
- Cost effective use of medicines;
- Integrated care models and better hospital management;
- Measuring and monitoring the effectiveness of health investments, (Council Conclusions, 2013).

In addition the Communication of the European Commission '' on effective, accessible and resilient health systems'' focuses on actions to:

1. Strengthen the effectiveness of health systems
2. Increase the accessibility of healthcare
3. Improve the resilience of health systems (COM, 2014-215).

The need for a shift to modern health systems is also highlighted by the European Union's draft 'Health for Growth Programme, the third multi-annual programme of EU action in the field of health for the period 2014-2020' (COM, 2011-709), which focuses on the links between economic growth and a healthy population. In line with Europe 2020 objectives and policy priorities, it is aimed at supporting Member States' efforts to improve the efficiency and financial sustainability of their health systems through the identification and implementation of innovative solutions for improving the quality, efficiency and sustainability of health systems. Specifically, the programme aims to encourage a shift of resources in the health care sector towards "the most innovative and valuable products and services" while also seeking to support a greater shift towards community care and integrated care. Monitoring of inequalities in health is an important public health task.

MAIN FOCUS OF THE CHAPTER

Addressing How Healthcare Policies Are Linked With Healthcare Service Quality

Citizens' health is a core EU priority (European Commission, 2013a).

WHO has introduced and recommended that *''Assuring the quality of health care in the European Union''* is a result of many factors, including movement of patients and professionals (facilitated by rulings of the European Court of Justice), common public expectations across Europe, dissemination of new medical technologies and techniques through information technology (IT), and the enlargement of the EU (WHO, 2008a).

In addition, Tallinn Chapter is a commitment of the Member States of the World Health Organisation (WHO) in the European Region to improve people's health by strengthening health systems, while acknowledging social, cultural and economic diversity across the Region. Improved health contributes to social well-being through its impact on economic development, competitiveness and productivity. High performing health systems contribute to economic development and wealth (WHO, 2008b).

EU health policy complements national policies to ensure that everyone living in the EU has access to quality healthcare (European Commission, 2013a).

The main objectives of EU health policy are to:

- Prevent disease,
- Promote healthier lifestyles,
- Promote well-being,
- Protect people from serious cross-border threats to health,
- Improve access to healthcare,
- Promote health information and education,
- Improve patient safety,
- Support dynamic health systems and new technologies,
- Set high quality and safety standards for organs and other substances of human origin,
- Ensure high quality, safety and efficacy for medicinal products and devices for medical use.

While the organisation and delivery of healthcare is the responsibility of individual countries, the EU brings added value in helping countries achieve common objectives. EU health policy generates economies of scale by pooling resources, and helps countries to tackle the common challenges, including health threats such as pandemics, the risk factors associated with chronic diseases or the impact of increased life expectancy on healthcare systems (European Commission, 2013a).

The European Union explained that one of the key challenges is health inequalities. Huge differences in health and healthcare exist between and within EU countries and regions. The level of disease and the age at which people die are strongly influenced by factors such as employment, income, education and ethnicity, as well as access to healthcare (European Commission, 2013b).

In particular, poverty and social exclusion continue to be serious challenges across the European Union and for health systems in Member States. People living in poverty or who are at risk of social exclusion are more likely to face health problems and there is evidence that they sometimes do not receive the care that best responds to their needs. There is therefore room for improvement of both health promotion and prevention strategies with these groups in mind, and for more active policies to tackle barriers of access to high-quality care. This has been recognised at an EU level. Achieving access for all to adequate healthcare and long-term care and tackling inequalities in access has been an objective for social protection and social inclusion to support EU policies (European Commission, 2008).

Addressing Health Inequalities in the EU

Health inequalities are largely due to the unequal distribution of health determinants between people with different positions at the social hierarchy. People in lower socioeconomic are more exposed to health hazards in the physical environment, they more often experience psychosocial stressors, and they are more likely to adhere to unhealthy behaviours, such as smoking, inadequate diet, excessive alcohol consumption, and lack of physical exercise. As a result of their greater exposure to such risk factors, people in lower socioeconomic groups more often suffer from disease and disability. Part of this association may be attributable to reverse "selection" effects of health of poor health on educational level or occupational position, e.g. due to health problems in early childhood on school attainment. However, these reverse effects have been found to play a minor role only (Mackenbach, 2007). Health inequalities thus are principally a problem of unequal distribution of risk factors and health risks affecting mostly lower socioeconomic groups:

- Health inequalities are caused by a wide range of other factors which are not necessarily discriminatory, but may be regarded as unfair. These include policies which contribute to systematic differences between social groups in income, education, living conditions, and access to services.
- Health inequalities are due to systematic differences in factors influencing the health of people from different social groups and people living in different places. Large health inequalities exist both between and within EU Member States.
- They impact both on access to appropriate and affordable health and social services, and also on the quality of services which need to be low threshold and targeted to the needs of vulnerable groups.

- Health inequalities are not solely related to access to healthcare. Mostly socio-economic factors and common lifestyle-related risk factors are at the basis to health inequalities.
- On the positive side the considerable differences in life expectancy and infant mortality between EU countries are narrowing.
- Available data on citizens' perception of their unmet needs for care (from the SILC survey) show that the cost of healthcare is an important barrier to access to care for citizens with low income. The same can be said regarding distance to healthcare, where populations in rural areas face the most serious problems of access.
- Measuring access to healthcare encompasses significant difficulties. Available indicators are based on survey or opinion poll where citizens are asked whether they face unmet needs for care but we have no tool allowing for an objective measurement of access. For instance, indicators for coverage, waiting times and affordability are either non-existent or inadequate. An improvement in the tools available to measure access to healthcare is needed (Mackenbach, 2007).

WHO targeted the reduction of health inequalities both within and between countries by launching the programmes "Health for All by the year 2000" and "Closing the Gap" (WHO, 2008c). The relevant WHO report reached to the conclusion that health inequalities should be a major concern of governmental policies in all countries and that it is a matter of social justice to combat poverty and health inequalities, particularly among the most disadvantaged. Some EU states, such as the UK, have developed over the last 40 years a growing concern to investigate and tackle socioeconomic inequalities in health. After the publication of the Black Report in 1977, the Acheson Report in 1998 and the Marmot report in 2010, several actions and public health policies have been implemented aiming at the improvement of the living standards of the poor and the reduction of overall health inequalities among regions and socio-economic groups.

Even if health inequalities have been addressed highlighting the fact that most analyses of the relationship between health and the economy focus on average health, but health is actually very unevenly distributed across society; the global financial crisis that began in 2007 can be classified as a health system shock – that is, an unexpected occurrence originating outside the health system that has a large negative effect on the availability of health system resources or a large positive effect on the demand for health services. In 2009, WHO's Regional Committee for Europe adopted a resolution (EUR/RC59/R3, 2009), urging Member States to ensure that their health systems would continue to protect and promote universal access to effective health services during a time of economic crisis. This policy summary aims to address a gap in the literature by presenting a framework for analysing health policy responses to economic shocks; summarizing the results of a survey of health policy responses to the financial crisis in the European Region's 53 Member States; and discussing the potential effects of these responses on health system performance (European Observatory, 2012).

To date, there has been no systematic cross-country analysis of health policy responses to the financial crisis in Europe, although some overviews of health system responses to the crisis have been published (European Observatory, 2012).

The Marmot report on heath inequalities in the EU was published in December 2013 highlights: "health inequalities are killing on a grand scale''. While the impact of the economic recession is likely to have increased these risks, the start of the recovery is an opportunity to begin to reduce them. There is now overwhelming evidence that everyone in Europe should and could live in better health for longer, provided all government policies prioritise reducing health' (European Commission, 2013b).

Overall, the Commission's action aims both to support policy development in EU countries and improve the contribution of EU policies to address health inequalities.

In 2009, the Commission adopted a strategy on health inequalities entitled "Solidarity in Health: Reducing Health Inequalities in the EU" (COM, 2009- 567). It aims to support Member States and develop the contribution of EU policies towards addressing health inequalities in areas such as public health, employment, social, research and regional policy. In September 2013 the Commission reported about implementation of the strategy by publishing the Staff Working Document (SWD) (SWD, 2013-328) which looks at how far we have come on the five main challenges laid out in the strategy: 1) an equitable distribution of health as part of overall social and economic development; 2) improving the data and knowledge base; 3) building commitment across society; 4) meeting the needs of vulnerable groups; and 5) developing the contribution of EU policies.

The main message from the SWD was that *Gaps in life expectancy and infant mortality narrow across the EU.* The report presented the following results:

Inequalities in infant mortality between EU countries went down by 32% between 2001 and 2011. Overall infant mortality fell from 5.7 to 3.9 over this period with the gap between the top and bottom Member State moving from 15.2 to 7.3.

People in different EU Member States now have a more similar life expectancy than in earlier years. The gap in male life expectancy at birth between the highest and lowest values for the EU-27 Member States was 11.8 years in 2011. However this gap has narrowed since 2007 when it was 14.2 years, an improvement of 17%. The gap in female life expectancy at birth between the highest and lowest values among the EU-27 Member States was 7.9 years in 2011, which is also below its peak of 8.2 years in 2006, an improvement of 4%.

However, health inequalities between and within Member States remain unacceptably high. The report confirms continued gaps in health between social groups, between rich and poor and between those with the highest and lowest levels of education. The report points to some positive developments in implementing the EU strategy on health inequalities, 'Solidarity in Health', but concludes that more action is needed at local, national and EU levels. More specifically health inequalities between countries, regions and social groups (2011 figures) were outlined:

- Sweden has the highest life expectancy for males – 79.9 years, and Lithuania the lowest 68.1 years – a difference of nearly 12 years.
- In 2011 life expectancy for women is highest in France – 85.7 years and lowest in Bulgaria – 77.8 years.
- When it comes to healthy life years in men, there is a difference of 19 years between the lowest and highest values in the EU. For women, this was nearly as high at 18.4 years.
- In 2010, the gap between life expectancy at birth between most and least advantaged regions in the EU was 13.4 years for men and 10.6 years for women.
- In the same year, there were seven EU regions with infant mortality rates greater than 10 per 1000 live births. This is more than 2.5 the EU average of 4.1/1000.
- In 2010, the estimated gap in life expectancy at age 30 for males between the least and the most educated varied from around three years up to 17 years in different Member States. For females the gap was slightly smaller, varying from 1 to 9 years.

The report examines various factors causing health inequalities and finds that social inequalities in health are due to a disparity in the conditions of daily life and drivers such as income, unemployment levels and levels of education. The review found many examples of associations between risk factors for health, including tobacco use and obesity, and socioeconomic circumstances. This reflects the influence that lack of control, stress and reduced capabilities – all strongly associated with social disadvantage – have on both health and health-related behaviours.

When the report was published the former European Health Commissioner, Tonio Borg, said:

It is encouraging that for overall life expectancy and infant mortality we have managed to reduce inequalities between EU countries. However, more progress is needed, particularly in narrowing the health gaps between social groups. Action on health inequalities must remain a public health priority for the EU. It is in everyone's interest to avoid the waste in human potential and the related economic loss, which is conservatively estimated at between 1.5% and 9.5% of GDP (European Commission press release, 2013).

More specifically:

Achieving the goals of Europe 2020 for inclusive growth is fundamental to addressing health inequalities. In February 2013, the Commission adopted a paper on Investing in Health (SWD, 2013-43), as part of the Social Investment package. The paper establishes the role of health as integral to the Europe 2020 strategy (COM, 2010-2020). It strengthens the link between EU health policies and national health system reforms and presents the case for: smart investments for sustainable health systems; investing in people's health; and investing in reducing inequalities in health. Investing in health helps the EU rise to the challenges identified in its Health Strategy (COM, 2007-630) that have been compounded by the economic crisis: an ageing population, an increase in chronic diseases, a greater demand for healthcare and the high cost of technological progress. More specifically the pillars are:

1. Investing in sustainable health systems combines innovative reforms aimed at improving cost-efficiency and reconciling fiscal consolidation targets with the continued provision of sufficient levels of public services.
2. Investing in people's health as human capital helps improve the health of the population in general and reinforces employability, thus making active employment policies more effective, helping to secure adequate livelihoods and contributing to growth.
3. Investing in reducing health inequalities contributes to social cohesion and breaks the vicious spiral of poor health contributing to, and resulting from, poverty and exclusion.
4. Investing in health through adequate support from EU funds (SWD, 2013-43).

The EU Health Program, the Cohesion and Structural Funds, as well as the Research and Innovation Funds (Horizon 2020) can support investment in health all across the European Union. In addition in the Commission Communication on health systems of April 2014, increasing accessibility of healthcare was presented as one of the three pillars of the EU agenda for effective, accessible and resilient health systems. Moreover this document complements the Commission Communication *Towards Social Investment for Growth and Cohesion* (COM, 2013-83) by showing how investing in health contributes to the Europe 2020 objective of smart, sustainable and inclusive growth.

Increasing the Accessibility in Quality Healthcare

Access to good quality healthcare services is a prerequisite for social integration and inclusive growth. It was recognised as a key objective of EU Member States' social protection systems as early as 1992 (Council Recommendations, 92/442/EEC).

Accessibility to health care is human right. This is one of the principles stated in the European Social Charter (Revised European Social Charter, 1996), which emphasises the importance of transparent criteria for access to medical treatment, and the obligation for Member States to have an adequate healthcare system which does not exclude parts of the population from receiving healthcare services (COM, 2014-215). However, access to healthcare is difficult to measure and there is no EU wide detailed methodology to monitor it and promote best practice. This would be an important step to reduce health inequalities (COM, 2009-567).

There has been increasing convergence of equity and health systems agendas as demonstrated by the reports of the Commission on Social Determinants of Health (WHO, 2008d) and the WHO reports on health financing and on health systems (WHO, 2010, 2000). Health equity, health governance, the economics of prevention, and health systems strengthening and public health form the four pillars (socio economic, environmental determinants, lifestyle and behavioural factors and capacity and efficiency of the health care systems) of the WHO European Health 2020 strategy (WHO Regional Office for Europe, 2011).

Equity and Choice: A Gender Issue

Men and women are biologically different because of differences that exist in their reproductive system, and this aspect, hence, forms the basis of differentiation of their health needs.

Equity in health also depends on the recognition by the health sector that men and women might be different in roles and responsibilities that society assigns to them (WHO, 2005a). The equity and choice discussion therefore has to include the gender discussion. The distinct roles and behaviours of men and women in a given society, dictated by that society's gender norms and values, give rise to gender inequalities – inequalities which so far systematically empowered one group over the other (Sen & Östlin, 2007). Besides, there are many other issues like access to health services, cost of recovery, distance to health facility, etc. have differential connotations and implications on the health of men and women.

In relation to health, women are often seen as the group having a natural disposition to health and care issues. They are most often the ones caring for the family – providing food, care as well as a warm and safe home. Women might have a higher sensitivity than men regarding health issues. Providing easy access to health information and care and facilitating system and market navigation for those almost exclusively assuming the sole responsibility for health is essential.

Gender differences are more relevant when considering the reasons for unmet medical needs: women are usually more likely than men to be constrained by barriers to access, such as the cost of medical care, time and geographical barriers (European Commission, 2010). In 2011, there was a more than one percentage point difference of self-reported unmet medical care between men (6.1%) and women (7.2%) in the European Union (EU27). This disadvantage to women comes from specific barriers of access to health care: too expensive, too far to travel or waiting list (3.9 vs. 2.8%). The countries with the lowest reported unmet needs for medical examination for reasons of barriers of access, by sex and age are Slovenia, Austria and Netherlands. Latvia has the highest percentage of unmet needs in EU27 (European Commission Conference Conclusions, 2014).

Women are more likely than men to report that they are unwell or that their imperfect health hampers their daily activities - partly attributable to women's lower socioeconomic status. There is considerable variation in reporting self-perceived health between Member States. While cultural differences in reporting are evident, controlling for all three socioeconomic indicators described above accounted for a significant part of the differences in reporting that exist between Member States (European Commission, 2013b).

The different roles and behaviours of men and women in a given culture, dictated by that culture's gender norms and values, give rise to gender differences between men and women in health status and access to health care. For example:

- A woman cannot receive needed health care because norms in her community prevent her from travelling alone to a clinic.
- A teenage boy dies in an accident because of trying to live up to his peers' expectations that young men should be "bold" risk-takers.
- A married woman contracts HIV because societal standards encourage her husband's promiscuity while simultaneously preventing her from insisting on condom use.
- A country's lung cancer mortality rate for men far outstrips the corresponding rate for women because smoking is considered an attractive marker of masculinity, while it is frowned upon in women (WHO, 2015).

In each of these cases, gender norms and values, and resulting behaviours, are negatively affecting health (WHO, 2015). In fact, the gender picture in a given time and place can be one of the major obstacles - sometimes the single most important obstacle - standing between men and women and the achievement of well-being.

These unfair and avoidable gender inequalities are resulting mainly from patriarchy, the systematic domination of women by men.

The good news is that gender norms and values are not fixed. They evolve over time, vary substantially from place to place, and are subject to change. Thus, the poor health consequences resulting from gender differences and gender inequalities are not static either (Sen & Östlin, 2007).

It is important for all health personnel especially the policy planners and those associated with implementation, to have knowledge and awareness of the ways in which gender issues affect the health differentially for men and women in any society. The process of creating this knowledge and awareness 'of' and responsibility 'for' gender among professionals enabling them to address gender issues in appropriate and most effective ways is called 'gender mainstreaming'. A key focus is given to raising awareness of gender inequalities. This is done by getting participants to challenge stereotypes, gender power relations and gendered assumptions about the factors that influence women's and men's health. Participants are encouraged to explore how services can be provided to women and men in gender-sensitive ways. It is not simply an 'add in' of a gender component in any policy, programme, reform or activity or viewed as a measure to act as 'watch dogs' in the domain of differentiation or inequalities emerging as a result of biological differences. Mainstreaming gender perspective in the health sector has to go beyond the feminist view, often construed with patriarchy to include aspects such as socially constructed discrimination, cultural construction of roles and status on the basis of sex, etc. The goal of gender mainstreaming is to transform health policy, planning and service delivery ensuring equal outcomes for women and men (Piang, Khattar & Nandan, 2010).

Gender mainstreaming is not just about women's health; it is a process for identifying and acting upon the gender-related factors that affect women's and men's health. This is important as gender norms, gender roles and gender relations impact on women's and men's health in different ways. Gender mainstreaming has implications for a whole range of health interventions. In this training guide the focus is given to providing gender sensitive health services (Pillinger, 2014).

There are other areas that potentially could be included, but are not the part of the content of the training. For example, women are often not included in clinical trials and clinical data is often not subject to a specific gender data analysis. Even if women are included in clinical trials the results are not always analysed by gender. This is also relevant for medical education and training. In gender mainstreaming, a broad approach is taken to health, so that the factors or determinants that influence health are addressed across the broad spectrum of inequalities in health. This is important because gender intersects with other population groups such as older people, minority ethic groups including travellers, and across other determinants such as poverty and disadvantage (Pillinger, 2014).

Core to this is bringing the experience, knowledge, interests and voice of women and men into policy making, service planning and service delivery. Gender mainstreaming requires a whole systems approach. This means policy makers, planners, managers and front-line service providers make a commitment to implementing gender mainstreaming in practice.

Except from the gender mainstreaming policies, the European Union has been active in promoting women's reproductive health, in particular through aid for actions on reproductive and sexual health and related rights - one of the two thematic areas of the EuropeAid Cooperation Office. The European Commission, through its Directorate-General for Development, has affirmed its conviction that the United Nations Millennium Development Goals should be linked to the health and rights of women and children, as well as its commitment to the implementation of the United Nations Millennium Declaration (Maastricht University, 2009).

Similarly, EU countries have affirmed, both at the global and regional level, their belief in reproductive health and rights as a development priority. At a meeting organized by the Swedish government and the United Nations Population Fund in Stockholm, in April 2005, over 20 developing and developed countries issued the 'Stockholm Call to Action: Investing in Reproductive Health and Rights as a Development Priority', by which they committed, among other things, to mobilize political commitment on this issue in national and global meetings, to strengthen health systems to support reproductive and sexual health, to invest in efforts to increase women's decision-making power in all aspects of their lives, and to continue to work towards improved aid effectiveness in this area. In January 2006, in the Latvian capital, Riga, parliamentarians from the new EU Baltic member states expressed similar concerns and their wish to contribute to increased awareness on the subject. Through the Riga parliamentary statement of commitment, they committed themselves, in particular, to give high priority to sexual and reproductive health and rights in international development policies at national level and in European institutions (Maastricht University, 2009).

The WHO has also prioritised a gender analysis approach to their work on health and implements gender mainstreaming activities at every level globally. The aim is to shift thinking and attitudes so that the gender-related causes of ill health can be addressed by health professionals. Core to this is providing gender sensitive services (Pillinger,_2014).

Chronic Diseases

The long-term nature of many chronic diseases, and in particular multiple conditions, calls for a comprehensive health system response that brings together a trained workforce with appropriate skills, affordable technologies, reliable supply of medicines, referral systems, and active engagement of people with chronic health problems to manage their own care, all acting over a sustained period of time. Major chronic diseases often result in premature morbidity and loss of healthy life years (WHO, 2005b). They are preventable through addressing their common risk factors, including unhealthy nutrition, lack of physical activity, tobacco use, and alcohol related harm. The prevalence and burden of chronic diseases is increasing worldwide. In the EU, 86% of all deaths, or 4 million per year are related to chronic diseases. 70% to 80% of all healthcare costs, about €700 billion, are currently spent on chronic diseases in the EU (EU Health Policy Forum Report, 2012).

Chronic diseases contribute to reduced economic productivity and labour market participation. 23.5% of employed people suffer from a chronic condition (ENWHP, 2011), and experience restrictions in their daily activities due to it, and absenteeism due to ill-health represents a yearly cost of an estimated 2.5% of GDP (SWD, 2013- 43).

The European Union has a number of activities in place to complement the efforts of Member States to address chronic diseases. Examples include (i) action on major risk factors: tobacco legislation, EU-strategies on nutrition and physical activity, and alcohol-related harm (ii) disease-specific initiatives e.g. on cancer and mental health (iii) funding of projects related to chronic diseases through the Health and Research Programmes (iv) the establishment of fora for the sharing best practices, such as the European Innovation Partnership on Active and Healthy ageing (Council Conclusions, 2010a).

The UN process on non-communicable diseases (NCDs) sets a political framework for action. The WHO action plan on NCDs sets global targets to be reached until 2020 (WHO, 2013).

The EU Reflection Process on chronic diseases (2012 – 2013) illustrated the importance of the issue and the need to take action to curb the rise of chronic diseases (Council Conclusions, 2013). As a first outcome of the process, a Chronic Diseases Summit took place in April 2014 (EU Summit on Chronic Diseases, 2014). It called for stronger political leadership, enhanced efforts to target key societal challenges including ageing; more efficient use of resources; greater involvement of citizens, patients and the health and social sectors in policy development and implementation; and stronger evidence and information on prevention, treatments, cost-effectiveness and demographic change. To take forward work, it called for the establishment of a "Coalition on chronic diseases". The "Coalition" would consist of voluntary members from Member States and stakeholders, and would work on the implementation of action plans around specific issues. This could include for example: early detection of atrial fibrillation, diagnosis and management of depression or effective self-care strategies for improved health outcomes, in order to produce recommendations which could be up-scaled in other settings (EU Summit on Chronic Diseases Conference Conclusions, 2014).

Migrant Health: A Critical Issue of Modern Societies

Migration is present all over the world, and especially in Europe it plays a major social and economic role. Mostly migrants are considered to seek better opportunities in other countries for themselves and their children (European Health Forum Badgastein, 2005).

Migration connects whole populations as well as societies. Migrants traveling for different reasons and surely not always of their own accord. In common with other lower socio-economic groups they frequently have more health problems. Furthermore, minority groups are most vulnerable and at a special risk of not receiving the same level of care and treatment than the average population (LBISHM, 2005). These problems, many times already existing before migrating to another than the home country – low socio-economic and educational level – are often intensified due to lacking or insufficient access to and understanding of healthcare options and treatments in home and destination countries (European Health Forum Badgastein, 2005).

Migrant health – the state of physical, mental and social well-being of migrants and mobile populations (International Organization for Migration, 2005). In general, migrants have greater difficulty maintaining their health and well-being. Ethnic minority groups and migrants are disproportionately more affected by disease and illnesses (Mladovsky, 2007).

Many experience mental or emotional vulnerability and low self-esteem, acquired in source or transit countries on the journey or as a result of their socio-economic conditions, lost family ties and safety networks characterizing their stay in the host country. Migrants with health problems entering European countries are having important implications for public health. They represent potential and possible risks to destination countries as migration is always concerned with transitioning diseases from one country to another. For the host countries, migrants are having special health and welfare priorities that are associated with their basic human rights, including the right to health and access to available health and welfare services. This puts destination countries in the position where they have to equilibrate between their responsibility to safeguard citizens' rights and security as well as their international obligation. The fact that migrants often do not fit in bureaucratic regulations and insurance systems puts an extra strain, both on patients and on professionals (European Health Forum Badgastein, 2005).

Migration has become a priority in the new Commission 2015-2020 (European Commission priorities, 2014). Access to health care for migrants is an issue which is not harmonised in the European level (EQUI-HEALTH, 2013). The right to healthcare is guaranteed under international and European human rights law. These standards apply to everyone regardless of their migration status (FRA report, 2011). Although this does not oblige EU Member States to guarantee access to all health services on an equal footing for citizens, it does impose some minimum requirements such as access to the emergency and necessary healthcare for all, equal access to healthcare. Currently the legal framework which applies is:

- The Return Directive 2008/115/EC covers access to healthcare of those irregular migrants who are subject of return procedures (both in detention centres and outside detention): The Return Directive obliges Member States to provide emergency health care and essential treatment of illness to illegally staying third country nationals who are subject of return procedures (Articles 14(1)(b) and 16(3) of the directive) (Directive, 2008/115/EC).
- The Charter of Fundamental Rights reinforces the EU commitment to equal opportunities and antidiscrimination and also guarantees access to health care (Official Journal of European Union, Chapter of Fundamental Rights of the EU, 2010/C 83/02).
- **Article 10 of the Treaty on the Functioning of the European Union:** The Union shall aim to combat discrimination when defining and implementing all its policies and activities (Official Journal of European Union, 2012/C 326/49).
- **European Parliament Resolution on "Undocumented Migrant Women in the EU (4 February 2014):** Underlining the need for equal access to justice and services for all women regardless of administrative status. The resolution calls on national and European authorities to ensure that a woman's immigration status does not prevent her from accessing decent housing, health care, education, and justice (European Parliament resolution on undocumented women migrants in the European Union, 2013/2115(INI)).
- Council Conclusions on the Common Values and Principles of EU Health Systems, June 2006. In their declaration, ministers agree that health services must be underpinned by the values of universality, access to good quality care, equity and solidarity (Council Conclusions, 2006/C 146/01).
- The European Union Council Conclusions on ''Equity and Health in all policies: Solidarity in Health'' (Madrid, 8 June 2010, Article 8), the European Parliament Resolution ''Reducing Health Inequalities in the EU (A7-0032/2011, 8 March 2011 points 5-22) address the issues of vulnerable groups (Council Conclusions, 2010b).
- The Commission, as part of its economic governance under the European Semester, highlighted the "twin aim of a more efficient use of public resourc-

es and access to high quality healthcare" in its 2013 Annual growth Survey (Priorities at EU level: the Annual Growth Survey, 2015). In follow-up, both under the 2013 and 2014 European Semester, the Commission proposed recommendations to improve or maintain the accessibility of health systems in selected Member States (in 2014 for Romania, Latvia, Spain as adopted by Council on 8 July 2014) (The European Semester, 2015).

- In its Communication on "Effective, Accessible and Resilient" health systems of 4 April 2014, the Commission presented the accessibility of health services as one of three key general topics on the EU's health systems agenda (COM, 2014-215).
- The Europe 2020 Strategy gives a new impetus to efforts addressing poverty and social exclusion in the EU (COM, 2010-2020).

The EU is committed to tackling all forms of discrimination. Specific antidiscrimination activities include the legal framework; support for the development and exchange of good practice; projects, studies and the work of agencies such as the Fundamental Rights Agency (FRA).

It is important to mention that Member States are responsible for the provision of health care such provision needs to comply with EU law. This includes the right for legal migrants to have access to health care on the same basis as nationals. Irregular migrants must have as a minimum access to emergency medical care and access to healthcare for children, as well as antenatal, delivery and postnatal healthcare for mothers.

Modern societies need migrant-friendly hospitals initiatives. An initiative exclusively addressing the urgency of migration is the "migrant-friendly hospitals" initiative. Increasing migration and ethno-cultural diversity due to migration in Europe is and important issue for health systems and services. Many of the problems related to migration and care are not only related to language barriers and cultural diversity, but include scarcities in hospital and care resources as well as low levels of minority purchasing power. These additional problems pose new challenges to health professionals, especially in hospitals, playing and particularly important role in serving the migrant segment of the population. The migrant-friendly hospitals initiative is composed of a group of hospitals from diverse European countries collaborating with a number of high-profile experts and a wide range of international and European organizations. The collaboration aims at putting migrant-friendly, culturally-competent health care and health promotion higher up on the European health policy agenda as well as to support new interested hospitals improving their migrant friendliness by providing practical knowledge and instruments. Participants are aiming at becoming migrant-friendly and culturally-competent organizations. The priorities of the collaboration are set on the following areas: (1) Improving interpreting services; (2) migrant friendly information and training for mother –and child care, and (3) staff training towards cultural competence (LBISHM, 2005).

Modern Hospitals in Europe

For several years, hospitals have been required to act more efficiently and to increase their performance. Yet, today healthcare systems are facing conflicting trends: increasing demand of an ever-expanding and ageing population: short and long-term impacts of an economic and financial crisis and increasing request/availability of technological innovations. To adapt to this situation, the role of hospitals is further evolving.

In practice, change has taken place with emerging trends involving the creation of chains and networks in countries such as Sweden, Slovenia and the Netherlands, the formation of integrated providers as in the UK and Hungary, the development of regional systems as for example in Denmark and France. Other trends include a rising trend towards mergers, with examples including the UK and Norway. Indeed, in Norway, mergers have presented the main approach to more than halving the number of hospitals from around 50 since 2002. This was accompanied by a number of configurational changes including for example the introduction of observational units next to Accident and Emergency (A&E) departments as a means to reduce admissions, as well as changes to management structures such as the involvement of physicians and nurses at the various levels of governance alongside investment in training of hospital managers (WHO, 2012).

These examples illustrate that change is possible although difficult questions remain such as trade-offs between centralization and decentralization, for example maternity wards; or the role of small hospitals in rural areas. It was recognized that hospitals form part of integrated population health management, and the hospital should be a full part of the pathway. However, especially in relation to the issue of geographical location discussants expressed concerns of whether the answer to multimorbidity indeed involved a shift from hospital to primary care, in particular in sparsely populated areas, or whether it might be more appropriate for training to accommodate generalist skills in the hospital setting. More broadly, this raises the general question about the appropriate 'delivery system' to respond to the challenge posed by chronic diseases (WHO, 2012).

In addition to the aforementioned discussion WHO is giving 3 possible different pillars:

At the macro-level, the need:

- For the development of a clear vision for system design regarding how future health care should look like

- The development of new incentives for hospitals
- To engage with the EU level (subsidiarity)

At the meso-level, the need:

- To identify and implement new ways of organising primary care
- To describe the level of population health coordination
- To better understand how hospital change in terms of the delivery model has been achieved

At the micro-level, the need:

- To invest in the workforce involving the development of new skills as well as redesigning the work of specialists to be better suited to chronic care
- To develop and strengthen the ability to describe and measure what is being produced
- To identify better ways of working between organizations (World Health Organisation Regional Office for Europe, 2010).

Emphasis should be given to the management of primary care, as well as ongoing work on the role of hospitals in the context of integrated health care delivery (European Observatory on Health Systems and Policies, 2009).

RECOMMENDATIONS

There is a need to rethink the role and function of the 'modern' health system. Causes of health inequalities vary between Member States and between specific population groups. Addressing health inequalities effectively requires policies which include both actions to address the gradient in health across the whole of society as well as actions which are specifically targeted to vulnerable groups. The primary responsibility for health systems rests with the Member States. Member States should aim to establish, in close collaboration with the European Commission, a common set of indicators to monitor health inequalities and a methodology to audit the health situation in Member States aimed to identify and prioritizing areas of improvement and best practices. The European Commission could support Member States to achieve their objectives by providing analysis and support on the basis of available information. This could prove to be a useful tool for Member States when designing, prioritizing and implementing more efficient and effective policies adjusted to their specific situation, and to better use the existing EU tools to support their actions. The EU has taken a number of actions that can support Member States, in particular by providing guidelines and as monitoring or evaluation tools. Member States' future ability to provide high quality care to all will depend on making health systems more resilient, more capable of coping with the challenges that lie ahead. Controlled investment in the health sector, particularly for health infrastructure and expensive equipment, public health measures to reduce the burden of disease, integration and coordination of primary care and secondary care, and of health and social care could be considered as opportunities to use structural funds and other funds.

FUTURE RESEARCH DIRECTIONS

Action on health inequalities is being taken forward as part of Europe 2020 initiative and through the Commission's communication on health inequalities. The reduction of health inequalities is part of the objective of 'inclusive growth'; to ensure that all Europeans can benefit from a smarter, more sustainable economy. Future research directions may include more visibility to best practices in specific health areas which will enable stakeholders to interact amongst each other, countries profile overview on health inequalities with up to date data, tools to encourage reform of health systems aiming at cost-efficiency and sustainability which will ensure patient access to healthcare in the long term and mechanisms to ensure quality health care to all.

CONCLUSION

National governments, regional authorities in many countries have an important role in public health and health services and thus need to be actively involved. The health sector has a leading role to play, with the local governments, workplaces, and other stakeholders also to have a vital contribution to make.

REFERENCES

Acheson Report. (1998). *Inequalities in health Report on inequalities in health did give priority for steps to be tackled*. Retrieved February 01, 2015, from http://www.ncbi.nlm.nih.gov/pmc/articles/PMC1114452/

Black Report. (1977). *The Black Report and the health divide*. Retrieved February 25, 2015, from http://history.lshtm.ac.uk/files/2013/07/The-Black-Report-and-the-Health-Divide-VB.pdf

COM. (2007). *630 final.* Commission White Paper: Together for Health: A Strategic Approach for the EU 2008-2013. Retrieved February 08, 2015, from http://ec.europa.eu/health/ph_overview/Documents/strategy_wp_en.pdf

COM. (2009). *567 final.* Solidarity in health, reducing health inequalities in the EU. Retrieved February 01, 2015, from http://eur-lex.europa.eu/legal-content/EN/TXT/PDF/?uri=CELEX:52009DC0567&from=EN

COM. (2010). *2020 final.* Commission Communication, Europe 2020 Strategy, A strategy for smart, sustainable and inclusive growth. Retrieved February 06, 2015, from file:///C:/Users/user/Downloads/COM_COM(2010)2020_EN.pdf

COM. (2011). *709 final.* European Commission. Proposal for a Regulation of the European Parliament and of the Council on establishing a Health for Growth Programme, the third multi-annual programme of EU action in the field of health for the period 2014-2020. Retrieved February 05, 2015, from http://ec.europa.eu/health/programme/docs/prop_prog2014_en.pdf

COM. (2013). *83 final.* Towards Social Investment for Growth and Cohesion – including implementing the European Social Fund 2014-2020. Retrieved February 24, 2015, from http://ec.europa.eu/social/main.jsp?catId=1044&langId=en&newsId=1807&moreDocuments=yes&tableName=news

COM. (2014). *215 final.* On effective, accessible and resilient health systems. Retrieved February 08, 2015, from http://ec.europa.eu/health/healthcare/docs/com2014_215_final_en.pdf

Council Conclusions. (2006). *C 146/01.* On Common values and principles in European Union Health Systems. Retrieved February 03, 2015, from http://eur-lex.europa.eu/LexUriServ/LexUriServ.do?uri=OJ:C:2006:146:0001:0003:EN:PDF

Council Conclusions. (2010a). *Innovative approaches for chronic diseases in public health and healthcare systems*, Retrieved February 08, 2015, from http://www.idf.org/sites/default/files/Council_conclusions_7%20Dec%202010_Chronic%20Disease.pdf

Council Conclusions. (2010b). *On Equity and Health in All Policies: Solidarity in Health.* Retrieved February 06, 2015, from http://www.consilium.europa.eu/uedocs/cms_data/docs/pressdata/en/lsa/114994.pdf

Council Conclusions. (2013). *On the Reflection process on modern, responsive and sustainable health systems.* Retrieved February 11, 2015, from http://www.consilium.europa.eu/uedocs/cms_data/docs/pressdata/en/lsa/140004.pdf

Council of the European Union. (2008). *Presidency conclusions.* Retrieved February 16, 2015, from http://www.consilium.europa.eu/uedocs/cms_data/docs/pressdata/en/ec/101346.pdf

Council of the European Union. (2011). *Council conclusions: Towards modern, responsive and sustainable health systems.* Retrieved February 11, 2015, from http://www.consilium.europa.eu/uedocs/cms_data/docs/pressdata/en/lsa/122395.pdf

Council Recommendations. (1992). *92/442/EEC: of 27 July.* On the convergence of social protection objectives and policies. Retrieved February 11, 2015, from http://eur-lex.europa.eu/legal-content/EN/TXT/PDF/?uri=CELEX:31992H0442&from=GA

Directive. (2008). *115/EC, of the European Parliament and of the Council of 16 December 2008, on common standards and procedures in Member States for returning illegally staying third-country nationals.* Retrieved February 11, 2015, from http://eur-lex.europa.eu/LexUriServ/LexUriServ.do?uri=OJ:L:2008:348:0098:0107:EN:PDF

ENWHP. (2011). *The 9th initiative by the European Network for Workplace Health promotion (ENWHP) and its campaign Work. Adapted for all. Move Europe, is co-funded by the European Commission under the Public Health Programme (2008-2013).* Retrieved February 21, 2015, from http://www.enwhp.org/enwhp-initiatives/9th-initiative-ph-work.html

EQUI-HEALTH. (2013). *Fostering health Fostering health provision for Migrants, the provision for Migrants, the Roma and other vulnerable groups Roma and other vulnerable groups.* Retrieved February 21, 2015, from http://ec.europa.eu/health/social_determinants/docs/ev_20130121_co06_en.pdf

European Parliament Resolution. (2014). *On undocumented women migrants in the European Union* (2013/2115(INI)). Retrieved February 01, 2015, from http://www.europarl.europa.eu/sides/getDoc.do?pubRef=-//EP//TEXT+TA+P7-TA-2014-0068+0+DOC+XML+V0//EN EUR/RC59/R3

European Commission. (2003). *The health status of the European Union: Narrowing the health gap.* Luxembourg: European Communities.

European Commission. (2008). *Quality in and Equality of access to health-care services.* Retrieved February 01, 2015, from http://www.euro.centre.org/data/1237457784_41597.pdf

European Commission. (2010). *Strategy for equality between women and men 2010-2015*. Retrieved February 10, 2015, from http://ec.europa.eu/justice/gender-equality/files/strategy_equality_women_men_en.pdf Access

European Commission Press Release. (2013). *Report on Health inequalities: gaps in life expectancy and infant mortality narrow across the EU*. Retrieved February 01, 2015, from http://europa.eu/rapid/press-release_IP-13-823_en.htm

European Commission. (2013a). *Public Health -Improving health for all EU citizens*. Retrieved February 01, 2015, from http://ec.europa.eu/health/health_policies/docs/improving_health_for_all_eu_citizens_en.pdf

European Commission. (2013b). *Report on Health Inequalities in the EU*. Retrieved February 21, 2015, from http://ec.europa.eu/health/social_determinants/docs/health-inequalitiesineu_2013_en.pdf

European Commission Conference Conclusions. (2014). *Health in Europe Making it Fairer*. Retrieved February 11, 2015, from http://ec.europa.eu/health/social_determinants/docs/ev_20140318_bkgr_note_en.pdf

European Commission Priorities. (2014). *A New Start for Europe: My Agenda for Jobs, Growth, Fairness and Democratic Change, Political Guidelines for the next European Commission*. Retrieved March 01, 2015, from http://ec.europa.eu/priorities/docs/pg_en.pdf#page=10

European Health Forum Badgastein. (2005). *Partnerships for Health Enabling healthy choices in modern health societies*. Retrieved March 05, 2015, from http://old.ilonakickbusch.com/health-literacy/Gastein_2005.pdf

European Observatory on Health Systems and Policies. (2009). *Investing in hospitals of the future, Observatory Studies Series, No.16*. Retrieved March 10, 2015, from http://www.euro.who.int/__data/assets/pdf_file/0009/98406/E92354.pdf

European Observatory. (2012). *Health policy responses to the financial crisis of Europe*. WHO. Retrieved March 01, 2015, from http://www.euro.who.int/__data/assets/pdf_file/0009/170865/e96643.pdf

EU Health Policy Forum Report. (2012). *Answer to DG SANCO consultation on chronic diseases*. Retrieved March 07, 2015, from http://ec.europa.eu/health/major_chronic_diseases/docs/hpf_response_consultation_cd_en.pdf

EU Summit on Chronic Diseases. (2014). *Addressing the medical, social and economic burden of chronic diseases in the EU*. Retrieved March 14, 2015, from http://ec.europa.eu/health/major_chronic_diseases/docs/ev_20140403_ag_en.pdf

EU Summit on Chronic Diseases Conference Conclusions. (2014). Retrieved March 01, 2015, from http://ec.europa.eu/health/major_chronic_diseases/docs/ev_20140403_mi_en.pdf

Fundamental Rights Agency (FRA) Report (2011). *EU: Right to healthcare not guaranteed in practice*. Retrieved March 05, 2015, from http://fra.europa.eu/en/press-release/2011/eu-right-healthcare-not-guaranteed-practice

International Organization for Migration. (2005). *Health and Migration: Bridging the Gap*. Geneva: Migration Policy and Research Programme.

LBISHM. (2005). *Project Summary on Migrant-Friendly Hospitals*. WHO Collaboration Centre for Health Promotion on Hospitals and Health Care, Institute for Sociology, University Vienna.

Maastricht University. (2009). *Europe, gender inequality and global health*. Retrieved February 01, 2015, from http://www.globalhealtheurope.org/index.php/resources/glossary/values/72-europe-gender-inequality-and-global-health

Mackenbach, J. (2007). *Economic implications of socio-economic inequalities in health in the European Union*. European Commission report. Retrieved February 05, 2015, from http://ec.europa.eu/health/ph_determinants/socio_economics/documents/socioeco_inequalities_en.pdf

Marmot Report. (2010). *Fair society healthy lifes*. Retrieved February 10, 2015, from http://www.instituteofhealthequity.org/projects/fair-society-healthy-lives-the-marmot-review

Mladovsky, P. (2007). *Research Note Migration and health in the EU*. London School of Economics and Political Science, European Commission. Retrieved February 10, 2015, from http://ec.europa.eu/employment_social/social_situation/docs/rn_migration_health.pdf

Official Journal of European Union. (2010). C 83/02. Chapter of Fundamental Rights of the EU. Retrieved February 11, 2015, from http://eur-lex.europa.eu/LexUriServ/LexUriServ.do?uri=OJ:C:2010:083:0389:0403:en:PDF

Official Journal of European Union. (2012). C 326/49. Consolidated Version of the Treaty on the Functioning of the European Union. Retrieved February 11, 2015, from http://eur-lex.europa.eu/legal-content/EN/TXT/PDF/?uri=CELEX:12012E/TXT&from=EN

Piang, L. K., Khattar, P., & Nandan, D. (2010). Mainstreaming Gender perspective in the National Health Programmes: the challenges ahead. *Health and Population, Perspectives and Issues, 33*(1), 34-41. Retrieved February 12, 2015, from http://medind.nic.in/hab/t10/i1/habt10i1p34.pdf

Pillinger, J. (2014). *Gender Mainstreaming in Health, training Handbook*. Retrieved February 13, 2015, from http://www.nwci.ie/images/uploads/NWCI_GM_Training_Manual_A4_WEB.pdf

Revised European Social Charter. (1996). *Strasbourg 3 May*. Retrieved February 13, 2015, from http://conventions.coe.int/Treaty/en/Treaties/Html/163.htm

Priorities at EU level: the Annual Growth Survey. (2015). Retrieved February 10, 2015, from http://ec.europa.eu/europe2020/making-it-happen/annual-growth-surveys/index_en.htm

Sen, G., & Östlin, P. (2007). *Women and Gender Equity Knowledge Network*. Retrieved February 13, 2015, from http://www.who.int/social_determinants/resources/csdh_media/wgekn_final_report_07.pdf

SWD. (2013). *43 final*. Investing in Health. Retrieved February 02, 2015, from http://www.europarl.europa.eu/meetdocs/2009_2014/documents/swd/com_swd%282013%290043_/com_swd%282013%290043_en.pdf

SWD. (2013). *328 final*. Report on Health inequalities in the EU. Retrieved February 06, 2015, from http://ec.europa.eu/health/social_determinants/docs/report_health-inequalities_swd_2013_328_en.pdf

The Lisbon Special European Council. (2000). *Towards a Europe of Innovation and Knowledge*. Retrieved February 09, 2015, from http://europa.eu/legislation_summaries/education_training_youth/general_framework/c10241_en.htm

The European Semester. (2015). *Economic Policies for Growth, Jobs and Investment*. Retrieved February 18, 2015, from http://ec.europa.eu/economy_finance/economic_governance/the_european_semester/index_en.htm

World Health Organisation (WHO). (2000). *The world health report 2000 - Health systems: improving performance*. Retrieved February 19, 2015, from http://www.who.int/whr/2000/en/

World Health Organization (WHO). (2005a). *Executive Board, Gender, women and health: incorporating a gender perspective into the mainstream of WHO's policies and programme*. Report by the Secretariat, 12th May, EB116/13.

World Health Organization (WHO). (2005b). *Preventing Chronic Diseases a vital investment*. Retrieved February 20, 2015, from http://www.who.int/chp/chronic_disease_report/contents/part2.pdf

World Health Organisation (WHO). (2008a). *Assuring the quality of health care in the European Union*. United Kingdom by MPG Books Ltd, Bodmin, Cornwall. Retrieved February 16, 2015, from http://www.euro.who.int/__data/assets/pdf_file/0007/98233/E91397.pdf

World Health Organisation (WHO). (2008b). *The Tallinn Charter: Health Systems for Health and Wealth. Tallinn*. Retrieved February 10, 2015, from http://www.euro.who.int/__data/assets/pdf_file/0008/88613/E91438.pdf

World Health Organisation (WHO). (2008c). *Closing the Gap: Health Equity through action on the social determinants of health*. Retrieved February 20, 2015, from http://www.who.int/social_determinants/final_report/csdh_finalreport_2008.pdf

World Health Organisation (WHO). (2008d). *Commission on Social Determinants of Health – final report*. Retrieved February 10, 2015, from http://www.who.int/social_determinants/thecommission/finalreport/en/index.html

World Health Organisation. (2010). *The world health report - Health systems financing: the path to universal coverage*. Retrieved February 15, 2015, from http://www.who.int/whr/2010/en/index.html

World Health Organisation Regional Office for Europe. (2010). *Primary Care Evaluation Tool (PCET)*. Retrieved February 20, 2015, from http://www.euro.who.int/__data/assets/pdf_file/0005/128849/e94554.pdf

World Health Organization Regional Office for Europe. (2011). *The new European policy for health – Health 2020*. EUR/RC61/Inf.Doc./4. Retrieved February 18, 2015, from http://www.euro.who.int/__data/assets/pdf_file/0005/148946/RC61_InfDoc4.pdf

World Health Organization (WHO). (2012). *Modern health care delivery systems, care coordination and the role of hospitals*. Retrieved February 13, 2015, from http://www.euro.who.int/__data/assets/pdf_file/0008/158885/BRU-report-Modern-health-care-delivery-systems.pdf?ua=1

World Health Organization (WHO). (2013). *Global action plan for the prevention and control of non-communicable diseases 2013-2020*. Retrieved February 10, 2015, from http://apps.who.int/iris/bitstream/10665/94384/1/9789241506236_eng.pdf

World Health Organization (WHO). (2015). *Gender, Women and Heath, Why gender and Health?* Retrieved February 12, 2015, from http://www.who.int/gender/genderandhealth/en/

Compilation of References

Abdel-Tawab, R., James, D. H., Fichtinger, A., Clatworthy, J., Horne, R., & Davies, G. (2011). Development and validation of the Medication-Related Consultation Framework (MRCF). *Patient Education and Counseling*, *83*(3), 451–457. doi:10.1016/j.pec.2011.05.005 PMID:21621944

AbuAlRub, R. F., & Al-Zaru, I. M. (2008). Job stress, recognition, job performance and intention to stay at work among Jordanian hospital nurses. *Journal of Nursing Management*, *16*(3), 227–236. doi:10.1111/j.1365-2834.2007.00810.x PMID:18324981

Acheson Report. (1998). *Inequalities in health Report on inequalities in health did give priority for steps to be tackled.* Retrieved February 01, 2015, from http://www.ncbi.nlm.nih.gov/pmc/articles/PMC1114452/

Adamakidou, T., & Kalokairinou-Anagnostopoulou, A. (2009). The methods of financing of hospital and primary health care in Greece. *Nosileutiki*, *48*(1), 37–49.

Alexander, F. E., & Boyle, P. (Eds.). (1996). Methods for investigating localized clustering of disease. IARC Scientific Publications.

Allscripts. (2014). *Solutions that round-out all the elements offinancial health*. Retrieved December 1, 2014 from https://www.allscripts.com/en/solutions/acute-solutions/performance-management/performancemanagement.html

Allwood, J. M., & Lee, W. L. (2004). The impact of job rotation on problem solving skills. *International Journal of Production Research*, *42*(5), 865–881. doi:10.1080/00207540310001631566

Alper, S., Tjosvold, D., & Law, K. S. (1998). Interdependence and controversy in-group decision-making: Antecedents to effective self-managing teams. *Organizational Behavior and Human Decision Processes*, *74*(1), 33–52. doi:10.1006/obhd.1998.2748 PMID:9719650

Al-Quteimat, O. M., & Amer, A. M. (2014). Evidence-based pharmaceutical care: The next chapter in pharmacy practice. *Saudi Pharmaceutical Journal*. doi:10.1016/j.jsps.2014.07.010

Alturkia, M., & Khanb, T. M. (2013). A study investigating the level of satisfaction with the health services provided by the Pharmacist at ENT hospital, Eastern Region Alahsah, Kingdom of Saudi Arabia. *Saudi Pharmaceutical Journal*, *21*(3), 255–260. doi:10.1016/j.jsps.2012.09.001 PMID:23960841

Amariles, P., Sabater-Hernández, D., García-Jiménez, E., Rodríguez-Chamorro, M. Á., Prats-Más, R., Marín-Magán, F., & Faus, M. J. et al. (2012). Effectiveness of Dader Method for pharmaceutical care on control of blood pressure and total cholesterol in outpatients with cardiovascular disease or cardiovascular risk: EMDADER-CV randomized controlled trial. *Journal of Managed Care Pharmacy*, *18*(4), 311–323. doi:10.18553/jmcp.2012.18.4.311 PMID:22548691

American Medical Informatics Association (AMIA). (2014). *Nursing Informatics*. Retrieved December 1, 2014 from http://www.amia.org/programs/working-groups/nursing-informatics

Amer, S. (2007). *Towards Spatial Justice in Urban Health Services Planning – A Spatial Analytic GIS based Approach Using Dares Salaam, Tanzania as a Case Study*. The Netherlands: International Institute for Geo-Information Science and Earth.

Andalleb, S. S., Siddiqui, N., & Shahjahan, K. (2007). Patient satisfaction with health services in Bangladesh. *Health Policy and Planning*, *2*(4), 263–273. doi:10.1093/heapol/czm017 PMID:17545252

Anderson, D. R., Sweeney, D. J., & Williams, T. A. (2005). *An introduction to management science: Quantitative approaches to decision making* (11th ed.). Mason, OH: South-Western.

Andrews, R. M. (2015). Statewide hospital discharge data: Collection, use, limitations, and improvements. *Health Services Research*, *50*(1), 1273–1299. doi:10.1111/1475-6773.12343 PMID:26150118

Appelbaum, S. H., & Kamal, R. (2000). An analysis of the utilization and effectiveness of non-financial incentives in small business. *Journal of Management Development*, *19*(9), 733–763. doi:10.1108/02621710010378200

Aringhieri, R., Landa, P., Soriano, P., Tànfani, E., & Testi, A. (2015). A two level metaheuristic for the operating room scheduling and assignment problem. *Computers & Operations Research*, *54*, 21–34. doi:10.1016/j.cor.2014.08.014

Armstrong, M., & Baron, A. (1998). *Performance Management: The New Realities*. London: Institute of Personnel and Development.

Asadi-Lari, M., Tamburini, M., & Gray, D. (2004). Patients' needs, satisfaction, and health related quality of life: Towards a comprehensive model. *Health and Quality of Life Outcomes*, *2*(1Suppl 32), 1–15. doi:10.1186/1477-7525-2-32 PMID:15225377

Ashford, S. J., Lee, C., & Bobko, P. (1989). Content, cause, and consequences of job insecurity: A theory-based measure and substantive test. *Academy of Management Journal*, *32*(4), 803–829. doi:10.2307/256569

Athanassopoulos, A. D., Gounaris, C., & Sissouras, A. (1999). A descriptive assessment of the production and cost efficiency of general hospitals in Greece. *Health Care Management (Philadelphia, Pa.)*, *2*(2), 97–106. doi:10.1023/A:1019023408924 PMID:10916606

Austin, C. J., & Boxerman, S. B. (1995). *Quantitative analysis for health services administration*. Chicago, IL: Health Administration Press.

Austin, C. J., & Boxerman, S. B. (1998). *Information systems for health services administration* (5th ed.). Chicago, IL: Health Administration Press.

Austin, Z., Gregory, P. A., & Martin, J. C. (2006). Characterizing the professional relationships of community Pharmacists. *Research in Social & Administrative Pharmacy*, *2*(4), 533–546. doi:10.1016/j.sapharm.2006.02.007 PMID:17161810

Azevedo, H., & Mateus, C. (2013). Cost effects of hospital mergers in Portugal. *The European Journal of Health Economics*, *15*(9), 999–1010. doi:10.1007/s10198-013-0552-6 PMID:24379130

Bakan, I., Suseno, Y., Pinnington, A., & Money, A. (2004). The influence of financial participation and participation in decision-making on employee job attitudes. *International Journal of Human Resource Management*, *15*(3), 587–616. doi:10.1080/09585192.2004.10057654

Baluch, A. M., Salge, T. O., & Piening, E. P. (2013). Untangling the relationship between HRM and hospital performance: The mediating role of attitudinal and behavioural HR outcomes. *International Journal of Human Resource Management*, *24*(16), 3038–3061. doi:10.1080/09585192.2013.775027

Barney, J. (1991). Firm resources and sustained competitive advantage. *Journal of Management*, *17*(1), 99–120. doi:10.1177/014920639101700108

Barrett, F. A. (2002). The role of French-language contributors to the development of medical geography (1782–1933). *Social Science & Medicine*, *55*(1), 155–165. doi:10.1016/S0277-9536(01)00210-6 PMID:12137184

Bartram, T., Casimir, G., Leggat, S. G., Stanton, P., Bonias, D., & Cheng, C. (2009). *Employee participation as a moderator on the high performance work systems and the perception of quality of care relationship in a large regional Australian health servicel NOVA*. The University of Newcastle's Digital Repository.

Bartram, T., Karimi, L., Leggat, S. G., & Stanton, P. (2014). Social identification: Linking high performance work systems, psychological empowerment and patient care. *International Journal of Human Resource Management*, *25*(17), 2401–2419. doi:10.1080/09585192.2014.880152

Bateman, T., & Snell, S. (2004). *Management The new Competitive landscape* (6th ed.). New York: McGraw- Hill/ Irwin.

Bates, D. W., & Bitton, A. (2010). The future of health information technology in the patient-centered medical home. *Health Affairs*, *29*(4), 614–621. doi:10.1377/hlthaff.2010.0007 PMID:20368590

Beardwell, J., & Claydon, T. (Eds.). (2007). *Human resource management: a contemporary approach*. Pearson Education.

Becker, B., & Gerhart, B. (1996). The impact of human resource management on organizational performance: Progress and prospects. *Academy of Management Journal*, *39*(4), 779–801. doi:10.2307/256712

Becker, G. S. (1975). *Human Capital*. New York: Columbia University Press.

Bédard, Y., & Henriques, W. (2002). Modern Information Technology in Environmental Health Surveil-lance: Overview and Analysis. *Canadian Journal of Public Health, 93*, S29–S33. PMID:12425172

Bennis, W. (1976). *The Unconscious Conspiracy: Why leaders can't lead.* New York: Amacon.

Berg, B. P., Denton, B. T., Erdogan, S. A., Rohleder, T., & Huschka, T. (2014). Optimal booking and scheduling in outpatient procedure centers. *Computers & Operations Research, 50*, 24–37. doi:10.1016/j.cor.2014.04.007

Bernstein, A. B., Hing, E., Moss, A. J., Allen, K. F., Siller, A. B., & Tiggle, R. B. (2003). *Health care in American: Trends in utilization.* National Center for Health Statistics. Retrieved from http://www.cdc.gov/nchs/data/misc/healthcare.pdf

Berwick, D. (2011). Launching Accountable Care Organizations — the proposed rule for the Medicare shared savings program. *The New England Journal of Medicine, 10*(1056), 1–4. PMID:21452999

Beven, K., & Binley, A. (1992). The future of distributed models: Model calibration and uncertainty prediction. *Hydrological Processes, 6*(3), 279–298. doi:10.1002/hyp.3360060305

Bitton, A., Filer, L. A., & Jha, A. K. (2012). Health information technology in the era of care delivery reform. *Journal of the American Medical Association, 307*(24), 2593–2594. doi:10.1001/jama.2012.6663 PMID:22735426

Black Report. (1977). *The Black Report and the health divide.* Retrieved February 25, 2015, from http://history.lshtm.ac.uk/files/2013/07/The-Black-Report-and-the-Health-Divide-VB.pdf

Bleich, S. N., Özaltin, E., & Murray, C. J. L. (2009). How does satisfaction with the health-care system relate to patient experience? *Bulletin of the World Health Organization, 87*(4), 271–278. doi:10.2471/BLT.07.050401 PMID:19551235

Blendon, R. J., Schoen, C., DesRoches, C., Osborn, R., & Zapert, K. (2003). Common concerns amid diverse systems: Health care experiences in five countries. *Health Affairs, 22*(3), 106–121. doi:10.1377/hlthaff.22.3.106 PMID:12757276

Bloomberg Business Week. (2014). *Company overview of Epic Systems Corporation.* Retrieved December 10, 2014 from http://investing.businessweek.com/research/stocks/private/snapshot.asp?privcapId=6479863

Blöschl, G., & Sivapalan, M. (1995). Scale issues in hydrological modelling: A review. *Hydrological Processes, 9*(3-4), 251–290. doi:10.1002/hyp.3360090305

Blumenthal, D. (2010). Launching HITECH. *The New England Journal of Medicine, 362*(5), 382–385. doi:10.1056/NEJMp0912825 PMID:20042745

Bonias, D., Bartram, T., Leggat, S. G., & Stanton, P. (2010). Does psychological empowerment mediate the relationship between high performance work systems and patient care quality in hospitals? *Asia Pacific Journal of Human Resources, 48*(3), 319–337. doi:10.1177/1038411110381667

Boselie, P. (2010). High performance work practices in the health care sector: A Dutch case study. *International Journal of Manpower*, *31*(1), 42–58. doi:10.1108/01437721011031685

Boselie, P., Dietz, G., & Boon, C. (2005). Commonalities and contradictions in HRM and performance research. *Human Resource Management Journal*, *15*(3), 67–94. doi:10.1111/j.1748-8583.2005.tb00154.x

Bouguerra, A., Sauvey, C., & Sauer, N. (2015, May). *Mathematical model for maximizing operating rooms utilization*. Paper presented at the 15th IFAC/IEEE/IFIP/IFORS Symposium on Information Control Problems in Manufacturing INCOM'2015, Ottawa, Canada. doi:10.1016/j.ifacol.2015.06.068

Bourandas, D. (2002). *Management: Background and Current Practices*. Athens: Publications Benou. [in Geek]

Boutsioli, Z. (2011). A promising Health Care Reform in Greece. *International Journal of Healthcare Delivery Reform Initiatives*, *3*(2), 23–27. doi:10.4018/jhdri.2011040102

Boxall, P. (1996). The strategic HRM debate and the resource-based view of the firm. *Human Resource Management Journal*, *6*(3), 59–75. doi:10.1111/j.1748-8583.1996.tb00412.x

Boxall, P. F., & Purcell, J. (2003). *Strategy and Human Resource Management*. Basingstoke: Palgrave Macmillan.

Boyer, L., François, P., Doutre, E., Weil, G., & Labarere, J. (2006). Perception and use of the results of patient satisfaction surveys by care providers in a French teaching hospital. *International Journal for Quality in Health Care*, *18*(5), 359–364. doi:10.1093/intqhc/mzl029 PMID:16931825

Breaugh, J. A. (2008). Employee recruitment: Current knowledge and important areas for future research. *Human Resource Management Review*, *18*(3), 103–118. doi:10.1016/j.hrmr.2008.07.003

Brown, L. D. (1983). *Managing conflict at Organizational Interfaces*. Massachusetts: Addition-Wesley.

Brun, J. P., & Dugas, N. (2008). An analysis of employee recognition: Perspectives on human resources practices. *International Journal of Human Resource Management*, *19*(4), 716–730. doi:10.1080/09585190801953723

Buchner, T. W. (2007). Performance management theory: A look from the performer's perspective with implications for HRD. *Human Resource Development International*, *10*(1), 59–73. doi:10.1080/13678860601170294

Burke, E. K., & Riise, A. (2008, August). *Surgery Allocation and Scheduling*. Paper presented at the 7th International Conference on the Practice and Theory of Automated Timetabling, Montreal, Canada.

Burrough, P. (1986). *Geographic Information Systems for Natural Resources Assessment*. New York: Oxford University Press.

Cadogan, C. A., & Ryder, S. A. (2015). Community Pharmacists' role in benzodiazepine supply in Ireland: A questionnaire of Pharmacists' views and experiences. *International Journal of Pharmacy Practice*, *23*(6), 415–422. doi:10.1111/ijpp.12182 PMID:25756294

Cain, D. M. (1982). Is the decision to merge really a question of access to capital? *Trustee*, *35*(7), 30–32, 34–35. PMID:10256858

Campbell, R. K., & Saulie, B. A. (1998). Providing pharmaceutical care in a physician office. *Journal of the American Pharmacists Association*, *38*, 495–499. PMID:9707960

Campion, M. A., Cheraskin, L., & Stevens, M. J. (1994). Career-related antecedents and outcomes of job rotation. *Academy of Management Journal*, *37*(6), 1518–1542. doi:10.2307/256797

Campion, M. A., Palmer, D. K., & Campion, J. E. (1998). Structuring employment interviews to improve reliability, validity, and users' reactions. *Current Directions in Psychological Science*, *7*(3), 77–82. doi:10.1111/1467-8721.ep10773001

Cappelli, P., & Neumark, D. (2001). Do "high-performance" work practices improve establishment-level outcomes? *Industrial & Labor Relations Review*, *54*(4), 737–775. doi:10.1177/001979390105400401

Cardoen, B., Demeulemeester, E., & Beliën, J. (2009). Operating room planning and scheduling: A literature review. *European Journal of Operational Research*, *1016*(10), 14–25.

Carey, M. A., & Appleby, J. (2013). *How do the health law's online exchanges work? What you need to know to get started.* Retrieved December 10, 2014 from http://www.washingtonpost.com/national/health-science/how-do-the-health-laws-online-exchanges-work-what-you-need-to-know-to-get-started/2013/09/16/ef7974c8-1988-11e3-a628-7e6dde8f889d_story.html

Casanova, J., Day, K., Dorpat, D., Hendricks, B., & Wiesman Theis, L. S. (2007). Nurse-physician work relations and role expectations. *The Journal of Nursing Administration*, *37*(2), 68–70. doi:10.1097/00005110-200702000-00007 PMID:17273025

Chae, Y. M., Kim, H. S., Tark, K. C., Park, H. J., & Ho, S. H. (2003). Analysis of healthcare quality indicator using data mining and decision support system. *Expert Systems with Applications*, *2*(24), 167–172. doi:10.1016/S0957-4174(02)00139-2

Charles, D., Gabriel, M., & Furukawa, M. F. (May2014). Adoption of Electronic Health Record Systems among U.S. Non-federal Acute Care Hospitals: 2008-2013. In *ONC Data Brief, no. 16*. Washington, DC: Office of the National Coordinator for Health Information Technology.

Chassin, M. R., & Loeb, L. M. (2013). High-reliability health care: Getting there from here. *The Milbank Quarterly*, *91*(3), 459–490. doi:10.1111/1468-0009.12023 PMID:24028696

Cheng, S.-H., Wei, Y.-J., & Chang, H.-J. (2006). Quality Competition Among Hospitals: The effects of Perceived Quality and perceived Expensiveness on Health Care Consumers. *American Journal of Medical Quality*, *21*(1), 68–75. doi:10.1177/1062860605283618 PMID:16401707

Cheng, Y., Raisch, D. W., Borrego, M. E., & Gupchup, G. V. (2013). Economic, clinical, and humanistic outcomes (ECHOs) of pharmaceutical care services for minority patients: A literature review. *Research in Social & Administrative Pharmacy*, *9*(3), 311–329. doi:10.1016/j.sapharm.2012.05.004 PMID:22835704

Cheng, Y., Raisch, D. W., Borrego, M. E., & Gupchup, G. V. (2015). Development of Patient-Reported Outcomes Measure of Pharmaceutical Therapy for Quality of Life (PROMPT-QoL): A novel instrument for medication management. *Research in Social & Administrative Pharmacy*, *11*(3), 315–338. doi:10.1016/j.sapharm.2014.10.002 PMID:25453539

Chen, H. C., Chiang, R. L., & Storey, V. C. (2012). Business intelligence and analytics: From big data to big impact. *Management Information Systems Quarterly*, *36*(4), 1165–1188.

Chen, L. C., & Wallace, M. (2011). Multiskilling of frontline managers in the five star hotel industry in Taiwan. *Research and Practice in Human Resource Management*, *19*(1), 25.

Cherrington, D. (1989). *Organizational Behavior*. Simon & Schuster Inc.

Cho, I., Kim, J. K., Park, H., & Cho, N. H. (2013). The relationship between organisational culture and service quality through organisational learning framework. *Total Quality Management*, *24*(7), 753–768. doi:10.1080/14783363.2013.791100

Cho, M. H., Yoo, K. B., Lee, H. I., Lee, K.-S., Kwon, J. A., Han, K.-T., & Park, E.-C. et al. (2015). The effect of new drug pricing systems and new reimbursement guidelines on pharmaceutical expenditures and prescribing behavior among hypertensive patients in Korea. *Health Policy (Amsterdam)*, *119*(5), 604–611. doi:10.1016/j.healthpol.2015.01.002 PMID:25630635

Christie, S., and Fone, D., (2003). Equity of access to tertiary hospitals in Wales: a travel time analysis. *Journal of Public Health Medicine, 25*(4), 344-350.

Chuang, C. H., & Liao, H. U. I. (2010). Strategic human resource management in service context: Taking care of business by taking care of employees and customers. *Personnel Psychology*, *63*(1), 153–196. doi:10.1111/j.1744-6570.2009.01165.x

Chumney, E. C., & Robinson, L. C. (2006). The effects of Pharmacist interventions on patients with polypharmacy. *Pharmacy Practice*, *4*, 103–109. PMID:25247007

Chung, K. H., & Ross, M. F. (1977). Differences in motivational properties between job enlargement and job enrichment. *Academy of Management Review*, *2*(1), 113–122.

Cipolle, R. J., Strand, L. M., & Morley, P. C. (1998). *Pharmaceutical Care Practice*. New York: McGraw-Hill.

Cipolle, R. J., Strand, L. M., & Morley, P. C. (2004). *Pharmaceutical Care Practice: the Clinicians Guide*. New York: McGraw-Hill.

Citrome, L. (2011). Evidence-based medicine: It's not just about the evidence. *International Journal of Clinical Practice*, *65*(6), 633–635. doi:10.1111/j.1742-1241.2011.02669.x PMID:21564431

Classen, D. C. M., Lloyd, R. C. P., Provost, L. P., Griffin, F. A. R., & Resar, R. M. (2008). Development and Evaluation of the Institute for Healthcare Improvement Global Trigger Tool. *Journal of Patient Safety*, *4*(3), 169–177. doi:10.1097/PTS.0b013e318183a475

Clemes, M. D., Ozanne, L. K., & Laurensen, W. L. (2001). Patients' perceptions of service quality dimensions: An empirical examination of health care in New Zealand. *Health Marketing Quarterly*, *19*(1), 3–22. doi:10.1300/J026v19n01_02 PMID:11727291

Cliff, A., & Haggett, P. (1988). *Atlas of disease distributions: analytic approaches to epidemiological data*. Oxford, UK: Blackwell Reference.

Cohen, S. G., & Bailey, D. E. (1997). What makes teams work: Group effectiveness research from the shop floor to the executive suite. *Journal of Management*, *23*(3), 239–290. doi:10.1177/014920639702300303

Cohen, V., Jellinek, S. P., Hatch, A., & Motov, S. (2009). Effect of clinical Pharmacists on care in the emergency department: A systematic review. *American Journal of Health-System Pharmacy*, *66*(15), 1353–1361. doi:10.2146/ajhp080304 PMID:19635771

Colantonio, A., Moldofsky, B., Escobar, M., Vernich, L., Chipman, M., McLellan, B. (2011). Using Geographical Information Systems Mapping to Identify Areas Presenting High Risk for Traumatic Brain Injury. *Emerg Themes Epidemiol*, *4*(1), 7.

COM. (2007). *630 final*. Commission White Paper: Together for Health: A Strategic Approach for the EU 2008-2013. Retrieved February 08, 2015, from http://ec.europa.eu/health/ph_overview/Documents/strategy_wp_en.pdf

COM. (2009). *567 final*. Solidarity in health, reducing health inequalities in the EU. Retrieved February 01, 2015, from http://eur-lex.europa.eu/legal-content/EN/TXT/PDF/?uri=CELEX:52009DC0567&from=EN

COM. (2010). *2020 final*. Commission Communication, Europe 2020 Strategy, A strategy for smart, sustainable and inclusive growth. Retrieved February 06, 2015, from file:///C:/Users/user/Downloads/COM_COM(2010)2020_EN.pdf

COM. (2011). *709 final*. European Commission. Proposal for a Regulation of the European Parliament and of the Council on establishing a Health for Growth Programme, the third multi-annual programme of EU action in the field of health for the period 2014-2020. Retrieved February 05, 2015, from http://ec.europa.eu/health/programme/docs/prop_prog2014_en.pdf

COM. (2013). *83 final*. Towards Social Investment for Growth and Cohesion – including implementing the European Social Fund 2014-2020. Retrieved February 24, 2015, from http://ec.europa.eu/social/main.jsp?catId=1044&langId=en&newsId=1807&moreDocuments=yes&tableName=news

COM. (2014). *215 final*. On effective, accessible and resilient health systems. Retrieved February 08, 2015, from http://ec.europa.eu/health/healthcare/docs/com2014_215_final_en.pdf

Combs, J., Liu, Y., Hall, A., & Ketchen, D. (2006). How much do high-performance work practices matter? A meta-analysis of their effects on organizational performance. *Personnel Psychology*, *59*(3), 501–528. doi:10.1111/j.1744-6570.2006.00045.x

Constantino, C. A., & Merchant, C. S. (1996). *Designing Conflict Management Systems: A Guide to Creating Productive and Healthy*. San Francisco: Publiser Jossey- Bass.

Cooke, G. S., Tanser, F. C., Barnighausen, T. W., & Newell, M. L. (2010). Population uptake of antiretroviral treatment through primary care in rural South Africa. *BMC Public Health*, *10*(1), 585. doi:10.1186/1471-2458-10-585 PMID:20920267

Cordery, J. L., Wright, B., & Wall, T. D. (1997, April). Towards a more comprehensive and integrated approach to work design: Production uncertainty and self-managing work team performance. In *12th Annual Conference of the Society for Industrial and Organisational Psychology*.

Council Conclusions. (2006). *C 146/01*. On Common values and principles in European Union Health Systems. Retrieved February 03, 2015, from http://eur-lex.europa.eu/LexUriServ/LexUriServ.do?uri=OJ:C:2006:146:0001:0003:EN:PDF

Council Conclusions. (2010a). *Innovative approaches for chronic diseases in public health and healthcare systems*, Retrieved February 08, 2015, from http://www.idf.org/sites/default/files/Council_conclusions_7%20Dec%202010_Chronic%20Disease.pdf

Council Conclusions. (2010b). *On Equity and Health in All Policies: Solidarity in Health*. Retrieved February 06, 2015, from http://www.consilium.europa.eu/uedocs/cms_data/docs/pressdata/en/lsa/114994.pdf

Council Conclusions. (2013). *On the Reflection process on modern, responsive and sustainable health systems*. Retrieved February 11, 2015, from http://www.consilium.europa.eu/uedocs/cms_data/docs/pressdata/en/lsa/140004.pdf

Council of the European Union. (2008). *Presidency conclusions*. Retrieved February 16, 2015, from http://www.consilium.europa.eu/uedocs/cms_data/docs/pressdata/en/ec/101346.pdf

Council of the European Union. (2011). *Council conclusions: Towards modern, responsive and sustainable health systems*. Retrieved February 11, 2015, from http://www.consilium.europa.eu/uedocs/cms_data/docs/pressdata/en/lsa/122395.pdf

Council Recommendations. (1992). *92/442/EEC: of 27 July*. On the convergence of social protection objectives and policies. Retrieved February 11, 2015, from http://eur-lex.europa.eu/legal-content/EN/TXT/PDF/?uri=CELEX:31992H0442&from=GA

Cranor, C. W., & Christensen, D. B. (2003). The Asheville Project: Short-term outcomes of a community pharmacy diabetes care program. *Journal of the American Pharmacists Association*, *43*(2), 149–159. doi:10.1331/108658003321480696 PMID:23945854

Cressie, N. A. (1993). *Statistics for Spatial Data* (revised edition). John Wiley & Sons.

Cullen, J. B., Parboteeah, K. P., & Victor, B. (2003). The effects of ethical climates on organizational commitment: A two-study analysis. *Journal of Business Ethics*, *46*(2), 127–141. doi:10.1023/A:1025089819456

Dagger, T. S., Sweeney, J. C., & Johnson, L. W. (2007). A hierarchical model of health service quality: Scale development and investigation of an integrated model. *Journal of Service Research*, *10*(2), 123–142. doi:10.1177/1094670507309594

Dagger, T., & Sweeney, J. C. (2006). The effects of service evaluation on behavioral intentions and quality of life. *Journal of Service Research*, *19*(1), 3–19. doi:10.1177/1094670506289528

Dale, M. R. T. (1999). *Spatial Pattern Analysis in Plant Ecology*. Cambridge University Press. doi:10.1017/CBO9780511612589

Damiani, M., Propper, C., & Dixon, J. (2005). Mapping choice in the NHS: Cross sectional study of routinely collected data. *British Medical Journal*, *330*(7486), 284–288. doi:10.1136/bmj.330.7486.284 PMID:15695275

Davenhall, W. F. (2003). *Redefining Quality of Patient Care and Patient Safety using GIS*. Directions Magazine.

Davis, D. D. (1995). Form, function, and strategy in boundaryless organizations. In A. Howard (Ed.), *The Changing Nature of Work* (pp. 112–138). San Franciso, CA: Jossey-Bass.

Davis, K., & Newstrom, J. (1989). *Human Behavior at work. Organizational Behavior at work* (5th ed.). USA: McGraw-Hill.

Day, E. A., Blair, C., Daniels, S., Kligyte, V., & Mumford, M. D. (2006). Linking instructional objectives to the design of instructional environments: The Integrative Training Design Matrix. *Human Resource Management Review*, *16*(3), 376–395. doi:10.1016/j.hrmr.2006.05.007

Delaney, J. T., & Huselid, M. A. (1996). The impact of human resource management practices on perceptions of organizational performance. *Academy of Management Journal*, *39*(4), 949–969. doi:10.2307/256718

Delery, J. E., & Doty, D. H. (1996). Modes of theorizing in strategic human resource management: Tests of universalistic, contingency, and configurational performance predictions. *Academy of Management Journal*, *39*(4), 802–835. doi:10.2307/256713

Denton, B., Viapiano, J., & Vogl, A. (2007). Optimization of surgery sequencing and scheduling decisions under uncertainty. *Health Care Management Science*, *10*(1), 13–24. doi:10.1007/s10729-006-9005-4 PMID:17323652

Dexter, F. (1999). An operation room scheduling strategy to maximize the use of operation rooms. *Anesthesia and Analgesia*, *89*(1), 7–20. PMID:10389771

Dexter, F., Macario, A., & Traub, R. D. (1999). Which algorithm for scheduling add-on elective cases maximizes operating room utilization? Use of bin packing algorithms and fuzzy constraints in operating room management. *Anesthesiology*, *91*(5), 1491–1500. doi:10.1097/00000542-199911000-00043 PMID:10551602

Dias-Souza, M. V., & Barros, G. C. (2012). Development of Drug Use Instructional Cards for Compounded Formulations as a Complementary Patient Education Tool. *Brazilian Journal of Hosptal Pharmacy and Health Services*, *3*, 6–9.

Dias-Souza, M. V., & Barros, G. C. (2012a). Pharmaceutical Care and Clinical Monitoring of the Allergic Patient: A Case Report. *Brazilian Journal of Hospital Pharmacy and Health Services*, *3*, 338–341.

Dias-Souza, M. V., & Barros, P. H. (2012b). For a Paperless Pharmaceutical Practice: Development and Implementation of FEEDPHARMA System. *Brazilian Journal of Hospital Pharmacy and Health Services*, *3*, 20–22.

Diez-Quevedo, C., Rangil, T., Sanchez-Planell, L., Kroenke, K., & Spitzer, R. L. (2001). Validation and utility of the patient health questionnaire in diagnosing mental disorders in 1003 general hospital Spanish inpatients. *Psychosomatic Medicine*, *63*(4), 679–686. doi:10.1097/00006842-200107000-00021 PMID:11485122

Diggle, P. J. (2003). *Spatial Analysis of Spatial Point Patterns* (2nd ed.). Arnold Publishers.

Diniz-Filho, J. A. F., Bini, L. M., & Hawkins, B. A. (2003). Spatial autocorrelation and red herrings in geographical ecology. *Global Ecology and Biogeography*, *12*(1), 53–64. doi:10.1046/j.1466-822X.2003.00322.x

Directive. (2008). *115/EC, of the European Parliament and of the Council of 16 December 2008, on common standards and procedures in Member States for returning illegally staying third-country nationals*. Retrieved February 11, 2015, from http://eur-lex.europa.eu/LexUriServ/LexUriServ.do?uri=OJ:L:2008:348:0098:0107:EN:PDF

Division of Adult and Community Health, National Center for Chronic Disease Prevention and Health Promotion, Centers for Disease Control and Prevention. (n.d.). *Chronic Disease Prevention - The Burden of Chronic Disease and the Future of Public Health,2005*. Retrieved from http://www.cdc.gov/nccdphp/burden_pres/

Donabedian, A. (1966). Evaluating the quality of medical care. *The Milbank Memorial Fund Quarterly, 44*(3), 166-206.

Donabedian, A. (1978). The quality of medical care. *Science, 200*(4344), 856-864.

Donabedian, A. (1983). The quality of care in a health maintenance organization: A personal view. *Inquiry*, *20*, 218–222. PMID:6226606

Donabedian, A. (1988). The quality of care: How can it be assessed? *Journal of the American Medical Association*, *260*(12), 1743–1748. doi:10.1001/jama.1988.03410120089033 PMID:3045356

Donaldson, L. (1995). *American anti-management theories of organization: A critique of paradigm proliferation*. Cambridge, UK: Cambridge University Press.

Donaldson, L. (2001). *The contingency theory of organizations*. Thousand Oaks, CA: Sage Publications. doi:10.4135/9781452229249

Dowse, R., Ramela, T., & Browne, S. H. (2011). An illustrated leaflet containing antiretroviral information targeted for low-literate readers: Development and evaluation. *Patient Education and Counseling*, *85*(3), 508–515. doi:10.1016/j.pec.2011.01.013 PMID:21306856

Driedger, S. M., Kothari, A., Morrison, J., Sawada, M., Crighton, E., & Graham, I. (2007). Using participatory design to develop (public) health decision support systems within GIS. *International Journal of Health Geographics*, *6*(1), 53. doi:10.1186/1476-072X-6-53 PMID:18042298

Dyer, L., & Reeves, T. (1995). Human resource strategies and firm performance: What do we know and where do we need to go? *International Journal of Human Resource Management*, *6*(3), 656–670. doi:10.1080/09585199500000041

ENWHP. (2011). *The 9th initiative by the European Network for Workplace Health promotion (ENWHP) and its campaign Work. Adapted for all. Move Europe, is co-funded by the European Commission under the Public Health Programme (2008-2013)*. Retrieved February 21, 2015, from http://www.enwhp.org/enwhp-initiatives/9th-initiative-ph-work.html

Epstein, R. M., Fiscella, K., Lesser, C. S., & Stange, K. C. (2010). Why the nation needs a policy push on patient-centered health care. *Health Affairs*, *29*(8), 1489–1495. doi:10.1377/hlthaff.2009.0888 PMID:20679652

EQUI-HEALTH. (2013). *Fostering health Fostering health provision for Migrants, the provision for Migrants, the Roma and other vulnerable groups Roma and other vulnerable groups*. Retrieved February 21, 2015, from http://ec.europa.eu/health/social_determinants/docs/ev_20130121_co06_en.pdf

Erdogan, S. A., & Denton, B. T. (2011). Surgery planning and scheduling. In J. J. Cochran, L. A. Cox, P. Keskinocak, J. Kharoufeh, & J. C. Smith (Eds.), *Wiley Encyclopedia of Operations Research and Management Science*. doi:10.1002/9780470400531.eorms0861

EU Health Policy Forum Report. (2012). *Answer to DG SANCO consultation on chronic diseases*. Retrieved March 07, 2015, from http://ec.europa.eu/health/major_chronic_diseases/docs/hpf_response_consultation_cd_en.pdf

EU Summit on Chronic Diseases Conference Conclusions. (2014). Retrieved March 01, 2015, from http://ec.europa.eu/health/major_chronic_diseases/docs/ev_20140403_mi_en.pdf

EU Summit on Chronic Diseases. (2014). *Addressing the medical, social and economic burden of chronic diseases in the EU*. Retrieved March 14, 2015, from http://ec.europa.eu/health/major_chronic_diseases/docs/ev_20140403_ag_en.pdf

European Commission Conference Conclusions. (2014). *Health in Europe Making it Fairer.* Retrieved February 11, 2015, from http://ec.europa.eu/health/social_determinants/docs/ev_20140318_bkgr_note_en.pdf

European Commission Press Release. (2013). *Report on Health inequalities: gaps in life expectancy and infant mortality narrow across the EU.* Retrieved February 01, 2015, from http://europa.eu/rapid/press-release_IP-13-823_en.htm

European Commission Priorities. (2014). *A New Start for Europe: My Agenda for Jobs, Growth, Fairness and Democratic Change, Political Guidelines for the next European Commission.* Retrieved March 01, 2015, from http://ec.europa.eu/priorities/docs/pg_en.pdf#page=10

European Commission. (2003). *The health status of the European Union: Narrowing the health gap*. Luxembourg: European Communities.

European Commission. (2008). *Quality in and Equality of access to healthcare services*. Retrieved February 01, 2015, from http://www.euro.centre.org/data/1237457784_41597.pdf

European Commission. (2010). Patient safety and quality of health care. Brussels, Belgium: Author.

European Commission. (2010). *Strategy for equality between women and men 2010-2015*. Retrieved February 10, 2015, from http://ec.europa.eu/justice/gender-equality/files/strategy_equality_women_men_en.pdf Access

European Commission. (2013a). *Public Health -Improving health for all EU citizens*. Retrieved February 01, 2015, from http://ec.europa.eu/health/health_policies/docs/improving_health_for_all_eu_citizens_en.pdf

European Commission. (2013b). *Report on Health Inequalities in the EU.* Retrieved February 21, 2015, from http://ec.europa.eu/health/social_determinants/docs/healthinequalitiesineu_2013_en.pdf

European Health Forum Badgastein. (2005). *Partnerships for Health Enabling healthy choices in modern health societies.* Retrieved March 05, 2015, from http://old.ilonakickbusch.com/health-literacy/Gastein_2005.pdf

European Observatory on Health Systems and Policies. (2009). *Investing in hospitals of the future, Observatory Studies Series, No.16*. Retrieved March 10, 2015, from http://www.euro.who.int/__data/assets/pdf_file/0009/98406/E92354.pdf

European Observatory. (2012). *Health policy responses to the financial crisis of Europe*. WHO. Retrieved March 01, 2015, from http://www.euro.who.int/__data/assets/pdf_file/0009/170865/e96643.pdf

European Parliament Resolution. (2014). *On undocumented women migrants in the European Union* (2013/2115(INI)). Retrieved February 01, 2015, from http://www.europarl.europa.eu/sides/getDoc.do?pubRef=-//EP//TEXT+TA+P7-TA-2014-0068+0+DOC+XML+V0//EN EUR/RC59/R3

European Union. (2004). *Official Journal of the European Union 47(C 310/01): 1480*. Retrieved from http://eurhttp://lex.europa.eu/LexUriServ/LexUriServ.do?uri=OJ:C:2004:310:FULL:EN:PDF

Evans, W. R., & Davis, W. D. (2005). High-performance work systems and organizational performance: The mediating role of internal social structure. *Journal of Management*, *31*(5), 758–775. doi:10.1177/0149206305279370

Fakhran, S., Alhilali, L., Kale, H., & Kanal, E. (2015). Assessment of rates of acute adverse reactions to gadobenate dimeglumine: Review of more than 130,000 administrations in 7.5 years. *AJR. American Journal of Roentgenology*, *204*(4), 703–706. doi:10.2214/AJR.14.13430 PMID:25794059

Fan, D., Cui, L., Zhang, M. M., Zhu, C. J., Härtel, C. E., & Nyland, C. (2014). Influence of high performance work systems on employee subjective well-being and job burnout: Empirical evidence from the Chinese healthcare sector. *International Journal of Human Resource Management*, *25*(7), 931–950. doi:10.1080/09585192.2014.876740

Farndale, E., Hope-Hailey, V., & Kelliher, C. (2011). High commitment performance management: The roles of justice and trust. *Personnel Review*, *40*(1), 5–23. doi:10.1108/00483481111095492

Fei, H., Chu, C., Meskens, N., & Artiba, A. (2008). Solving surgical cases assignment problem by a branch-and-price approach. *International Journal of Production Economics*, *112*(1), pp, 96-108.

Fei, H., Meskens, N., & Chu, C. (2010). A planning and scheduling problem for an operating theatre using an open scheduling strategy. *Computers & Industrial Engineering*, *58*(2), 221–230. doi:10.1016/j.cie.2009.02.012

Ferguson, E. C., Maheswaran, R., & Daly, M. (2004). Road-traffic pollution and asthma – using modeled exposure assessment for routine public health surveillance. *International Journal of Health Geographics*, *3*(1), 24. doi:10.1186/1476-072X-3-24 PMID:15485575

Ferris, L. E., Williams, J. I., Llewellyn-Thomas, H. A., Basinski, A. S. H., Cohen, M. M., & Naylor, C. D. (1992). A guide to direct measures of patient satisfaction in clinical practice. *Canadian Medical Association Journal*, *146*(10), 1727–1731. PMID:1596808

Fisher, J. A., Cottingham, M. D., & Kalbaugh, C. A. (2015). Peering into the pharmaceutical "pipeline": Investigational drugs, clinical trials, and industry priorities. *Social Science & Medicine*, *131*, 322–330. doi:10.1016/j.socscimed.2014.08.023 PMID:25159693

Fitzpatrick, R., & Hopkins, A. (1983). Problems in the conceptual framework of patient satisfaction research: An empirical exploration. *Sociology of Health & Illness*, *5*(3), 297–311. doi:10.1111/1467-9566.ep10491836 PMID:10265564

Fiz, J., Duran, M., Capella, D., Carbonell, J., & Farre, M. (2011). *Cannabis* Use in Patients with Fibromyalgia: Effect on Symptoms Relief and Health-Related Quality of Life. *PLoS ONE*, *6*(4), e18440. doi:10.1371/journal.pone.0018440 PMID:21533029

Fleurant, M., Kell, R., Love, J., Jenter, C., Volk, L. A., Zhang, F., & Simon, S. R. et al. (2011). Massachusetts e-Health Project increased physicians' ability to use registries, and signals progress toward better care. *Health Affairs (Project Hope)*, *30*(7), 1256–1264. doi:10.1377/hlthaff.2010.1020 PMID:21734198

Fontenot, S. F. (2014). The affordable care act and electronic health care records: Can technology help reduce the cost of health care? *Physician Executive*, *40*(1), 68–72. PMID:24575706

Ford, P. (2013). *The Obamacare website didn't have to fail. How to do better next time.* Retrieved December 10, 2014 from http://www.businessweek.com/articles/2013-10-16/open-source-everything-the-moral-of-the-healthcare-dot-gov-debacle#p3

Forte, P. S. (1997). The High Cost of Conflict. *Nursing Economics*, *15*(3), 119–123. PMID:9305111

Fortin, M.-J., & Dale, M. R. T. (2005). *Spatial analysis: a guide for ecologists*. Cambridge: Cambridge University Press.

Fottler, M. D. (2005). Job analysis and job design. In B. J. Fried, M. D. Fottler, & J. A. Johnson (Eds.), *Human resources in healthcare* (2nd ed.; pp. 133–161). Chicago, IL: Health Administration Press.

Fottler, M. D., Ford, R. C., & Heaton, C. P. (2002). *Achieving Service Excellence*. Chicago, IL: Health Administration Press.

Fox, J. G., & Storms, D. M. (1981). A different approach to sociodemographic predictors of satisfaction with health care. *Social Science & Medicine. Part A, Medical Sociology*, *15*(5), 557–564. doi:10.1016/0271-7123(81)90079-1 PMID:6976620

Frank, L. D., Andresen, M. A., & Schmid, T. L. (2004). Obesity relationships with community design, physical activity, and time spent in cars. *American Journal of Preventive Medicine*, *27*(2), 87–96. doi:10.1016/j.amepre.2004.04.011 PMID:15261894

Frank, L. D., Engelke, P. O., & Schmidt, T. L. (2003). *Health and community design. The impact of the built environment on physical activity*. Washington, DC: Island Press.

Freedman, L. P. (2005). Achieving the MDGs: Health systems as core social institutions. *Development*, *48*(1), 19–24. doi:10.1057/palgrave.development.1100107

Freudenheim, M. (2012). Digitizing health records before it was cool. *The New York Times*. Retrieved December 10, 2014 from http://www.nytimes.com/2012/01/15/business/epic-systems-digitizing-health-records-before-it-was-cool.html?pagewanted=all&_r=1&

Fried, Y., & Ferris, G. R. (1987). The validity of the job characteristics model: A review and meta-analysis. *Personnel Psychology*, *40*(2), 287–322. doi:10.1111/j.1744-6570.1987.tb00605.x

Fronstin, P., & Roebuck, C. (2014). The cost of spousal health coverage. *Employee Benefit Research Institute*, *35*(1), 2-7. Retrieved December 1, 2014 from http://www.ebri.org/pdf/notespdf/EBRI_Notes_01_Jan-14_SpslCvg-RetPlns1.pdf

Fundamental Rights Agency (FRA) Report (2011). *EU: Right to healthcare not guaranteed in practice.* Retrieved March 05, 2015, from http://fra.europa.eu/en/press-release/2011/eu-right-healthcare-not-guaranteed-practice

Funtowwicz, S., & Ravetz. (1990). Uncertainty and Quality in Science for Policy. Kluwer Academic Publishers.

Furnham, A. (2008). *Personality and intelligence at work: Exploring and explaining individual differences at work.* Routledge. doi:10.4324/9780203938911

Gabriel, M. H., Jones, E. B., Samy, L., & King, J. (2014). Progress and challenges: Implementation and use of health information technology among critical-access hospitals. *Health Affairs*, *33*(7), 1262–1270. doi:10.1377/hlthaff.2014.0279 PMID:25006155

Gabr, W. M., & Shams, M. E. E. (2015). Adherence to medication among outpatient adolescents with epilepsy. *Saudi Pharmaceutical Journal*, *23*(1), 33–40. doi:10.1016/j.jsps.2014.05.003 PMID:25685041

Galbraith, J. R..(1973). *Designing complex organizations.* Reading, MA: Addison-Wesley Pub. Co.

Gant, J., Ichniowski, C., & Shaw, K. (2002). Social capital and organizational change in high-involvement and traditional work organizations. *Journal of Economics & Management Strategy*, *11*(2), 289–328. doi:10.1162/105864002317474576

Garets, D., & Davis, M. (2006). Electronic medical records vs. electronic health records: Yes, there is a difference. *HIMSS Analytics*. Retrieved December 10, 2014 from http://www.himss.org/files/HIMSSorg/content/files/WP_EMR_EHR.pdf

Garmon, C. (2013). Employer-provided health insurance and hospital mergers. *Health Economics, Policy, and Law*, *8*(3), 365–384. doi:10.1017/S1744133112000357 PMID:23347566

Garrett, D. G., & Bluml, B. M. (2005). Patient self-management program for diabetes: First-year clinical, humanistic, and economic outcomes. *Journal of the American Pharmacists Association*, *45*(2), 130–137. doi:10.1331/1544345053623492 PMID:15868754

Gatrell, A. C., & Löytönen, M. (Eds.). (1998). GIS and Health. Taylor and Francis.

Gaynor, M., Laudicella, M., & Propper, C. (2011). *Can governments do it better? Merger mania and hospital outcomes in the English NHS.* National Bureau of Economic Research, Working Paper No. 17608.

Gerardi, D. (2004). Using mediation techniques to manage conflict and create healthy work environments. *AACN Clinical Issues*, *15*(2), 182–195. doi:10.1097/00044067-200404000-00003 PMID:15461035

Gerard, R. (1984). Use of Location-Allocation Models for Improving Geographic Accessibility of Rural Services in Developing Countries. *International Regional Science Review*, *9*(3), 217–240. doi:10.1177/016001768400900303

Gerchak, Y., Gupta, D., & Henig, M. (1996). Reservation planning for elective surgery under uncertain demand for emergency surgery. *Management Science*, *42*(3), 321–334. doi:10.1287/mnsc.42.3.321

Gerhart, B., & Rynes, S. (2003). *Compensation: Theory, evidence, and strategic implications.* SAGE publications.

Gesler, W. M., Hayes, M., Arcury, T., Skelly, A. H., Nash, S., & Soward, A. C. M. (2004). Use of mapping technology in health intervention research. *Nursing Outlook*, *52*(3), 142–146. doi:10.1016/j.outlook.2004.01.009 PMID:15197363

Gilbert, G. R., Veloutsou, C., Goode, M. M. H., & Moutinho, L. (2004). Measuring customer satisfaction in the fast food industry: A cross-national approach. *Journal of Services Marketing*, *18*(4/5), 371–383. doi:10.1108/08876040410548294

Gill, L., & White, L. (2009). A critical review on patient satisfaction. *Leadership in Health Services*, *22*(1), 8–19. doi:10.1108/17511870910927994

GIS Lounge. (2012). Retrieved from http://www.gislounge.com/history-of-gis/

Gittell, J. H., Seidner, R., & Wimbush, J. (2010). A relational model of how high-performance work systems work. *Organization Science*, *21*(2), 490–506. doi:10.1287/orsc.1090.0446

Glass, G. E., Schwartz, B. S., Morgan, J. M. I. III, Johnson, D. T., Noy, P. M., & Israel, E. (1995). Environmental risk factors for Lyme disease identified with geographic information systems. *American Journal of Public Health*, *85*(7), 944–948. doi:10.2105/AJPH.85.7.944 PMID:7604918

Glassop, L. I. (2002). The organizational benefits of teams. *Human Relations*, *55*(2), 225–249. doi:10.1177/0018726702055002184

Golden, B. (2006). Transforming healthcare organizations. *Healthcare Quarterly*, *10*(sp), 10–19. doi:10.12927/hcq..18490 PMID:17163111

Goleman, D. (1995). *Emotional intelligence*. New York: Bantam Books.

Goleman, D. (1997). *Emotional Intelligence*. Athens, Greece: Editions Ellinika Grammata. (in Greek)

Goleman, D. (1998). *Working with emotional intelligence*. London: Bloomsbury.

Gonzalez, N., Quintana, J. M., Bilbao, A., Escobar, A., Aizpuru, F., Thompson, A., & de la Sierra, E. et al. (2005). Development and validation of an in-patient satisfaction questionnaire. *International Journal for Quality in Health Care*, *17*(6), 465–472. doi:10.1093/intqhc/mzi067 PMID:16100222

Goode, C. J., Ibarra, V., Blegen, M. A., Boshart-Yoder, T., Cram, E., Finn, L., & Anderson-Bruner, J. et al. (1993). What kind of recognition do staff nurses want? *AJN The American Journal of Nursing*, *93*(5), 64–68. PMID:8488903

Goodwin, P. J., Black, J. T., Bordeleau, L. J., & Ganz, P. A. (2003). Health-related quality-of-life measurement in randomized clinical trials in breast cancer--taking stock. *Journal of the National Cancer Institute*, *95*(4), 263–281. doi:10.1093/jnci/95.4.263 PMID:12591983

Goovaerts, P. (1998). Geostatistical tools for characterizing the spatial variability of microbiological and physico-chemical soil properties. *Biology and Fertility of Soils*, *27*(4), 315–334. doi:10.1007/s003740050439

Goovaerts, P. (2001). Geostatistical modelling of uncertainty in soil science. *Geoderma*, *103*(1), 3–26. doi:10.1016/S0016-7061(01)00067-2

Gourley, G. A., Portner, T. S., Gourley, D. R., Rigolosi, E. L., Holt, J. M., & Solomon, D. K. (1998). Humanistic outcomes in the hypertension and COPD arms of a multicenter outcomes study. *Journal of the American Pharmacists Association*, *38*, 586–597. PMID:9782692

Gourley, G. K., Gourley, D. R., Rigolosi, E., Reed, P., Solomon, D. K., & Washington, E. (2001). Development and validation of the pharmaceutical care satisfaction questionnaire. *The American Journal of Managed Care*, *7*, 461–466. PMID:11388126

Grauman, D. M., & Tam, M. P. (2012). The urge to merge. *Healthcare Financial Management*, *66*(11), 76–82, 84, 86. PMID:23173365

Greek Gazette, Law 1397/1983. National Health System. Gazette 143A / 1983.

Guinet, A., & Chaabane, S. (2003). Operating theatre planning. *International Journal of Production Economics*, *85*(1), 69–81. doi:10.1016/S0925-5273(03)00087-2

Hackman, J. R., & Oldham, G. R. (1975). Development of the job diagnostic survey. *The Journal of Applied Psychology*, *60*(2), 159–170. doi:10.1037/h0076546

Hackman, J. R., & Oldham, G. R. (1976). Motivation through the design of work: Test of a theory. *Organizational Behavior and Human Performance*, *16*(2), 250–279. doi:10.1016/0030-5073(76)90016-7

Hall, W. (n.d.). *Just another Medical Geography*. Retrieved from http://healthcybermap.org/HGeo/pg1_1.htm

Hall, J. A., Milburn, M. A., & Epstein, A. M. (1993). A Causal Model of Health Status and Satisfaction With Medical Care. *Medical Care*, *31*(1), 84–94. doi:10.1097/00005650-199301000-00007 PMID:8417273

Hamrosi, K. K., Raynor, D. K., & Aslani, P. (2014). Pharmacist, general practitioner and consumer use of written medicine information in Australia: Are they on the same page? *Research in Social & Administrative Pharmacy*, *10*(4), 656–668. doi:10.1016/j.sapharm.2013.10.002 PMID:24239213

Hans, E. W., Wullink, G., Van Houdenhoven, M., & Kazemier, G. (2008). Robust surgery loading. *European Journal of Operational Research*, *185*(3), 1038–1050. doi:10.1016/j.ejor.2006.08.022

Han, T. S., Chiang, H. H., & Chang, A. (2010). Employee participation in decision making, psychological ownership and knowledge sharing: Mediating role of organizational commitment in Taiwanese high-tech organizations. *International Journal of Human Resource Management*, *21*(12), 2218–2233. doi:10.1080/09585192.2010.509625

Harmon, J., Scotti, D. J., Behson, S., Farias, G., Petzel, R., Neuman, J. H., & Keashly, L. (2003). Effects of high-involvement work systems on employee satisfaction and service costs in veterans healthcare. *Journal of Healthcare Management*, *48*(6), 393–405. PMID:14671948

Hart, A., & McCulloch, B. (2004). *Dengue and Data Management. In Empowering Business For Tomorrow*. Brisbane: Spatial Sciences Institute.

Hawkins, L. A., & Firek, C. J. (2014). Testing a novel pictorial medication sheet to improve adherence in veterans with heart failure and cognitive impairment. *Heart & Lung: The Journal of Acute and Critical Care*, *43*(6), 486–493. doi:10.1016/j.hrtlng.2014.05.003 PMID:24928185

Hawthorne, G. (2006). *Review of Patient Satisfaction Measures*. Canberra: Australian Government Department of Health and Ageing.

Health Care Financial Management Association. (2005). *Achieving operating room efficiency through process integration*. Technical Report, US National Library of Medicine, National Institutes of Health. *PubMed*, *57*(3), 113–119.

Hearld, L., Alexander, J., Fraser, I., & Jiang, H. (2008). How do hospital organizational structure and processes affect quality of care? *Medical Care Research and Review*, *65*(3), 259–299. doi:10.1177/1077558707309613 PMID:18089769

Heidegger, T., Saal, D., & Nuebling, M. (2006). Patient satisfaction with anaesthesia care: What is patient satisfaction, how should it be measured, and what is the evidence for assuring high patient satisfaction. *Best Practice & Research. Clinical Anaesthesiology*, *20*(2), 331–346. doi:10.1016/j.bpa.2005.10.010 PMID:16850781

Hendel, T., Fish, M., & Galon, V. (2005). Leadership style and choice of strategy in conflict management among Israeli nurse managers in general hospitals. *Journal of Nursing Management*, *13*(2), 137–146. doi:10.1111/j.1365-2934.2004.00525.x PMID:15720483

Hepler, C. D. (1996). Pharmaceutical Care. *Pharmacy World & Science*, *18*(6), 233–236. doi:10.1007/BF00735965 PMID:9010887

Hepler, C. D., & Strand, L. M. (1990). Opportunities and responsibilities in pharmaceutical care. *American Journal of Hospital Pharmacy*, *47*, 533–543. PMID:2316538

Herzberg, F. I. (1966). *Work and the nature of man*. Cleveland: World.

Hillestad, R., Bigelow, J., Bower, A., Girosi, F., Meili, R., Scoville, R., & Taylor, R. E. M. R. (2005). Can electronic medical record systems transform health care? Potential health benefits, savings, and costs. *Health Affairs*, *24*(5), 1103–1117. doi:10.1377/hlthaff.24.5.1103 PMID:16162551

Historica Canada. (1965). Retrieved from The Canada Geographic Information System (CGIS): http://www.thecanadianencyclopedia.ca/en/article/geographic-information-systems/

Hjalmars, U., Kulldorff, M., & Gustafsson, G. (1994). Risk of acute childhood leukaemia in Sweden after the Chernobyl reactor accident. *BMJ (Clinical Research Ed.)*, *309*(6948), 154–157. doi:10.1136/bmj.309.6948.154 PMID:8044093

Hjalmars, U., Kulldorff, M., Gustafsson, G., & Nagarwalla, N. (1996). Childhood leukaemia in Sweden: Using GIS and a spatial scan statistic for cluster detection. *Statistics in Medicine*, *15*(7-9), 707–715. doi:10.1002/(SICI)1097-0258(19960415)15:7/9<707::AID-SIM242>3.0.CO;2-4 PMID:9132898

Hjalmars, U., Kulldorff, M., Wahlqvist, Y., & Lannering, B. (1999). Increased incidence rates but no space-time clustering of childhood astrocytoma in Sweden, 1973-1992: A population-based study of pediatric brain tumors. *Cancer*, *85*(9), 2077–2090. doi:10.1002/(SICI)1097-0142(19990501)85:9%3C2077::AID-CNCR27%3E3.0.CO;2-4 PMID:10223251

Holroyd-Leduc, J., Lorenzetti, D., Straus, S. E., Sykes, L., & Quan, H. (2011). The impact of the electronic medical record on structure, process, and outcomes within primary care: A systematic review of the evidence. *Journal of the American Medical Informatics Association: JAMIA*, *18*(6), 732–737. doi:10.1136/amiajnl-2010-000019 PMID:21659445

Holtzman, C. W., Brady, K. A., & Yehia, B. R. (2015). Retention in Care and Medication Adherence: Current Challenges to Antiretroviral Therapy Success. *Drugs*, *75*(5), 445–454. doi:10.1007/s40265-015-0373-2 PMID:25792300

Hood, C. (1995). The new public management in the 1980s: Variations on a theme. *Journal of Accounting. Organizations and Society*, *20*(2/3), 93–109. doi:10.1016/0361-3682(93)E0001-W

Ho, W. H., Chang, C. S., Shih, Y. L., & Liang, R. D. (2009). Effects of job rotation and role stress among nurses on job satisfaction and organizational commitment. *BMC Health Services Research*, *9*(1), 8. doi:10.1186/1472-6963-9-8 PMID:19138390

Hsiao, C. J., & Hing, E. (2014). *Use and characteristics of electronic health record systems among office-based physician practices: United States, 2001-2013. NCHS data brief, no. 143*. Hyattsville, MD: National Center for Health Statistics.

Huang, C.-W., Lin, Y.-P., Chiang, L.-C., & Wang, Y.-C. (2013). *Using CV-GLUE Procedure in Analysis of Wetland Model Predictive Uncertainty*. Submiited.

Huh, W. T., Liu, N., & Truong, V. A. (2013). Multi-resource allocation scheduling in dynamic environments. *Manufacturing & Service Operations Management*, *15*(2), 280–291. doi:10.1287/msom.1120.0415

Hulin, C. L., & Blood, M. R. (1968). Job enlargement, individual differences, and worker responses. *Psychological Bulletin*, *69*(1), 41–55. doi:10.1037/h0025356

Hulka, B., Zyzanski, S., Cassel, J., & Thompson, S. (1970). Scale for the measurement of attitudes towards physicians and primary medical care. *Medical Care*, *8*(5), 429–436. doi:10.1097/00005650-197009000-00010 PMID:4920640

Huselid, M. A. (1995). The impact of human resource management practices on turnover, productivity, and corporate financial performance. *Academy of Management Journal*, *38*(3), 635–672. doi:10.2307/256741

Huselid, M. A., Jackson, S. E., & Schuler, R. S. (1997). Technical and strategic human resources management effectiveness as determinants of firm performance. *Academy of Management Journal*, *40*(1), 171–188. doi:10.2307/257025

Huynen, M. M., Martens, P., & Hilderink, H. B. (2005). The health impacts of globalization: A conceptual framework. *Globalization and Health*, *1*(1), 14. doi:10.1186/1744-8603-1-14 PMID:16078989

Hyde, P., Sparrow, P., Boaden, R., & Harris, C. (2013). High performance HRM: NHS employee perspectives. *Journal of Health Organization and Management*, *27*(3), 296–311. doi:10.1108/JHOM-10-2012-0206 PMID:23885395

Iacobuţă, A. O. (2012). Patients' evaluation of access and quality of healthcare in EU countries: A comparative analysis. *Procedia: Social and Behavioral Sciences*, *62*, 896–900. doi:10.1016/j.sbspro.2012.09.151

iHealthBeat. (2011). *Texas curbs spending by $1B by deploying EHRs, telehealth in prisons.* Retrieved December 1, 2014 from http://www.ihealthbeat.org/articles/2011/8/26/texas-curbs-spending-by-1b-by-deploying-ehrs-telehealth-in-prisons

Institute of Medicine (U.S.). (2001). Crossing the quality chasm: A new health system for the 21st century. Washington, DC: National Academy Press.

International Organization for Migration. (2005). *Health and Migration: Bridging the Gap.* Geneva: Migration Policy and Research Programme.

Isetts, B. J., Brown, L. M., Schondelmeyer, S. W., & Lenarz, L. A. (2003). Quality Assessment of a Collaborative Approach for Decreasing Drug-Related Morbidity and Achieving Therapeutic Goals. *Archives of Internal Medicine*, *163*(15), 1813–1820. doi:10.1001/archinte.163.15.1813 PMID:12912717

Iversen, L., & Sabroe, S. (1988). Psychological weil-being among unemployed and employed people after a company closedown: A longitudinal study. *The Journal of Social Issues*, *44*(4), 141–152. doi:10.1111/j.1540-4560.1988.tb02096.x

Jameson, J. K. (1999). Toward a comprehensive model for the assessment and management of intraorganizational conflict: Developing the framework. *The International Journal of Conflict Management*, *10*(3), 268–294. doi:10.1108/eb022827

Jankauskienė, D., & Jankauskaitė, I. (2011). Access and quality of health care system by opinion of patients in ten European countries. *Management in Health, 25*(3), 31–39.

Janssen, O., & Van de Vliert, E. (1996). Concern For the Other's Goals: Key to (DE-) Escalation of Conflict. *The International Journal of Conflict Management, 7*(2), 99–120. doi:10.1108/eb022777

Jehn, K. A. (1997). A Qualitative Analysis of Conflict Types and Dimensions in Organizational Groups. *Administrative Science Quarterly, 42*(3), 530–557. doi:10.2307/2393737

Jensen, J. B. (2003). Parameter and Uncertainty Estimation in Groundwater Modelling. Aalborg: Aalborg University.

Johns, G. (1993). Constraints on the adoption of psychology-based personnel practices: Lessons from organizational innovation. *Personnel Psychology, 46*(3), 569–592. doi:10.1111/j.1744-6570.1993.tb00885.x

Jordan, H., Roderick, P., Martin, D., & Barnett, S. (2004). Distance, reality and the need for care: Access to health services in South West England. *International Journal of Health Geographics, 3*(1), 21. doi:10.1186/1476-072X-3-21 PMID:15456514

Jung, J. Y., & Lim, S. G. (2007). Project categorization, prioritization, and execution based on six sigma concept: A case study of operational improvement project. *Project Management Journal, 38*(1), 55–60.

Kaiser Family Foundation. (2013). Employer Health Benefits: 2013 Summary of Findings. *The Kaiser Family Foundation and Health Research and Educational Trust*. Retrieved December 1, 2014 from http://kaiserfamilyfoundation.files.wordpress.com/2013/08/8466-employer-health-benefits-2013_summary-of-findings2.pdf

Kalogirou, S., & Foley, R. (2006). Health, Place & Hanly: Modelling Accessibility to Hospitals in Ireland. *Irish Geography, 39*(1), 52–68. doi:10.1080/00750770609555866

Kaló, Z., Holtorf, A. P., Alfonso-Cristancho, R., Shen, J., Ágh, T., Inotai, A., & Brixner, D. (2015). Need for multicriteria evaluation of generic drug policies. *Value in Health, 18*(2), 346–351. doi:10.1016/j.jval.2014.12.012 PMID:25773570

Kanigel, R. (1997). Taylor-made. *The Sciences, 37*(3), 1–5. doi:10.1002/j.2326-1951.1997.tb03309.x

Kaplan, R., & Norton, D. (1992). The balanced scorecard: Measures that drive performance. *Harvard Business Review, 70*(1), 71–79.

Kaplan, R., & Norton, D. (1996). *The balanced scorecard: Translating strategy into action.* Boston: Harvard Business School Press.

Kash, B. A., Spaulding, A., Johnson, C. E., & Gamm, L. (2014). Success factors for strategic change initiatives: A qualitative study of healthcare administrators' perspectives. *Journal of Healthcare Management, 59*(1), 65–80. PMID:24611428

Kassardjian, C. D., Gardner-Nix, J., Dupak, K., Barbati, J., & Lam-McCullock, J. (2008). Validating PRISM (Pictorial Representation of Illness and Self Measure) as a Measure of Suffering in Chronic Non-Cancer Pain Patients. *The Journal of Pain*, *9*(12), 1135–1143. doi:10.1016/j.jpain.2008.06.016 PMID:18755635

Katona, K., & Canoy, M. (2013). Welfare standards in hospital mergers. *The European Journal of Health Economics*, *14*(4), 573–586. doi:10.1007/s10198-012-0403-x PMID:22688439

Katz, R. W. (2002). Techniques for estimating uncertainty in climate change scenarios and impact studies. *Climate Research*, *20*, 167–185. doi:10.3354/cr020167

Kaufmann, C. P., Stämpfli, D., Hersberger, K. E., & Lampert, M. L. (2015). Determination of risk factors for drug-related problems: A multidisciplinary triangulation process. *BMJ Open*, *5*(3), e006376. doi:10.1136/bmjopen-2014-006376 PMID:25795686

Kaushal, R., Shojania, K. G., & Bates, D. W. (2003). Effects of computerized physician order entry and clinical decision support systems on medication safety: A systematic review. *Archives of Internal Medicine*, *163*(12), 1409–1416. doi:10.1001/archinte.163.12.1409 PMID:12824090

Kaymaz, K. (2010). The effects of job rotation practices on motivation: A research on managers in the automotive organizations. *Business and Economics Research Journal*, *1*(3), 69–85.

Khan, M. U., Khan, A. N., Ahmed, F. R., Feroz, Z., Rizvi, S. A., Shah, S., & Adil, Z. et al. (2013). Patients' opinion of Pharmacists and their roles in healthcare system in Pakistan. *Journal of Young Pharmacists*, *5*(3), 90–94. doi:10.1016/j.jyp.2013.08.001 PMID:24396248

Kheir, N. M., van Mil, J. W. F., Shaw, J. P., & Sheridan, J. L. (2004). Health-related quality of life measurement in pharmaceutical care - Targeting an outcome that matters. *Pharmacy World & Science*, *26*(3), 125–128. doi:10.1023/B:PHAR.0000026811.37414.4f PMID:15230357

Kiel, P. J., & McCord, A. D. (2005). Pharmacist impact on clinical outcomes in a diabetes disease management program via collaborative practice. *The Annals of Pharmacotherapy*, *39*(11), 1828–1832. doi:10.1345/aph.1G356 PMID:16219894

Kinnunen, U., & Nätti, J. (1994). Job insecurity in Finland: Antecedents and consequences. *European Journal of Work and Organizational Psychology*, *4*(3), 297–321. doi:10.1080/13594329408410490

Kitano, H. (2004). Biological robustness. *Nature Reviews. Genetics*, *5*(11), 826–837. doi:10.1038/nrg1471 PMID:15520792

Kitano, H. (2007). Innovation: A robustness-based approach to systems-oriented drug design. *Nature Reviews. Drug Discovery*, *4*(3), 202–210. doi:10.1038/nrd2195 PMID:17318209

Kjekshus, L.E., Bernstrom, V.H., Dahl, E., & Lorentzen, T. (2014). The effect of hospital mergers on long-term sickness absence among hospital employees: a fixed effects multivariate regression analysis using panel data. *BMC Health Serv Res, 3*(14), 50. doi:.10.1186/1472-6963-14-50

Klepper, O. (1997). Multivariate aspects of model uncertainty analysis: Tools for sensitivity analysis and calibration. *Ecological Modelling*, *101*(1), 1–13. doi:10.1016/S0304-3800(96)01922-9

Knapp, K. K., Okamoto, M. P., & Black, B. L. (2005). ASHP survey of ambulatory care pharmacy practice in health systems – 2004. *American Journal of Health-Systems Pharmacists*, *62*, 274–284. PMID:15719585

Koch, R. (2015). From business intelligence to predictive analytics. *Strategic Finance*, *97*(1), 56–57.

Koksalmis, E., Hancerliogullari, K. O., & Hancerliogullari, G. (2014, May). *How to schedule surgical operations into operating rooms? An application in Turkey*. Paper presented at the IIE Industrial and Systems Engineering Research Conference, Montreal, Canada.

Koutis, X. (2011). *Notes to the Postgraduate Studies Program "Applied Public Health"*. Athens, Greece: National School of Public Health. (in Greek)

Kraimer, M. L., Wayne, S. J., Liden, R. C., & Sparrowe, R. T. (2005). The role of job security in understanding the relationship between employees' perceptions of temporary workers and employees' performance. *The Journal of Applied Psychology*, *90*(2), 389–398. doi:10.1037/0021-9010.90.2.389 PMID:15769247

Krakauer, J. (2012). *The business intelligence competency center: Enabling continuous improvement in performance management*. Oracle Corporation. Retrieved from www.oracle.com/.../bicc-white-paper-1-2012-148691

Kraut, A. I. (2006). *Getting action from organizational surveys: New concepts, technologies, and applications*. San Francisco, CA: Jossey-Bass.

Kripalani, S., Robertson, R., Love-Ghaffari, M., Henderson, L. E., Praska, J., Strawder, A., & Jacobson, T. A. et al. (2007). Development of an illustrated medication schedule as a low-literacy patient education tool. *Patient Education and Counseling*, *66*(3), 368–377. doi:10.1016/j.pec.2007.01.020 PMID:17344015

Kroenke, K., Spitzer, R. L., & Williams, J. B. (2001). The PHQ-9: Validity of a brief depression severity measure. *Journal of General Internal Medicine*, *16*(9), 606–613. doi:10.1046/j.1525-1497.2001.016009606.x PMID:11556941

Kruk, M. E., & Freedman, L. P. (2008). Assessing health system performance in developing countries: A review of the literature. *Health Policy (Amsterdam)*, *85*(3), 263–276. doi:10.1016/j.healthpol.2007.09.003 PMID:17931736

Krumholz, H. M. (2014). Big data and new knowledge in medicine: The thinking, training, and tools needed for a learning health system. *Health Affairs*, *33*(7), 1163–1170. doi:10.1377/hlthaff.2014.0053 PMID:25006142

Krupinski, E. A. (2008). Telemedicine for home health and the new patient: When do we really need to go to the hospital? *Studies in Health Technology and Informatics*, *29*(4), 614–621. PMID:18305331

Kuhmmer, R., Lima, K. M., Ribeiro, R. A., Hammes, L. S., Bastos, G., & Cotta de Souza, M. et al. (2015). Effectiveness of pharmaceutical care at discharge in the emergency department: Study protocol of a randomized controlled trial. *Trials*, *16*(1), 579. doi:10.1186/s13063-015-0579-3 PMID:25888343

Ku, L., Jones, E., Finnegan, B., Shin, P., & Rosenbaum, S. (2009). *How is the primary care safety net faring in Massachusetts? Community health centers in the midst of health reform (Issue paper no. 7878)*. Washington, DC: Kaiser Commission on Medicaid and the Uninsured.

Kulldorff, M. (1998). Statistical methods for spatial epidemiology: Tests for randomness. In GIS and Health. Taylor and Francis.

Lada, P., & Delgado, G. (2007). Documentation of Pharmacists' interventions in an emergency department and associated cost avoidance. *American Journal of Health-System Pharmacy*, *64*(1), 63–68. doi:10.2146/ajhp050213 PMID:17189582

Lamiri, M., Xie, X., Dolgui, A., & Grimaud, F. (2008). A stochastic model for operating room planning with elective and emergency demand for surgery. *European Journal of Operational Research*, *185*(3), 1026–1037. doi:10.1016/j.ejor.2006.02.057

Lang, L. (2000). *GIS for Health Organisations*. ESRI Press.

Larsen, D. L., Attkisson, C. C., Hargreaves, W. A., & Nguyen, T. D. (1979). Assessment of client/patient satisfaction: Development of a general scale. *Evaluation and Program Planning*, *2*(3), 197–207. doi:10.1016/0149-7189(79)90094-6 PMID:10245370

Latkin, C., Glass, G. E., & Duncan, T. (1998). Using geographic information systems to assess spatial patterns of drug use, selection bias and attrition among a sample of injection drug users. *Drug and Alcohol Dependence*, *50*(2), 167–175. doi:10.1016/S0376-8716(98)00025-8 PMID:9649968

Lawrence, P. R., & Lorsch, J. W. (1967). Organization and environment; managing differentiation and integration. Boston: Harvard University.

LBISHM. (2005). *Project Summary on Migrant-Friendly Hospitals*. WHO Collaboration Centre for Health Promotion on Hospitals and Health Care, Institute for Sociology, University Vienna.

Leana, C. R., & Van Buren, H. J. (1999). Organizational social capital and employment practices. *Academy of Management Review*, *24*(3), 538–555.

Lee, P.-M., Khong, P., & Ghista, D. N. (2006). Impact of deficient healthcare service quality. *The TQM Magazine*, *18*(6), 563–571. doi:10.1108/09544780610707075

Lee, R. L. (2009). *Economics for healthcare managers* (2nd ed.). Chicago, IL: Health Administration Press.

Lee, S. M., Lee, D., & Kang, C. Y. (2012). The impact of high-performance work systems in the health-care industry: Employee reactions, service quality, customer satisfaction, and customer loyalty. *Service Industries Journal*, *32*(1), 17–36. doi:10.1080/02642069.2010.545397

Leininger, C. J., & Seaman, L. H. (2000). Selecting clinical quality improvement projects: Getting a bigger return for your investment. *Topics in Health Information Management*, *20*(3), 27–34. PMID:10747432

Lemieux-Charles, L. (1994). Physicians in health care management: 10 Managing conflict through negotiation. *Health Care Management. Canadian Medical Association Journal*, *151*(8), 1129–1132. PMID:7922944

Leplege, A., & Hunt, S. (1997). The problem of quality of life in medicine. *Journal of the American Medical Association*, *278*(1), 47–50. doi:10.1001/jama.1997.03550010061041 PMID:9207338

Lettieri, E., Bartoli, L., & Masella, C. (2013). Coordinating intra-sector services in healthcare: Requirements and elements that managers should take into account. *European Management Journal*, *31*(6), 591–601. doi:10.1016/j.emj.2013.05.004

Levin, D. Z., & Cross, R. (2004). The strength of weak ties you can trust: The mediating role of trust in effective knowledge transfer. *Management Science*, *50*(11), 1477–1490. doi:10.1287/mnsc.1030.0136

Leviss, J., Kremsdorf, R., & Mohaideen, M. (2006). The CMIO – A new leader for health systems. *Journal of the American Medical Informatics Association*, *13*(5), 573–578. doi:10.1197/jamia.M2097 PMID:16799119

Lewicki, R., Saunders, D., & Minton, J. (2004). The nature of the negotiations. Athens Publications Kritiki. (In Greek)

Lewin, B. (2013). Patient satisfaction with physician responses during interactions prompted by pharmaceutical advertisements. *The Social Science Journal*, *50*(4), 491–500. doi:10.1016/j.soscij.2013.03.002

Liaropoulos, L. (2007). *Organization of Health Services and Health Systems*. Athens, Greece: Publication Bita. (In Greek)

Liaropoulos, L. (2010). *International Health Systems. Organization of Health Services and Health Systems*. Athens, Greece: Publication Bita. (In Greek)

Li, J. M., Yang, J. S., & Wu, H. H. (2008). Improving service quality and organisation performance through human resource practices. *Total Quality Management*, *19*(9), 970–985.

Likert, R., & Likert, J. G. (1976). *New ways of managing conflict*. New York: McGraw-Hill.

Lin, B., & Kelly, E. (1995). Methodological issues in patient satisfaction surveys. *International Journal of Health Care Quality Assurance*, *8*(6), 32–37. doi:10.1108/09526869510098840 PMID:10165404

Linder-Pelz, S. (1982). Toward a theory of patient satisfaction. *Social Science & Medicine*, *16*(5), 577–582. doi:10.1016/0277-9536(82)90311-2 PMID:7100990

Lin, G., Allen, D., & Penning, M. (2002). Examining distance effects on hospitalizations using GIS: A study of three health regions in British Columbia, Canada. *Environment & Planning A*, *34*(11), 2037–2053. doi:10.1068/a3528

Lin, Y. P., Yeh, M. S., Deng, D. P., & Wang, Y. C. (2008a). Geostatistical approaches and optimal additional sampling schemes for spatial patterns and future sampling of bird diversity. *Global Ecology and Biogeography*, *17*(2), 175–188. doi:10.1111/j.1466-8238.2007.00352.x

Lin, Y.-P., Chang, T.-K., & Teng, T.-P. (2001). Characterization of soil lead by comparing of sequential Gaussian simulation, simulated annealing simulation and kriging methods. *Environmental Geology*, *41*(1-2), 189–199. doi:10.1007/s002540100382

Lin, Y.-P., Chu, H.-J., Huang, Y.-L., Cheng, B.-Y., & Chang, T.-K. (2011). Modeling spatial uncertainty of heavy metal content in soil by conditional Latin hypercube sampling and geostatistical simulation. *Environmental Earth Sciences*, *62*(2), 299–311. doi:10.1007/s12665-010-0523-5

Lin, Y.-P., Wu, P.-J., & Hong, N.-M. (2008b). The effects of changing the resolution of land-use modeling on simulations of land-use patterns and hydrology for a watershed land-use planning assessment in Wu-Tu, Taiwan. *Landscape and Urban Planning*, *87*(1), 54–66. doi:10.1016/j.landurbplan.2008.04.006

Locke, E., Alavi, M., & Wagner, J. (1997). Participation in deci sion-making: An information exchange perspective. In G. Ferris (Ed.), *Research in personal and human re sources management* (Vol. 15, pp. 293–331). Greenwich, CT: JAI Press.

Loi, R., Ngo, H. Y., Zhang, L., & Lau, V. P. (2011). The interaction between leader–member exchange and perceived job security in predicting employee altruism and work performance. *Journal of Occupational and Organizational Psychology*, *84*(4), 669–685. doi:10.1348/096317910X510468

Lovett, A., Haynes, R., Sünnenberg, G., & Gale, S. (2002). Car travel time and accessibility by bus to general practitioner services: A study using patient registers and GIS. *Social Science & Medicine*, *55*(1), 97–111. doi:10.1016/S0277-9536(01)00212-X PMID:12137192

Lovett, A., Poots, A. J., Clements, J. T. C., Green, S. A., Samarasundera, E., & Bell, D. (2014). Using geographical information systems and cartograms as a health service quality improvement tool. *Spatial and Spatio-temporal Epidemiology*, *10*, 67–74. doi:10.1016/j.sste.2014.05.004 PMID:25113592

Maastricht University. (2009). *Europe, gender inequality and global health.* Retrieved February 01, 2015, from http://www.globalhealtheurope.org/index.php/resources/glossary/values/72-europe-gender-inequality-and-global-health

MacDuffie, J. P. (1995). Human resource bundles and manufacturing performance: Organizational logic and flexible production systems in the world auto industry. *Industrial & Labor Relations Review*, *48*(2), 197–221. doi:10.1177/001979399504800201

Mackenbach, J. (2007). *Economic implications of socio-economic inequalities in health in the European Union*. European Commission report. Retrieved February 05, 2015, from http://ec.europa.eu/health/ph_determinants/socio_economics/documents/socioeco_inequalities_en.pdf

Mackintosh, M. (2001). Do health care systems contribute to inequalities. In D. A. Leon & G. Walt (Eds.), *Poverty, inequality and health: an international perspective*. Oxford: Oxford University Press.

Magerlein, J. M., & Martin, J. B. (1978). Surgical demand scheduling: A review. *Health Services Research*, *13*, 418–433. PMID:367987

Maher, A. R., Maglione, M., Bagley, S., Suttorp, M., Hu, J.-H., Ewing, B., & Shekelle, P. G. et al. (2011). Efficacy and comparative effectiveness of atypical antipsychotic medications for off-label uses in adults: A systematic review and metaanalysis. *Journal of the American Medical Association*, *306*(12), 1359–1369. doi:10.1001/jama.2011.1360 PMID:21954480

Malewski, D. F., Ream, A., & Gaither, C. A. (2015). Patient satisfaction with community pharmacy: Comparing urban and suburban chain-pharmacy populations. *Research in Social & Administrative Pharmacy*, *11*(1), 121–128. doi:10.1016/j.sapharm.2014.05.001 PMID:24933533

Malone, D. C., Carter, B. L., Billups, S. E., Valuck, R. J., Barnette, D. J., Sintek, C. D., & Amato, M. G. et al. (2001). Can clinical Pharmacists affect SF-36 scores in veterans at high risk for medication-related problems? *Journal of Medical Care*, *39*(2), 113–122. doi:10.1097/00005650-200102000-00002 PMID:11176549

Malone, M., & Alger-Mayer, S. A. (2003). Pharmacist intervention enhances adherence to Orlistat therapy. *The Annals of Pharmacotherapy*, *37*(11), 1598–1602. doi:10.1345/aph.1D183 PMID:14565841

Mapping the 1854 Broad Street Pump Outbreak. (2003). *John Snow and the Broad Street Pump on the Trial of an Epidemic*. Retrieved from http://www.ph.ucla.edu/epi/snow.html#YOUTH

Marchington, M., & Grugulis, I. (2000). 'Best practice'human resource management: Perfect opportunity or dangerous illusion? *International Journal of Human Resource Management*, *11*(6), 1104–1124. doi:10.1080/09585190050177184

March, J. G., & Simon, H. A. (1993). *Organizations* (2nd ed.). Cambridge, MA: Blackwell.

Marmot Report. (2010). *Fair society healthy lifes*. Retrieved February 10, 2015, from http://www.instituteofhealthequity.org/projects/fair-society-healthy-lives-the-marmot-review

Martin, D., Wrigley, H., Barnett, S., & Roderick, P. (2002). Increasing the sophistication of access measurement in a rural healthcare study. *Health & Place*, *8*(1), 3–13. doi:10.1016/S1353-8292(01)00031-4 PMID:11852259

Matysiewicz, J., & Smyczek, S. (2013). Relations between healthcare organizations and their patients: Three-factors models in the e-healthcare market. *Review of Business*, *33*(2), 7–25.

Mayer, R. C., & Schoorman, F. D. (1998). Differentiating antecedents of organizational commitment: A test of March and Simon's model. *Journal of Organizational Behavior*, *19*(1), 15–28. doi:10.1002/(SICI)1099-1379(199801)19:1<15::AID-JOB816>3.0.CO;2-C

McAlearney, A. S., Garman, A. N., Song, P. H., McHugh, M., Robbins, J., & Harrison, M. I. (2011). High-performance work systems in health care management, part 2: Qualitative evidence from five case studies. *Health Care Management Review*, *36*(3), 214–226. doi:10.1097/HMR.0b013e3182100dc4 PMID:21646881

McGregor, D. (1960). *The human side of enterprise*. New York.

McGuinness, S., & Bennett, J. (2006). Examining the link between skill shortages, training composition and productivity levels in the construction industry: Evidence from Northern Ireland 1. *International Journal of Human Resource Management*, *17*(2), 265–279. doi:10.1080/09585190500405538

McMichael, A. J., & Beaglehole, R. (2000). The changing global context of public health. *Lancet*, *356*(9228), 495–499. doi:10.1016/S0140-6736(00)02564-2 PMID:10981904

McNeese-Smith, D. K. (1997). The influence of manager behavior on nurses' job satisfaction, productivity, and commitment. *The Journal of Nursing Administration*, *27*(9), 47–55. doi:10.1097/00005110-199709000-00011 PMID:9300015

Meade, M. S., & Earickson, R. J. (2000). *Medical geography* (2nd ed.). New York: Guilford Press.

Mekhjian, H. S., Kumar, R. R., Kuehn, L., Bentley, T. D., Teater, P., Thomas, A., & Ahmad, A. et al. (2002). Immediate benefits realized following implementation of physician order entry at an academic medical center. *Journal of the American Medical Informatics Association*, *9*(5), 529–539. doi:10.1197/jamia.M1038 PMID:12223505

Menachemi, N., & Collum, T. (2011). Benefits and drawbacks of electronic health record systems. *Risk Management and Healthcare Policy*, *4*, 47–55. doi:10.2147/RMHP.S12985 PMID:22312227

Menon, A., Bharadwaj, G. S., & Howell, R. (1996). The quality and effectiveness of marketing strategy: Effects of functional and dysfunctional conflict in intraorganizational relationships. *Journal of the Academy of Marketing Science*, *24*(4), 299–313. doi:10.1177/0092070396244002

Menon, N. M., & Kohli, R. (2013). Blunting Damocles' Sword: A longitudinal model of healthcare IT impact on malpractice insurance premium and quality of patient care. *Information Systems Research*, *24*(4), 918–932, 1164–1165. doi:10.1287/isre.2013.0484

Michie, J., & Sheehan, M. (2005). Business strategy, human resources, labour market flexibility and competitive advantage. *International Journal of Human Resource Management*, *16*(3), 445–464. doi:10.1080/0958519042000339598

Min, D., & Yih, Y. (2010a). An elective surgery scheduling problem considering patient priority. *Computers & Operations Research*, *37*(6), 1091–1099. doi:10.1016/j.cor.2009.09.016

Min, D., & Yih, Y. (2010b). Scheduling elective surgery under uncertainty and downstream capacity constraints. *European Journal of Operational Research, 206*(3), 642–652. doi:10.1016/j.ejor.2010.03.014

Mladovsky, P. (2007). *Research Note Migration and health in the EU.* London School of Economics and Political Science, European Commission. Retrieved February 10, 2015, from http://ec.europa.eu/employment_social/social_situation/docs/rn_migration_health.pdf

Mohr, G. B. (2000). The changing significance of different stressors after the announcement of bankruptcy: A longitudinal investigation with special emphasis on job insecurity. *Journal of Organizational Behavior, 21*(3), 337–359. doi:10.1002/(SICI)1099-1379(200005)21:3<337::AID-JOB18>3.0.CO;2-G

Mohrman, S. A., & Cohen, S. G. (1995). When people get out of the box: New relationships, new systems. In A. Howard (Ed.), *The Changing Nature of Work* (pp. 365–410). San Francisco, CA: Jossey-Bass.

Molina-Pariente, J. M., Fernandez-Viagas, V., & Framinan, J. M. (2015). Integrated operating room planning and scheduling problem with assistant surgeon dependent surgery durations. *Computers & Industrial Engineering, 82*, 8–20. doi:10.1016/j.cie.2015.01.006

Montana, P., & Charnov, B. (2002). *Management: Management classical theory, organizations structures Management staff and dynamic working groups.* Athens, Greece: Publication Klidarithmos. (in Greek)

Montgomery, A. T., Kalvemark-Sporrong, S., Tully, M. P., & Kettis-Lindblad, A. (2008). Follow-up of patients receiving a pharmaceutical care service in Sweden. *Journal of Clinical Pharmacy and Therapeutics, 33*(6), 653–662. doi:10.1111/j.1365-2710.2008.00965.x PMID:19138243

Moore, D. A., & Carpenter, T. E. (1999). Spatial analytical methods and geographical information systems: Use in health research and epidemiology[Review]. *Epidemiologic Reviews, 21*(2), 143–161. doi:10.1093/oxfordjournals.epirev.a017993 PMID:10682254

Moore, T. J., Psaty, B. M., & Furberg, C. D. (1998). Time to act on drug safety. *Journal of the American Medical Association, 27919*(19), 1571–1573. doi:10.1001/jama.279.19.1571 PMID:9605903

Morello, C. M., Zadvorny, E. B., Cording, M. A., Suemoto, R. T., Skog, J., & Harari, A. (2006). Development and clinical outcomes of Pharmacist-managed diabetes care clinics. *American Journal of Health-System Pharmacy, 63*(14), 1325–1231. doi:10.2146/ajhp050430 PMID:16809752

Morgan, M. G., & Henrion, M. (1990). *Uncertainty: A Guide to Dealing with Uncertainty in Quantitative Risk and Policy Analysis*. Cambridge, UK: Cambridge University Press. doi:10.1017/CBO9780511840609

Moukheiber, Z. (2012). *Epic systems' tough billionaire*. Retrieved December 10, 2014 from http://www.forbes.com/sites/zinamoukheiber/2012/04/18/epic-systems-tough-billionaire/

Mueller, K., Voelkle, M. C., & Hattrup, K. (2011). On the relationship between job satisfaction and non-response in employee attitude surveys: A longitudinal field study. *Journal of Occupational and Organizational Psychology*, *84*(4), 780–798. doi:10.1348/096317910X526777

Murray, R. L., Bauld, L., Hackshaw, L. E., & McNeill, A. (2009). Improving access to smoking cessation services for disadvantaged groups: A systematic review. *Journal of Public Health*, *31*(2), 258–277. doi:10.1093/pubmed/fdp008 PMID:19208688

Najaftorkaman, M., Ghapanchi, A. H., Talaei-Khoei, A., & Ray, P. (2015). A taxonomy of antecedents to user adoption of health information systems: A synthesis of thirty years of research. *Journal of the Association for Information Science and Technology*, *66*(3), 576–598. doi:10.1002/asi.23181

Nandan, D., & Agarwal, D. (2012). Human Resources for Health in India: Urgent Need for Reforms. *Indian Journal of Community Medicine*, *37*(4), 205.

Nathan, J. (2004). Investigating Access to Reproductive Health Services Using GIS: Proximity to Services and the Use of Modern Contraceptives in Malawi. *African Journal of Reproductive Health*, *8*(2), 164–179. doi:10.2307/3583189 PMID:15623130

Niehoff, B. P., Moorman, R. H., Blakely, G., & Fuller, J. (2001). The influence of empowerment and job enrichment on employee loyalty in a downsizing environment. *Group & Organization Management*, *26*(1), 93–113. doi:10.1177/1059601101261006

Nikolaou, I. (2011). Core processes and applicant reactions to the employment interview: An exploratory study in Greece. *International Journal of Human Resource Management*, *22*(10), 2185–2201. doi:10.1080/09585192.2011.580187

Nkansah, N. T., Brewer, J. M., Connors, R., & Shermock, K. M. (2008). Clinical outcomes of patients with diabetes mellitus receiving medication management by Pharmacists in an urban private physician practice. *American Journal of Health-System Pharmacy*, *65*(2), 145–149. doi:10.2146/ajhp070012 PMID:18192260

Norman, G. R., Sloan, J. A., & Wyrwich, K. W. (2003). Interpretation of changes in health-related quality of life: The remarkable universality of half a standard deviation. *Medical Care*, *41*(5), 582–592. doi:10.1097/01.MLR.0000062554.74615.4C PMID:12719681

Nussbaum, A., Tirrell, M., Wechsler, P., & Randall, T. (2010, April 5). Obamacare's cost scalpel. *Business Week*, 64-65.

O'Connor, S. J., & Shewchuk, R. (2003). Commentary – patient satisfaction: What is the point? *Health Care Management Review*, *28*(1), 21–24. doi:10.1097/00004010-200301000-00003 PMID:12638370

O'Brien, M. S. (2006). Implementation of the EPIC Electronic Medical Record/Physician Order-Entry System. *Journal of Healthcare Management*, *51*(5), 338–343. PMID:17039692

Odedina, F. T., & Segal, R. (1996). Behavioural pharmaceutical care scale for measuring Pharmacists' activities. *American Journal of Health-System Pharmacy*, *53*, 855–865. PMID:8728382

Official Journal of European Union. (2010). C 83/02. Chapter of Fundamental Rights of the EU. Retrieved February 11, 2015, from http://eur-lex.europa.eu/LexUriServ/LexUriServ.do?uri=OJ:C:2010:083:0389:0403:en:PDF

Official Journal of European Union. (2012). C 326/49. Consolidated Version of the Treaty on the Functioning of the European Union. Retrieved February 11, 2015, from http://eur-lex.europa.eu/legal-content/EN/TXT/PDF/?uri=CELEX:12012E/TXT&from=EN

Ofili, O. U. (2014). Patient satisfaction in healthcare delivery – a review of current approaches and methods. *European Scientific Journal*, *10*(25), 25–39.

Oja, P. I., Kouri, T. T., & Pakarinen, A. J. (2006). From customer satisfaction survey to corrective actions in laboratory services in a university hospital. *International Journal for Quality in Health Care*, *18*(6), 422–428. doi:10.1093/intqhc/mzl050 PMID:17003077

Ojasalo, J. (2001). Managing customers expectations in professional services. *Managing Service Quality*, *11*(3), 200–212. doi:10.1108/09604520110391379

Olian, J. D., & Rynes, S. L. (1984). Organizational staffing: Integrating practice with strategy. *Industrial Relations*, *23*(2), 170–183. doi:10.1111/j.1468-232X.1984.tb00895.x

O'Neill, R. V., & Gardner, R. H. (1979). Sources of uncertainty in ecological models. In B. P. M. Zeigles, M. S. Elzas, G. J. Klir, & T. I. Oren (Eds.), Methodology in Systems Modelling and Simulation. North Holland.

Orpen, C. (1979). The effects of job enrichment on employee satisfaction, motivation, involvement, and performance: A field experiment. *Human Relations*, *32*(3), 189–217. doi:10.1177/001872677903200301

Ortega, J. (2001). Job rotation as a learning mechanism. *Management Science*, *47*(10), 1361–1370. doi:10.1287/mnsc.47.10.1361.10257

Osse, B. H., Vernooij-Dassen, M. J., de Vree, B. P., Schade, E., & Grol, R. P. (2000). Assessment of the need for palliative care as perceived by individual cancer patients and their families: A review of instruments for improving patient participation in palliative care. *Cancer*, *88*, 900–911. doi:10.1002/(SICI)1097-0142(20000215)88:4<900::AID-CNCR22>3.0.CO;2-2 PMID:10679661

Osterberg, L., & Blaschke, T. (2005). Adherence to medication. *The New England Journal of Medicine*, *353*(5), 487–497. doi:10.1056/NEJMra050100 PMID:16079372

Ostroff, C., & Bowen, D. E. (2000). Moving HR to a higher level: Human resource practices and organizational effectiveness. In K. J. Klein & S. W. J. Kozlowski (Eds.), *Multilevel theory, research, and methods*.

Owen, N. (2004). A Spatially-Based Approach to Cancer Prevention: The *PLACE* (Physical Activity in Localities and Community Environments) Study.*4th Annual Queensland Health and Medical Scientific Meeting*. BrisbaneConvention and Exhibition Centre.

Ozcan, Y. A. (2005). *Quantitative methods in health care management: Techniques and applications*. San Francisco, CA: Jossey-Bass.

Papadopoulou, D. (2009). Violence in the workplace nurses. *Nosileutiki*, *48*(4), 379–387.

Papanis, E. (2011). *Online counseling and Communication*. Athens, Greece: Publications Kyriakidis. (in Greek)

Papanis, E., & Rondos, K. (2005). *Psychology-Sociology of Labour and Human Resource Management*. Athens, Greece: Publications Sideri. (in Greek)

Parasuraman, A., Zeithanl, V. A., & Berry, L. L. (1988). SERVQUAL: A multiple-item scale for measuring consumer perceptions of service quality. *Journal of Retailing*, *64*(1), 12–40.

Parker, S. K. (1998). Enhancing role breadth self-efficacy: The roles of job enrichment and other organizational interventions. *The Journal of Applied Psychology*, *83*(6), 835–852. doi:10.1037/0021-9010.83.6.835 PMID:9885197

Pascoe, G. C. (1983). Patient satisfaction in primary health care: A literature review and analysis. *Evaluation and Program Planning*, *6*(3/4), 185–210. doi:10.1016/0149-7189(83)90002-2 PMID:10299618

Patil, P.R., & Mishra, N. (2014, November). Multipronged approach. *Quality Progress,* 22-29.

Patwardhan, P. D., Amin, M. E., & Chewning, B. A. (2014). Intervention research to enhance community Pharmacists' cognitive services: A systematic review. *Research in Social & Administrative Pharmacy*, *10*(3), 475–493. doi:10.1016/j.sapharm.2013.07.005 PMID:24071523

Paulus, P. (2000). Groups, Teams, and Creativity: The Creative Potential of Idea-generating Groups. *Applied Psychology*, *49*(2), 237–262. doi:10.1111/1464-0597.00013

Pauwels, K., Simoens, S., Casteels, M., & Huys, I. (2015). Insights into European drug shortages: A survey of hospital Pharmacists. *PLoS ONE*, *10*(3), e0119322. doi:10.1371/journal.pone.0119322 PMID:25775406

Pavlakis, A., Kateilidou, D., Theodorou, M., Galanis, P., Sourtzi, P., & Siskou, O. (2011). Conflict management in public hospitals: The Cyprus case. *International Nursing Review*, *58*(2), 242–248. doi:10.1111/j.1466-7657.2011.00880.x PMID:21554299

Penm, J., Chaar, B., Rose, G., & Moles, R. (2015). Pharmacists' influences on prescribing: Validating a clinical pharmacy services survey in the Western Pacific Region. *Research in Social & Administrative Pharmacy*, *11*(1), 63–73. doi:10.1016/j.sapharm.2014.04.001 PMID:25042568

Penna, R. P. (1990). Pharmaceutical Care: Pharmacists mission for the 1990s. *American Journal of Hospital Pharmacy*, *47*, 543–549. PMID:2316539

Petersen, A. C. (2000). Philosophy of climate science. *Bulletin of the American Meteorological Society*, *81*(2), 265–271. doi:10.1175/1520-0477(2000)081<0265:POCS>2.3.CO;2

Petrillo, J., van Nooten, F., Jones, P., & Rutten-van Mölken, M. (2011). Utility estimation in chronic obstructive pulmonary disease: A preference for change? *PharmacoEconomics*, *29*(11), 917–932. doi:10.2165/11589280-000000000-00000 PMID:21988291

Phillips, R., Kinman, E., Schnitzer, P., Lindbloom, E., & Ewigman, B. (2000). Using Geographic Information Systems to understand health care access. *Archives of Family Medicine*, *9*(10), 971–978. doi:10.1001/archfami.9.10.971 PMID:11115195

Piang, L. K., Khattar, P., & Nandan, D. (2010). Mainstreaming Gender perspective in the National Health Programmes: the challenges ahead. *Health and Population, Perspectives and Issues*, *33*(1), 34-41. Retrieved February 12, 2015, from http://medind.nic.in/hab/t10/i1/habt10i1p34.pdf

Pillinger, J. (2014). *Gender Mainstreaming in Health, training Handbook*. Retrieved February 13, 2015, from http://www.nwci.ie/images/uploads/NWCI_GM_Training_Manual_A4_WEB.pdf

Pispati, P. K. (2003). Evidence-based practice in rheumatology. *APLAR Journal of Rheumatology*, *6*(1), 44–49. doi:10.1046/j.0219-0494.2003.00026.x

Pitt, L. F., Watson, R. T., & Kavan, C. G. (1995). Service quality: A measure of information system effectiveness. *Management Information Systems Quarterly*, *19*(2), 173–187. doi:10.2307/249687

Pizzi, R. (2014). Nursing Informatics Adds Value as Healthcare is Transforming. *Healthcare IT News*. Retrieved December 1, 2014 from http://www.healthcareitnews.com/news/nursing-informatics-adds-value-healthcare-transforming

Polychroniou, P. (2008a). Styles of Handling Conflict in Greek Organizations: The impact of Transformation Leadership and Emotional Intelligence. *International Journal of Organizational Behavior*, *13*(1), 52–67.

Porter, L. (1996). Conflict. *Seminars in Perioperative Nursing*, *5*(3), 119–126. PMID:8718405

Porter, L. W., & Lawler, E. E. (1968). *Managerial attitudes and performance*. Homewood, IL: Irwin-Dorsey.

Posthuma, R. A., Campion, M. C., Masimova, M., & Campion, M. A. (2013). A high performance work practices taxonomy integrating the literature and directing future research. *Journal of Management*, *39*(5), 1184–1220. doi:10.1177/0149206313478184

Poulstrup, A., & Hansen, H. L. (2004). Use of GIS and exposure modeling as tools in a study of cancer incidence in a population exposed to airborne dioxin. *Environmental Health Perspectives*, *112*(9), 1032–1036. doi:10.1289/ehp.6739 PMID:15198924

Priorities at EU level: the Annual Growth Survey . (2015). Retrieved February 10, 2015, from http://ec.europa.eu/europe2020/making-it-happen/annual-growth-surveys/index_en.htm

Puntillo, K. A., & Mc Adam, J. L. (2006). Communication between physicians and nurses as a target for improving end-of-life care in the intensive care unit: Challenges and opportunities for moving forward. *Critical Care Medicine*, *34*(11Suppl), 332–340. doi:10.1097/01.CCM.0000237047.31376.28 PMID:17057595

Purcell, J. (1999). Best practice and best fit: Chimera or cul-de-sac? *Human Resource Management Journal*, *9*(3), 26–41. doi:10.1111/j.1748-8583.1999.tb00201.x

Raftopoulos, V. (2005). A grounded theory for patients' satisfaction with quality of hospital care. *ICUs & Nursing Web Journal*, *22*, 1–15.

Rahim, A., & Magner, R. (1995). Confirmatory factor analysis of the styles of handling interpersonal conflict: First- Order factor model and its invariance across groups. *The Journal of Applied Psychology*, *80*(1), 122–132. doi:10.1037/0021-9010.80.1.122 PMID:7706190

Rahman, S., & Smith, D. K. (2000). Use of location-allocation models in health service development planning in developing nations. *European Journal of Operational Research*, *123*(3), 437–452. doi:10.1016/S0377-2217(99)00289-1

Rahurkar, S., Vest, J., & Menachemi, N. (2015). Despite the spread of health information exchange, there is little evidence of its impact on cost, use, and quality of care. *Health Affairs*, *34*(3), 477-483.

Rangel, T. F., Diniz-Filho, J. A., & Bini, L. M. (2006). Towards an integrated computational tool for spatial analysis in macroecology and biogeography. *Global Ecology and Biogeography*, *15*(4), 321–327. doi:10.1111/j.1466-822X.2006.00237.x

Rannan-Eliya, R. (2004). *Affordable healthcare: how has Sri Lanka achieved low mortality rates at such low cost?* Sri Lanka: Institute of Policy Studies.

Rao, K. D., Peters, D. H., & Bandeen-Roche, K. (2006). Toward patient-centered health services in india-a scale to measure patient perceptions of quality. *International Journal for Quality in Health Care*, *18*(6), 414–421. doi:10.1093/intqhc/mzl049 PMID:17012306

Razzaque, A., Eldabi, T., & Jalal-Karim, A. (2013). Physician virtual community and medical decision making: Mediating role of knowledge sharing. *Journal of Enterprise Information Management*, *26*(5), 500–515. doi:10.1108/JEIM-07-2013-0047

Reader, T. W., Flin, R., Mearns, K., & Cuthbertson, B. H. (2007). Interdisciplinary communication in the intensive care unit. *British Journal of Anaesthesia*, *98*(3), 347–352. doi:10.1093/bja/ael372 PMID:17272386

Reeves, R., & Secombe, I. (2007). Do patient surveys work? The influence of a national survey programma on local quality-improvement initiatives. *Quality & Safety in Health Care*, *17*(6), 437–441. doi:10.1136/qshc.2007.022749 PMID:19064659

Regan, H., Colyvan, M., & Burgman, M. A. (2002). A taxonomy and treatment of uncertainty for ecology and conservation biology. *Ecological Applications*, *12*(2), 618–628. doi:10.1890/1051-0761(2002)012[0618:ATATOU]2.0.CO;2

Revised European Social Charter. (1996). *Strasbourg 3 May*. Retrieved February 13, 2015, from http://conventions.coe.int/Treaty/en/Treaties/Html/163.htm

Richardson, J. M. (1991). Management of conflict in organizations. *Physician Executive*, *17*(1), 39–42. PMID:10110137

Rigby, J. E., Skelly, C., Tate, N. J., Brabyn, L., King, R., & Borman, B. (2005). Inequalities in geographical access to healthcare services: using GIS to inform policy planning and implementation. *Proceedings of 10th International Symposium on Health Information Management Research*. SEERC.

Ritsema Van Eck, J.R., & Huguenin, P. (1993). *Conflicthantering en onderhandelen; een praktische inleiding*. Houten/Diegem: Bohn Stafleu van Loghum.

Roberts, N. J., Evans, G., Blenkhorn, P., & Partridge, M. R. (2010). Development of an electronic pictorial asthma action plan and its use in primary care. *Patient Education and Counseling*, *80*(1), 141–146. doi:10.1016/j.pec.2009.09.040 PMID:19879092

Robertson, I. T., & Smith, M. (2001). Personnel selection. *Journal of Occupational and Organizational Psychology*, *74*(4), 441–472. doi:10.1348/096317901167479

Robertson, J. G. W., & Wier, K. R. (1998). Using geographical information systems to enhance community-based child welfare services. *Child Maltreatment*, *3*(3), 224235. doi:10.1177/1077559598003003002

Rogelberg, S. G., Luong, A., Sederburg, M. E., & Cristol, D. S. (2000). Employee attitude surveys: Examining the attitudes of noncompliant employees. *The Journal of Applied Psychology*, *85*(2), 284–293. doi:10.1037/0021-9010.85.2.284 PMID:10783544

Romano, M. J., & Stafford, R. S. (2011). Electronic health records and clinical decision support systems: Impact on national ambulatory care quality. *National Library of Medicine. Archives of Internal Medicine*, *171*(10), 897–903. doi:10.1001/archinternmed.2010.527 PMID:21263077

Romzek, B. S. (1985). The effects of public service recognition, job security and staff reductions on organizational involvement. *Public Administration Review*, *45*(2), 282–291. doi:10.2307/976149

Rosenbaum, S., & Margulies, R. (2011). Tax-exempt hospitals and the Patient Protection and Affordable Care Act: Implications for public health policy and practice. *National Library of Medicine. Public Health Reports*, *126*(2), 283–286. PMID:21387959

Ross, E. L., Heizer, J., Mixon, M. A., Jorgensen, J., Valdez, C. A., Czaja, A. S., & Reiter, P. D. (2015). Development of recommendations for dosing of commonly prescribed medications in critically ill obese children. *American Journal of Health-System Pharmacy*, *72*(7), 542–556. doi:10.2146/ajhp140280 PMID:25788508

Ross, J. W., Beath, C. M., & Quaadgras, A. (2013). You may not need big data after all. *Harvard Business Review*, *91*(12), 90–98. PMID:23593770

Roth, K. (2004). Defending Economic, Social and Cultural Rights: Practical Issues Faced by an International Human Rights Organization. *Human Rights Quarterly*, *26*(1), 63–73. doi:10.1353/hrq.2004.0010

Rotter, T., Popa, D., Riley, B., Ellermann, T., Ryll, U., Burazeri, G., & Brand, H. et al. (2012). Methods for the evaluation of hospital cooperation activities (Systematic review protocol). *Syst Rev*, *1*(1), 11. doi:10.1186/2046-4053-1-11 PMID:22587989

Ruchlin, H., Dubbs, N., & Callahan, M. (2004).The role of leadership in instilling a culture of safety: lessons from the literature. *Journal of Healthcare Management*, *49*(1), 47-58.

Runde, C. E., & Flanagan, T. A. (2007). *Becoming a Conflict Competent Leader: How You and Your Organization Can Manage Conflict Effectively*. Jossey-Bass.

Rynes, S. L., Gerhart, B., & Parks, L. (2005). Personnel psychology: Performance evaluation and pay for performance. *Annual Review of Psychology*, *56*(1), 571–600. doi:10.1146/annurev.psych.56.091103.070254 PMID:15709947

Rytkonen, M. J. (2004). Not all maps are equal: GIS and spatial analysis in epidemiology. *International Journal of Circumpolar Health*, *63*(1), 9–24. doi:10.3402/ijch.v63i1.17642 PMID:15139238

Safaeian, L., Mahdanian, A. R., Salami, S., Pakmehr, F., & Mansourian, M. (2015). Seasonality and Physician-related Factors Associated with Antibiotic Prescribing: A Cross-sectional Study in Isfahan, Iran. *International Journal of Preventive Medicine*, *6*(1), 1. doi:10.4103/2008-7802.151431 PMID:25789136

Sakharkar, P., Bounthavong, M., Hirsch, J. D., Morello, C. M., Chen, T. C., & Law, A. V. (2015). Development and validation of PSPSQ 2.0 measuring patient satisfaction with Pharmacist services. *Research in Social & Administrative Pharmacy*, *11*(4), 487–498. doi:10.1016/j.sapharm.2014.10.006 PMID:25481330

Salgado, J. F. (1999). Personnel selection methods. In C. L. Cooper & I. T. Robertson (Eds.), *International Review of Industrial & Organizational Psychology*. New York: Wiley.

Sancar, M., Yalcin, B., & Mutlu, B. (2011). Determination of geriatric patients' drug profile and identify their pharmaceutical care requirements by determining potential risk factors. *European Geriatric Medicine*, *2*(5), 280–283. doi:10.1016/j.eurger.2011.07.011

Sankaranarayanan, J., Murante, L. J., & Moffett, L. M. (2014). A retrospective evaluation of remote Pharmacist interventions in a telepharmacy service model using a conceptual framework. *Telemedicine and E-Health Journal*, *20*(10), 893–901. doi:10.1089/tmj.2013.0362 PMID:24611489

Santacroce, R. (2014). A case study of a high functioning management engineering department. In J. A. Larson (Ed.), *Management engineering: A guide to best practices for industrial engineering in health care* (pp. 33–39). Boca Raton, FL: CRC Press.

Santibáñez, P., Begen, M., & Atkins, D. (2007). Surgical block scheduling in a system of hospitals: An application to resource and wait list management in a British Columbia health authority. *Health Care Management Science*, *10*(3), 269–282. doi:10.1007/s10729-007-9019-6 PMID:17695137

Saremi, A., Jula, P., ElMekkawy, T., & Wang, G. G. (2013). Appointment scheduling of outpatient surgical services in a multistage operating room department. *International Journal of Production Economics*, *141*(2), 646–658. doi:10.1016/j.ijpe.2012.10.004

Saunderson, R. (2004). Survey findings of the effectiveness of employee recognition in the public sector. *Public Personnel Management*, *33*(3), 255–275. doi:10.1177/009102600403300302

Schermerhorn, J. R., Hunt, J. G., & Osborn, R. (2007). *Organizational Behavior* (10th ed.). Hoboken, NJ: Wiley.

Schijndel van Strack, J. M. R., & Burchardi, H. (2007). Bench-to-bedside review: Leadership and conflict management in the intensive care unit. *Critical Care (London, England)*, *11*(6), 1–7. PMID:18086322

Schlundt, D. G., Mushi, C., Larson, C. O., & Marrs, M. (2001). Use of innovative technologies in the evaluation of Nashville''s REACH 2010 community action plan: Reducing disparities in cardiovascular disease and diabetes in the African American community. *The Journal of Ambulatory Care Management*, *24*(3), 51–60. doi:10.1097/00004479-200107000-00009 PMID:11433556

Schmelz, A. N., Nixon, B., McDaniel, A., Hudmon, K. S., & Zillich, A. J. (2010). Evaluation of an online tobacco cessation course for health professions students. *American Journal of Pharmaceutical Education*, *74*(2), 36. doi:10.5688/aj740236 PMID:20414451

Schmidt, I. K., & Svarstad, B. L. (2002). Nurse-physician communication and quality of drug use in Swedish nursing homes. *Social Science & Medicine*, *54*(12), 1767–1777. doi:10.1016/S0277-9536(01)00146-0 PMID:12113434

Schoemaker, P. J. H., & Russo, J. E. (1993). A pyramid of decision approaches. *California Management Review*, *36*(1), 9–31. doi:10.2307/41165732

Schoen C., Osborn R., Huynh P.T., Doty M. Zapet K., Peugh J. Davis K. (2005). Taking the Pulse of Health Care Systems: Experiences Of Patients With Health problems In Six Countries. *Health Affairs, Supl Web Exclusives*, (W5), 509-525.

Schoen, C., Osborn, R., Squires, D., Doty, M., Rasmussen, P., Pierson, R., & Applebaum, S. (2012). A survey of primary care doctors in ten countries shows progress in use of health information technology, less in other areas. *Health Affairs*, *31*(12), 2805–2816. doi:10.1377/hlthaff.2012.0884 PMID:23154997

Schulz, M., Verheyen, F., Muhlig, S., Müller, J. M., Mühlbauer, K., Knop-Schneickert, E., & Bergmann, K.-C. et al. (2001). Pharmaceutical care services for asthma patients: A controlled intervention study. *Journal of Clinical Pharmacology*, *41*(6), 668–676. doi:10.1177/00912700122010438 PMID:11402636

Schuurman, N., Bell, N. J., L'Heureux, R., & Hameed, S. M. (2009). Modelling optimal location for pre-hospital helicopter emergency medical services. *BMC Emergency Medicine*, *9*(6). PMID:19426532

Schuurman, N., Fiedler, R. S., Grzybowski, S. C., & Grund, D. (2006). Defining rational hospital catchments for non-urban areas based on travel-time. *International Journal of Health Geographics*, *5*(43). PMID:17018146

Schwartz, S. M., Bansal, V. P., Hale, C., Rossi, M., & Engle, J. P. (2008). Compliance, behavior change and weight loss with Orlistat in an overthe- counter setting. *Obesity (Silver Spring, Md.)*, *16*(3), 623–629. doi:10.1038/oby.2007.96 PMID:18239553

Schweiger, D. M., & Leana, C. R. (1986). Participation in decision making. *Generalizing from laboratory to field settings, 147*, 166.

Sciomachen, A., Tànfani, E., & Testi, A. (2005). Simulation models for optimal schedules of operating theatres. *International Journal of Simulation, 6*, 26–34.

Scott-Ladd, B., Travaglione, A., & Marshall, V. (2006). Causal inferences between participation in decision making, task attributes, work effort, rewards, job satisfaction and commitment. *Leadership and Organization Development Journal, 27*(5), 399–414. doi:10.1108/01437730610677990

Scott, W. R. (1990). Technology and structure: An organizational-level perspective. In P. S. Goodman & L. S. Sproull (Eds.), *Technology and organizations* (1st ed.; p. 109). San Francisco, CA: Jossey-Bass.

Scott, W. R., & Davis, G. F. (2007). *Organizations and organizing: Rational, natural, and open systems perspectives*. Upper Saddle River, NJ: Pearson Prentice Hall.

Scuffham, P. A., Yelland, M. J., Nikles, J., Pietrzak, E., & Wilkinson, D. (2008). Are N-of-1 Trials an Economically Viable Option to Improve Access to Selected High Cost Medications? The Australian Experience. *International Society for Pharmacoeconomics and Outcomes Research, 11*(1), 97–109. doi:10.1111/j.1524-4733.2007.00218.x PMID:18237364

Segel, J. E. (2006). *Cost-of-illness studies—a primer.* RTI International, RTI-UNC Center of Excellence in Health Promotion Economics. Retrieved from https://www.rti.org/pubs/coi_primer.pdf

Selgelid, M. J. (2007). The importance of "throwing money at" the problem of global health. *Ind J Med Ethics, 4*, 73–75. PMID:18630228

Sen, G., & Östlin, P. (2007). *Women and Gender Equity Knowledge Network*. Retrieved February 13, 2015, from http://www.who.int/social_determinants/resources/csdh_media/wgekn_final_report_07.pdf

Seybert, A. L., Kobulinsky, L. R., & McKaveneya, T. P. (2008). Human patient simulation in a pharmacotherapy course. *American Journal of Pharmaceutical Education, 72*(2), 37. doi:10.5688/aj720237 PMID:18483603

Shemeikka, T., Bastholm-Rahmner, P., Elinder, C. G., Vég, A., Törnqvist, E., Cornelius, B., & Korkmaz, S. (2015). A health record integrated clinical decision support system to support prescriptions of pharmaceutical drugs in patients with reduced renal function: Design, development and proof of concept. *International Journal of Medical Informatics, 84*(6), 387–395. doi:10.1016/j.ijmedinf.2015.02.005 PMID:25765963

Sheppard, E., McMaster, R., Leitner, H., & Tian, H. (1999). GIS-based Measures of Environmental Equity: Exploring Their Sensitivity and Significance. *Journal of Exposure Analysis and Environmental Epidemiology, 9*(1), 18–28. doi:10.1038/sj.jea.7500023 PMID:10189624

Shipton, H., West, M. A., Dawson, J., Birdi, K., & Patterson, M. (2006). HRM as a predictor of innovation. *Human Resource Management Journal, 16*(1), 3–27. doi:10.1111/j.1748-8583.2006.00002.x

Shortell, S. M. (1990). *Effective Hospital-Physician Relationships, Hospital Administration United States*. Ann Arbor, MI: Administration Press Prespectives.

Shortliffe, E. H. (2005). Strategic action in health information technology: Why the obvious has taken so long. *Health Affairs, 44*(5), 1222–1233. doi:10.1377/hlthaff.24.5.1222 PMID:16162567

Simarro, P. P., Cecchi, G., Paone, M., Franco, J. R., Diarra, A., Ruiz, J. A., & Jannin, J. G. et al. (2010). The Atlas of human African trypanosomiasis: A contribution to global mapping of neglected tropical diseases. *International Journal of Health Geographics, 9*(1), 57. doi:10.1186/1476-072X-9-57 PMID:21040555

Singer, T., Heifetz, B., & Morrissey, T.S. (2012). The benefits of mergers. Hospital mergers can increase competition through access to capital and economies of scale. *Trustee, 65*(10), 1-43.

Singleton, C., Weeks, S., & Flatt, S. (1998). Bully tactics. How can trust bosses combat bullying? *Nursing Standard, 12*(31), 21. PMID:9653231

Smither, R. D. (1994). *The Psychology of Work and Human Performance* (2nd ed.). New York: Harper Collins College Publishers.

Smythe, M. A., Shah, P. P., Spiteri, T. L., Lucarotti, R. L., & Begle, R. L. (1998). Pharmaceutical care in medical progressive care patients. *The Annals of Pharmacotherapy, 32*(3), 294–299. doi:10.1345/aph.17068 PMID:9533058

Sobal, J. (2001). Commentary: Globalization and the epidemiology of obesity. *International Journal of Epidemiology, 30*(5), 1136–1137. doi:10.1093/ije/30.5.1136 PMID:11689535

Sokka, T., & Pincus, T. (2001). Markers for work disability in rheumatoid arthritis. *The Journal of Rheumatology, 28*, 1718–1722. PMID:11469487

Somashekhar, S., & Sun, L. H. (2013). *HealthCare.gov meets deadline for fixes Obama administration says*. Retrieved December 10, 2014 from http://www.washingtonpost.com/national/health-science/healthcaregov-meets-deadline-for-fixes-white-house-says/2013/12/01/a3885612-5a13-11e3-ba82-16ed03681809_story.html

Spencer, J. (2004). Establishment of a national surveillance system to provide early warning of disease outbreaks - Discussion Document. In Commonwealth Department of Health and Ageing. Biosecurity and Disease Control Branch, Population Health Division.

Spencer, M., Briggs, A. H., Grossman, R. F., & Rance, L. (2005). Development of an economic model to assess the cost effectiveness of treatment interventions for chronic obstructive pulmonary disease. *PharmacoEconomics, 23*(6), 619–637. doi:10.2165/00019053-200523060-00008 PMID:15960557

Srivastava, D., & McGuire, A. (2015). Patient access to healthcare and medicines across low-income countries. *Social Science & Medicine, 133*, 21–27. doi:10.1016/j.socscimed.2015.03.021 PMID:25829195

Stathopoulou, Ch. (2006). Resolving conflicts in a hospital environment. *Nosileutiki, 45*(1), 50–58.

Stewart, M., Brown, J. B., & Weston, W. W. (1995). *Patient-centered Medicine: Transforming the Clinical Method*. California, USA: SAGE Publications Inc.

Stiglitz, J. E. (2010). A new capitalist order. In J. E. Stiglitz (Ed.), *Freefall: America, free markets, and the sinking of the world economy* (1st ed.). New York: W.W. Norton & Co.

Strasser, S., Aharony, L., & Greenberger, D. (1993). The patient satisfaction process: Moving toward a comprehensive model. *Medical Care Review*, *50*(2), 219–245. doi:10.1177/107755879305000205 PMID:10127084

Straus, S. E. (2002). Individualizing treatment decisions. The likelihood of being helped or harmed. *Evaluation & the Health Professions*, *25*(2), 210–224. doi:10.1177/016327870202500206 PMID:12026754

Streiner, D. L., & Norman, G. R. (1995). *Health measurement scales: a practical guide to their development and use* (2nd ed.). Oxford, UK: Oxford University Press.

Sullivan, E. J., & Decker, P. J. (1988). *Effective Management in Nursing* (2nd ed.). Addition Wesley.

Sverke, M., & Hellgren, J. (2002). The nature of job insecurity: Understanding employment uncertainty on the brink of a new millennium. *Applied Psychology*, *51*(1), 23–42. doi:10.1111/1464-0597.0077z

Swansburg, R. C., & Swansburg, R. J. (2003). *Introductory Management and Leadership for Clinical Nurses* (2nd ed.). Athens, Greece: Publication Iatrikes Lagos Dimitrios. (in Greek)

SWD. (2013). *328 final*. Report on Health inequalities in the EU. Retrieved February 06, 2015, from http://ec.europa.eu/health/social_determinants/docs/report_healthinequalities_swd_2013_328_en.pdf

SWD. (2013). *43 final*. Investing in Health. Retrieved February 02, 2015, from http://www.europarl.europa.eu/meetdocs/2009_2014/documents/swd/com_swd%282013%290043_/com_swd%282013%290043_en.pdf

Tabar, P. (2012). Data analytics: Marrying compliance and strategy. *Long-Term Living: For the Continuing Care Professional, 61*(7), 66-71.

Takeuchi, R., Lepak, D. P., Wang, H., & Takeuchi, K. (2007). An empirical examination of the mechanisms mediating between high-performance work systems and the performance of Japanese organizations. *The Journal of Applied Psychology*, *92*(4), 1069–1083. doi:10.1037/0021-9010.92.4.1069 PMID:17638466

Tanser, F. (2006). Methodology for optimising location of new primary health care facilities in rural communities: A case study in KwaZulu-Natal, South Africa. *Journal of Epidemiology and Community Health*, *60*(10), 846–850. doi:10.1136/jech.2005.043265 PMID:16973529

Taormina, R. J. (1997). Organizational socialization: A multidomain, continuous process model. *International Journal of Selection and Assessment*, *5*(1), 29–47. doi:10.1111/1468-2389.00043

Taylor, R. (1998). Small Area Epidemiological Analysis. In C. Kerr (Ed.), *Handbook of Public Health Methods* (pp. 627–637). Sydney: McGraw-Hill Book Company Australia Pty Ltd.

Tenglilimoglu, D., & Kisa, A. (2005). Conflict management in public university hospitals in Turkey: A pilot study. *Health Care Management (Philadelphia, Pa.)*, *24*(1), 55–60. PMID:15825820

The European Semester. (2015). *Economic Policies for Growth, Jobs and Investment.* Retrieved February 18, 2015, from http://ec.europa.eu/economy_finance/economic_governance/the_european_semester/index_en.htm

The Lisbon Special European Council. (2000). *Towards a Europe of Innovation and Knowledge.* Retrieved February 09, 2015, from http://europa.eu/legislation_summaries/education_training_youth/general_framework/c10241_en.htm

Their, S. O., Kelley, W. N., Pardes, H., Knight, A. W., & Wietecha, M. (2014). Success factors in merging teaching hospitals. *Academic Medicine*, *89*(2), 219–223. doi:10.1097/ACM.0000000000000094 PMID:24362373

Thibodeau, P., & Gross, G. (2013). HealthCare.gov had "no chance in hell". *Computerworld*, *47*(19), 6.

Thomas, B., Richards, C., Croner, G., Rushton, C., & Brown, K. (1999). Littleton Fowler. *Public Health Reports (Washington, D.C.)*, *114*(4), 359–373.

Thomas, E., Sexton, J., & Helmreich, R. (2003). Discrepant attitudes about teamwork among critical care nurses and physicians. *Critical Care Medicine*, *31*(3), 956–959. doi:10.1097/01.CCM.0000056183.89175.76 PMID:12627011

Thomas, K. W. (1992). Conflict and Conflict Management: Reflections and Update. *Journal of Organizational Behavior*, *13*(3), 265–274. doi:10.1002/job.4030130307

Thompson, A. E., Goldszmidt, M. A., Schwartz, A. J., & Bashook, P. G. (2010). A randomized trial of pictorial versus prose-based medication information pamphlets. *Patient Education and Counseling*, *78*(3), 389–393. doi:10.1016/j.pec.2010.01.010 PMID:20153597

Thompson, J. D. (1967). *Organizations in action; social science bases of administrative theory.* New York: McGraw-Hill.

Thorsteinson, T. J., & Ryan, A. M. (1997). The effect of selection ratio on perceptions of the fairness of a selection test battery. *International Journal of Selection and Assessment*, *5*(3), 159–168. doi:10.1111/1468-2389.00056

Toms, J. (2004). Project Summary - BSS Scoping Study Stakeholder Consultation October/November 2004. In Commonwealth Department of Health and Ageing. Population Health Division, Biosecurity and Disease Control Branch.

Torrington, D., Hall, L., Taylor, S., & Atkinson, C. (2009). *Fundamentals of Human Resourse Management Managing People at Work* (1st ed.). Edinburgh, UK: Prentice Hall.

Toubro, S., Dahlager, L., Hermansen, L., Herborg, H., & Astrup, A. (1999). Weight loss maintenance at one year follow-up after initial 12 weeks course in fat reduction on Danish pharmacies. *Ugeskrift for Laeger*, *161*, 5308–5313. PMID:10536516

Truven Health Analytics. (2014). *Disease Management Analytics*. Retrieved December 1, 2014 from http://truvenhealth.com/your-healthcare-focus/life-sciences/disease-management-analytics

Tsavalias, K., Siskou, O., & Liaropoulos, L. (2012). Hospital Mergers in Europe Lessons and prospects for Greece. *Arxia Ellinikis Iatrikis*, *29*(2), 233–239.

Tsui, A. S., Pearce, J. L., Porter, L. W., & Tripoli, A. M. (1997). Alternative approaches to the employee-organization relationship: Does investment in employees pay off? *Academy of Management Journal*, *40*(5), 1089–1121. doi:10.2307/256928

Turner, M. G., Dale, V. H., & Gardner, R. H. (1989). Predicting across scales: Theory development and testing. *Landscape Ecology*, *3*(3-4), 245–252. doi:10.1007/BF00131542

Turris, S. A. (2005). Unpacking the concept of patient satisfaction: A feminist analysis. *Journal of Advanced Nursing*, *50*(3), 293–298. doi:10.1111/j.1365-2648.2005.03392.x PMID:15811108

Tyler, D. C., Pasquariello, C. A., & Chen, C. H. (2003). Determining Optimum Operating Room Utilization. *Anesthesia and Analgesia*, *96*(4), 1114–1121. doi:10.1213/01.ANE.0000050561.41552.A6 PMID:12651670

Tzeng, H. M. (2002). The influence of nurses' working motivation and job satisfaction on intention to quit: An empirical investigation in Taiwan. *International Journal of Nursing Studies*, *39*(8), 867–878. doi:10.1016/S0020-7489(02)00027-5 PMID:12379304

U.S. Department of Health & Human Services. (2014). What is a medical home? Why is it important? *Health Resources and Services Administration (HRSA) - Health Information Technology*. Retrieved December 10, 2014 from http://www.hrsa.gov/healthit/toolbox/Childrenstoolbox/BuildingMedicalHome/whyimportant.html

U.S. Department of Health & Human Services. (2015). *Summary of the HIPAA security rule*. Retrieved April 20, 2015 from http://www.hhs.gov/ocr/privacy/hipaa/understanding/srsummary.html

Ury, W., Brett, J., & Goldberg, S. (1993). *Getting disputes resolved. Designing systems to cut the costs of conflict. The program of Negotiation at Harvard Law School, Cambridge* (2nd ed.). Jossey- Bass.

Valentine, P. E. (2001). A gender perspective on conflict management strategies of nurses. *Journal of Nursing Scholarship*, *33*(1), 69–74. doi:10.1111/j.1547-5069.2001.00069.x PMID:11253585

Van De Graaf, J., & Cameron, A. (2013). Quest for business intelligence in healthcare. *HFM*, *67*(2), 44–48. PMID:23413668

Van Houdenhoven, M., Van Oostrum, J. M., Hans, E. W., Wullink, G., & Kazemier, G. (2007). Improving operating room efficiency by applying bin-packing and portfolio techniques to surgical case scheduling. *Anesthesia and Analgesia, 105*(3), 707–714. doi:10.1213/01.ane.0000277492.90805.0f PMID:17717228

Van Oostrum, J. M., Van Houdenhoven, M., Hurink, J. L., Hans, E. W., Wullink, G., & Kazemier, G. (2008). A master surgical scheduling approach for cyclic scheduling in operating room departments. *OR-Spektrum, 30*(2), 355–374. doi:10.1007/s00291-006-0068-x

Vazirani, S., Hays, R. D., Shapiro, M. F., & Cowan, M. (2005). Effect of a multidisciplinary intervention on communication and collaboration among physicians and nurses. *American Journal of Critical Care, 14*(1), 71–77. PMID:15608112

Vijayanarayana, K., Sekhar, M. S., Surulivelrajan, M., Rajesh, R., Suhaj, A., Kumar, S. P., & Sreedharan, N. et al. (2014). Bridging pharmaceutical education. *Currents in Pharmacy Teaching and Learning, 6*(5), 745–747. doi:10.1016/j.cptl.2014.05.017

Vinks, T. H., de Koning, F. H., de Lange, T. M., & Egberts, T. C. (2006). Identification of potential drug-related problems in the elderly: The role of the community Pharmacist. *Pharmacy World & Science, 28*(1), 33–38. doi:10.1007/s11096-005-4213-4 PMID:16703267

Vo, A., & Bhaskar, R. (2012). Health Care Reform Requires Rethinking on the IT Strategy. *Journal of Cases on Information Technology, 14*(2), 65–72. doi:10.4018/jcit.2012040105

Vora, K. S., Yasobant, S., Patel, A., Upadhyay, A., & Mavalankar, D. V. (2015). Has Chiranjeevi Yojana changed the geographic availability of free Comprehensive Emergency Obstetric Care Services in Gujarat, India? *Global Health Action, 8*(0). doi:10.3402/gha.v8.28977 PMID:26446287

Wait, S. (2005). Cost sharing for medications: To what end? *Evidence-Based Healthcare & Public Health, 9*(3), 261–262. doi:10.1016/j.ehbc.2005.03.033

Wan, D., Ong, C. H., & Kok, V. (2002). Strategic human resource management and organizational performance in Singapore. *Compensation and Benefits Review, 34*(4), 33–42. doi:10.1177/0886368702034004006

Wang, Y.-C., Lin, Y.-P., Huang, C.-W., Chiang, L.-C., Chu, H.-J., & Ou, W.-S. (2012). A System Dynamic Model and Sensitivity Analysis for Simulating Domestic Pollution Removal in a Free-Water Surface Constructed Wetland. *Water, Air, and Soil Pollution, 223*(5), 2719–2742. doi:10.1007/s11270-011-1062-8

Ware, J. E. Jr, & Snyder, M. K. (1975). Dimensions of patient attitudes regarding doctors and medical care services. *Medical Care, 13*(8), 669–682. doi:10.1097/00005650-197508000-00006 PMID:1152557

Ware, J. E. Jr, Snyder, M. K., Wright, W. R., & Davies, A. R. (1983). Defining and measuring patient satisfaction with medical care. *Evaluation and Program Planning, 6*(3/4), 247–263. doi:10.1016/0149-7189(83)90005-8 PMID:10267253

Weick, K. E., & Sutcliffe, K. M. (2007). Managing the Unexpected (2nd ed.). Academic Press.

Weiss, M. C., Grey, E., Harris, M., & Rodham, K. (2015). Dispensing doctor practices and community pharmacies: Exploring the quality of pharmaceutical services. *Primary Health Care Research and Development*, *17*, 1–14. PMID:25777160

Wen, H. W. (2000). Generalized Linear Models. Department of Statistics, Tunghai University.

West, M. A., Borrill, C., Dawson, J., Scully, J., Carter, M., Anelay, S., & Waring, J. et al. (2002). The link between the management of employees and patient mortality in acute hospitals. *International Journal of Human Resource Management*, *13*(8), 1299–1310. doi:10.1080/09585190210156521

West, M. A., Guthrie, J. P., Dawson, J. F., Borrill, C. S., & Carter, M. (2006). Reducing patient mortality in hospitals: The role of human resource management. *Journal of Organizational Behavior*, *27*(7), 983–1002. doi:10.1002/job.396

Whetten, D. A., & Cameron, K. S. (1991). *Developing Management Skills* (2nd ed.). New York: Harper Collins.

WHO document in TELEMEDICINE: Opportunities and developments in Member States, 2010. (n.d.). Available at: http://www.who.int/goe/publications/goe_telemedicine_2010.pdf

WHO. (2000). *World Health Report: health systems improving performance*. Geneva, Switzerland: World Health Organization.

Wilde, B., Starrin, B., Larsson, G., & Larsson, M. (1993). Quality of Care from a Patient Perspective. A Grounded Theory Study. *Scandinavian Journal of Caring Sciences*, *7*(2), 113–120. doi:10.1111/j.1471-6712.1993.tb00180.x PMID:8248668

Wiley, M. T., Jin, C., Hristidis, V., & Esterling, K. M. (2014). Pharmaceutical drugs chatter on Online Social Networks. *Journal of Biomedical Informatics*, *49*, 245–254. doi:10.1016/j.jbi.2014.03.006 PMID:24637141

Wilkinson, D., & Tanser, F. (1999). GIS/GPS to document increased access to community based treatment for tuberculosis in Africa. Geographic information system/global positioning system. *Lancet*, *354*(9176), 394–395. doi:10.1016/S0140-6736(99)01893-0 PMID:10437874

Williams, A. (1998). Trust mergers. Turning threates into opportunities. *The Health Service Journal*, *108*(5604), 30–31. PMID:10180008

Williams, B. (1994). Patient Satisfaction: A Valid Concept? *Social Science & Medicine*, *38*(4), 509–516. doi:10.1016/0277-9536(94)90247-X PMID:8184314

Wilmot, W., & Hocker, G. L. (2001). *Interpersonal Conflict* (6th ed.). New York: McGraw-Hill Higher Edukation.

Winston, S., & Albright, S. C. (2001). *Practical management science* (2nd ed.). Pacific Grove, CA: Duxbury.

Wirtz, J., & Bateson, J. E. G. (1995). An experimental investigation of halo effects in satisfaction measures of service attributes. *International Journal of Service Industry Management*, *6*(3), 84–102. doi:10.1108/09564239510091358

Witte, H. D. (1999). Job insecurity and psychological well-being: Review of the literature and exploration of some unresolved issues. *European Journal of Work and Organizational Psychology*, *8*(2), 155–177. doi:10.1080/135943299398302

Wolfstadt, J. I., Gurwitz, J. H., Field, T. S., Lee, M., Kalkar, S., Wu, W., & Rochon, P. A. (2008). The effect of computerized physician order entry with clinical decision support on the rates of adverse drug events: A systematic review. *Journal of General Internal Medicine*, *23*(4), 451–458. doi:10.1007/s11606-008-0504-5 PMID:18373144

Wong, H., Legnini, M., & Whitmore, H. (2000). The diffusion of decision support systems in healthcare: are we there yet?. *Journal of Healthcare Management*, *45*(4), 240-249.

World Health Organisation (WHO). (2000). *The world health report 2000 - Health systems: improving performance*. Retrieved February 19, 2015, from http://www.who.int/whr/2000/en/

World Health Organisation (WHO). (2008a). *Assuring the quality of health care in the European Union*. United Kingdom by MPG Books Ltd, Bodmin, Cornwall. Retrieved February 16, 2015, from http://www.euro.who.int/__data/assets/pdf_file/0007/98233/E91397.pdf

World Health Organisation (WHO). (2008b). *The Tallinn Charter: Health Systems for Health and Wealth. Tallinn*. Retrieved February 10, 2015, from http://www.euro.who.int/__data/assets/pdf_file/0008/88613/E91438.pdf

World Health Organisation (WHO). (2008c). *Closing the Gap: Health Equity through action on the social determinants of health*. Retrieved February 20, 2015, from http://www.who.int/social_determinants/final_report/csdh_finalreport_2008.pdf

World Health Organisation (WHO). (2008d). *Commission on Social Determinants of Health – final report*. Retrieved February 10, 2015, from http://www.who.int/social_determinants/thecommission/finalreport/en/index.html

World Health Organisation Regional Office for Europe. (2010). *Primary Care Evaluation Tool (PCET)*. Retrieved February 20, 2015, from http://www.euro.who.int/__data/assets/pdf_file/0005/128849/e94554.pdf

World Health Organisation. (2010). *The world health report - Health systems financing: the path to universal coverage*. Retrieved February 15, 2015, from http://www.who.int/whr/2010/en/index.html

World Health Organization (WHO). (2000). *The world health report 2000, Health systems Improving performance*. Geneva: WHO.

World Health Organization (WHO). (2005a). *Executive Board, Gender, women and health: incorporating a gender perspective into the mainstream of WHO's policies and programme*. Report by the Secretariat, 12th May, EB116/13.

World Health Organization (WHO). (2005b). *Preventing Chronic Diseases a vital investment*. Retrieved February 20, 2015, from http://www.who.int/chp/chronic_disease_report/contents/part2.pdf

World Health Organization (WHO). (2012). *Modern health care delivery systems, care coordination and the role of hospitals*. Retrieved February 13, 2015, from http://www.euro.who.int/__data/assets/pdf_file/0008/158885/BRU-report-Modern-health-care-delivery-systems.pdf?ua=1

World Health Organization (WHO). (2013). *Global action plan for the prevention and control of non-communicable diseases 2013-2020*. Retrieved February 10, 2015, from http://apps.who.int/iris/bitstream/10665/94384/1/9789241506236_eng.pdf

World Health Organization (WHO). (2015). *Gender, Women and Heath, Why gender and Health?* Retrieved February 12, 2015, from http://www.who.int/gender/genderandhealth/en/

World Health Organization Regional Office for Europe. (2011). *The new European policy for health – Health 2020*. EUR/RC61/Inf.Doc./4. Retrieved February 18, 2015, from http://www.euro.who.int/__data/assets/pdf_file/0005/148946/RC61_InfDoc4.pdf

Worley-Louis, M. M., Schommer, J. C., & Finnegan, J. R. (2003). Construct-identification and measure development for investigating Pharmacist–patient relationships. *Patient Education and Counseling*, *51*(3), 229–238. doi:10.1016/S0738-3991(02)00222-7 PMID:14630379

Worley, M. M., Schommer, J. C., Brown, L. M., Hadsall, R. S., Ranelli, P. L., Stratton, T. P., & Uden, D. L. (2007). Pharmacists' and patients' roles in the Pharmacist–patient relationship: Are Pharmacists and patients reading from the same relationship script? *Research in Social & Administrative Pharmacy*, *3*(1), 47–69. doi:10.1016/j.sapharm.2006.03.003 PMID:17350557

Wright, P. M., & McMahan, G. C. (1992). Theoretical perspectives for strategic human resource management. *Journal of Management*, *18*(2), 295–320. doi:10.1177/014920639201800205

Wu, J. (1999). Hierarchy and scaling: Extrapolating information along a scaling ladder. *Canadian Journal of Remote Sensing*, *25*(4), 367–380. doi:10.1080/07038992.1999.10874736

Wu, J., & Li, H. (2006). *Scaling and uncertainty analysis in ecology*. Springer. doi:10.1007/1-4020-4663-4

Wullink, G., Van Houdenhoven, M., Hans, E. W., Van Oostrum, J. M., Van der Lans, M., & Kazemier, G. (2007). Closing emergency operating rooms improves efficiency. *Journal of Medical Systems*, *31*(6), 543–546. doi:10.1007/s10916-007-9096-6 PMID:18041289

Xiang, W., Yin, J., & Lim, G. (2015). A short-term operating room surgery scheduling problem integrating multiple nurses' roster constraints. *Artificial Intelligence in Medicine*, *63*(2), 91–106. doi:10.1016/j.artmed.2014.12.005 PMID:25563674

Yang, S. B., & Lee, K. H. (2009). Linking empowerment and job enrichment to turnover intention: The influence of job satisfaction. *International Review of Public Administration*, *14*(2), 13–24. doi:10.1080/12294659.2009.10805152

Yasobant, S., Vora, K. S., Hughes, C., Upadhyay, A., & Mavalankar, D. V. (2015). Geovisualization: A Newer GIS Technology for Implementation Research in Health. *Journal of Geographic Information System*, *7*(01), 20–28. doi:10.4236/jgis.2015.71002

Young, G. J., Meterko, M., & Desai, K. R. (2000). Patient satisfaction with hospital care: Effects of demographic and institutional characteristics. *Medical Care*, *38*(3), 325–334. doi:10.1097/00005650-200003000-00009 PMID:10718357

Young, S., Bartram, T., Stanton, P., & Leggat, S. G. (2010). High performance work systems and employee well-being: A two stage study of a rural Australian hospital. *Journal of Health Organization and Management*, *24*(2), 182–199. doi:10.1108/14777261011047345 PMID:20698193

Zai, A. H., Grant, R. W., Estey, G., Lester, W. T., Andrews, C. T., Yee, R., & Chueh, H. et al. (2008). Lessons from implementing a combined workflow-informatics system for diabetes management. *Journal of the American Medical Informatics Association*, *15*(4), 524–533. doi:10.1197/jamia.M2598 PMID:18436907

Zavlanos, M. (2002). *Organizational behavior*. Athens, Greece: Publication Stamouli. (in Greek)

Zhang, M., Zhu, C. J., Dowling, P. J., & Bartram, T. (2013). Exploring the effects of high-performance work systems (HPWS) on the work-related well-being of Chinese hospital employees. *International Journal of Human Resource Management*, *24*(16), 3196–3212. doi:10.1080/09585192.2013.775026

Zhang, Y., & Li, L. (2009, May). Study on balanced scorecard of commercial bank in performance management system. In *Proceedings of the 2009 International Symposium on Web Information Systems and Applications (WISA'09)*(pp. 22-24).

Zhao, Z., & Li, X. (2014). Scheduling elective surgeries with sequence-dependent setup times to multiple operating rooms using constraint programming. *Operations Research for Health Care*, *3*(3), 160–167. doi:10.1016/j.orhc.2014.05.003

Zimeras, S. (1997). *Statistical models in medical imaging*. (Ph. D. Thesis). Leeds University.

Zimeras, S., & Matsinos, Y. (2011). *Spatial Uncertainty*. Paper presented at the 4th International Conference in Geography and Geology, Corfu, Greece.

Zimeras, S., & Matsinos, Y. (2012). *Bayesian Spatial Uncertainty Analysis*. Paper presented at the 7th IASME/WSEAS International Conference on Energy & Environment (EE '12), Kos Island, Greece.

Zimeras, S. (2007). In E. A. Zoeller (Ed.), *Spatial Pattern Recognition Models with Application in Image Analysis. In Pattern Recognition Theory and Application* (pp. 201–219). Nova Publishers.

Zimeras, S., & Aykroyd, R. G. (1999). Neighbourhood structure estimation of images using hierarchical testing. *Electronics Letters*, *35*(25), 2188–2189. doi:10.1049/el:19991476

Zimeras, S., & Georgiakodis, F. (2005). Bayesian models for medical image biology using Monte Carlo Markov Chain techniques. *Mathematical and Computer Modelling*, *42*(7-8), 759–768. doi:10.1016/j.mcm.2005.09.005

Zimeras, S., & Matsinos, Y. (2013). Uncertainty analysis in ecological systems System. *International Journal of Systems Biology and Biomedical Technologies*, *2*, 14–24. doi:10.4018/ijsbbt.2013010102

Zineldin, M. (2006). The quality of health care and patient satisfaction: An exploratory investigation of the 5Qs model at some Egyptian and Jordanian medical clinics. *International Journal for Quality in Health Care*, *19*(1), 60–99. doi:10.1108/09526860610642609 PMID:16548402

Zlabek, J. A., Wickus, J. W., & Mathiason, M. A. (2011). Early cost and safety benefits of an inpatient electronic health record. *Journal of the American Medical Informatics Association*, *18*(2), 169–172. doi:10.1136/jamia.2010.007229 PMID:21292703

About the Contributors

Panagiotis Manolitzas is a researcher at the Decision Support Systems Laboratory of Technical University of Crete. He holds a Bachelor in Public Administration (specialization in Management Science) from the University of Athens, a MSc in Public Management (specialization in Management Science) from the University of Athens and a PhD in Operational Research from the Technical University of Crete. He taught Management Information Systems, Health Management at University of Athens, Management Information Systems and Principles of Business Administration at Technological Educational institute of Piraeus, Decision Support Systems at Technical University of Crete, Health Care Management and Health Information Systems at European Cyprus University. He has over 50 publications in International, National Scientific Conferences and scientific journals. He is a Member of Hellenic Operational Research Society. His research interests lie in the areas of Simulation, Decision Support Systems for the health care organizations, health services research, process mining and multiple criteria analysis.

Evangelos Grigoroudis is an Assistant Professor at the Department of Production Engineering and Management, Technical University of Crete, Chania, Greece. He received the diploma in production and management engineering from the Technical University of Crete, in 1991 and M.S. and Ph.D. degrees from the same University, in 1996 and 1999, respectively. His research interests are in service quality, operational research, and customer behavioral analysis. He acts as reviewer for more than 50 scientific journals and he is an Assistant Editor of Operational Research: An International Journal and International Journal of Decision Support Systems, and a member of the Editorial Board International Journal of Information and Decision Sciences, International Journal of Information Systems in the Service Sector, and International Journal of Multicriteria Decision Making.

Nikolaos Matsatsinis is a Professor of Information and Intelligent Decision Support Systems at the Department of Production Engineering and Management of the Technical University of Crete, Greece. He is Chairman of the Department,

Director of Decision Support Systems Lab and President of Hellenic Operational Research Society (HELORS). He also has over twenty eight years of experience in Information and Decision Systems development. He has coordinate or/and contribute on over of thirty projects. He is the author or co-author of fifteen books and over of sixty six articles in international scientific journals and books. He is member of the international advisory board of three scientific journals. His research interests fall into the areas of Decision Support Systems, Artificial Intelligent and Multi-Agent Systems, Multicriteria Decision Analysis, Group Decision Support Systems, Workflow Management Systems, e-Business, e-Marketing, Consumer Behaviour Analysis.

Denis Yannacopoulos is Professor of Management Information Systems in the Business Administration Department of the Piraeus University of Applied Sciences. He holds a BSc in Chemistry, a MSc and a PhD in Information Systems. His research interests are in Operational Research, Multicriteria Analysis and Decision Support Systems. His expertise in training issues and EU projects is utilized by the Ministry of Employment and Education and he has been a consultant of numerous public and private organisations in Greece and Cyprus. He is an active member of editorial boards and a referee of many scientific journals. He was Dean of the Administration and Economy School of the TEI of Piraeus from 2006 to 2010 and 2014 to 2016 and also President of the Hellenic Operational Research Society (HELORS) from 2005 to 2009.

* * *

Foulvia Adroutsou is a PhD student in Gender and Politics – University of Creta, with a MSc in Political Science and History – Panteion University Athens.

Lorena Androutsou has a PhD in Health Economics – University of Thessaly, MSc in health management – Imperial College London, and MSc in contemporary health and social care policy – City University London.

Edward T. Chen is a professor of Management Information Systems of Operations and Information Systems Department in the Manning School of Business at University of Massachusetts Lowell. Dr. Chen has published over sixty refereed research articles in scholarly journals and reference books. Dr. Chen has served as vice-president, board director, track chair, and session chair of many professional associations and conferences. Professor Chen has also served as journal editor, editorial reviewer, and ad hoc reviewer for various academic journals. Dr. Chen has received the Irwin Distinguished Paper Award at the Southwestern Federation of Administrative Disciplines conference and the Best Paper Award at the International

Conference on Accounting and Information Technology. His main research interests are in the areas of Social Media, Project Management, Knowledge Management, and Software Development.

Fatah Chetouane is a Professor in Industrial Engineering, associated with the Electrical Engineering Department at Université de Moncton. Fatah Chetouane is a senior IEEE member, a senior IIE member, and a registered professional engineer in Canada. His research interests include industrial engineering, automatic control, computer-aided manufacturing, healthcare process management, and discrete event simulation.

Marcus Vinícius Dias-Souza is from the Federal University of Minas Gerais, Brazil, and Integrated Pharmacology and Drug Interactions Research Group (GPq-FAR), the Steel Valley Pharmaceutical Association, Minas Gerais, Brazil.

Panagiotis Gkorezis has completed his post-doctoral research in organizational behavior and his Ph.D. in Human Resource Management from Aristotle University of Thessaloniki at the department of Business Administration. In addition, he holds a postgraduate degree in Human Resource and Knowledge Management from Lancaster University. He has published in various academic journals, such as The International Journal of Human Resource Management, Management Decision, Leadership and Organization Development Journal, Health Services Management Research. He currently teaches as an adjunct lecturer at the Open University of Cyprus and the Hellenic Open University. He is also a research fellow at Aristotle University of Thessaloniki. His research interests include human resource management, empowering leadership and psychological empowerment, organizational identification and humor in organizations whereas his teaching interests include organizational behavior and human resource management.

Eman Ibraheem earned her Bachelor's degree in Industrial Engineering from the University of Jordan, Jordan, in 2001, and her Master of Applied Science in Industrial Engineering, from the Université de Moncton, Canada, in 2011. She is a Registered Professional Engineer in Jordan, since 2001. Her professional experience is in the broad area of management and service engineering, where she accomplished several projects involving, lean manufacturing tools, strategic sourcing, supply chain management and optimization.

Yiannis G. Matsinos is an Associate Professor at the Department of Environment, School of Environment, University of the Aegean, Greece. He received the diploma in Mathematics from the University of Athens, in 1986 and M.S. and

Ph.D. degrees from the University of Tennessee, Knoxville, USA in 1990 and 1994, respectively. His research interests are ecological modelling, cellular automata in ecology, biostatistics and Population Viability Analysis. He acts as an editor and reviewer for more than 50 scientific journals and has published 55 articles in peer reviewed ISI journals.

Christopher L. Pate is an Adjunct Professor in the George Herbert Walker School of Business and Technology at Webster University (San Antonio Campus). He has more than 30 years of experience in academic and federal healthcare management. He received his doctoral degree in Health Policy and Administration at The Pennsylvania State University in 2001 and his Master of Public Administration from Syracuse University in 1994. His research interests include quantitative methods in healthcare settings, organizational design, and civility in work environments. He is affiliated with the American Economic Association, the Association of Military Surgeons of the United States, the American Society for Quality and the Healthcare Financial Management Association. He also serves on the International Editorial Review Board of the International Journal of Reliable and Quality E-Healthcare (IJRQEH).

Athanasia Stamatopoulou studied at the School of Administration and Economics in Accounting and Finance department of Piraeus University of Applied Sciences (Technological Education Institute of Piraeus). Additionally she acquired MSc Master in International Human Resource Management, and MSc Master of Science in Management of Health and Social Welfare Services. From 2004 to 2005 she worked at the Economic department of an Insurance Company. She also served as Administrator in Section employer contributions to IKA Piraeus St.Sophia. From then on she has been working at Administrative Personnel in Iatropolis Medical Group of companies, Greece. She is a member of the Economic Chamber of Greece and since 2008 a Deputy member of the Greek Medical Association of study of psychosomatic problems. Her research interests refer to the Administration in Human Resource Management, in Economics and Health Policy, where she has written extensively and has presented a significant number of research papers in Greek and International conferences.

Eleni Stamatopoulou is an Officer of Public Health, MSc National School of Public Health and Graduate Nurse of A.T.E.I. Athens and Head of "School Asthma" in the (H.C.) of Peristeri, and Researcher. She holds extensive experience in ICU as she has worked in the Central Administration of the Ministry of Health at the Center for Disease Control (H.C.D.C.P.), in the department of Epidemiological Surveillance and Intervention. This period provides services to H.C.D.C.P., placed in the Administration of Primary Health Care in 'Model' Health Center of Peristeri, implementing preventive medicine programs, education of asthmatic patients, and with COPD. Also she has conducted training courses in Nursing students of A.T.E.I. of Athens in the Urban Model Health Center Peristeri. She is distinguished in the scientific health care representing the H.C.D.C.P., and her 'Model' Health Center Peristeri world conferences on research has been rewarded. She is a member of the Greek Society for the Study of Medicine of psychosomatic problems, of cultural educational movement EE (PO.KE.PE), of the Association of Nurses Greece, Greek Society for Disease Control, the Greek Company Prehospital Emergency Care, the European Resuscitation Council, the Asthma Group Greek Respiratory Society and Research Associate, General Hospital Nafplio. She is certified by the Prehospital Trauma Live Support, American Heart Association in "Airway Management", Advanced Trauma Live Support and ILS Provider Course.

Mark Swofford is a Colonel in the United States Army and currently serves as the Chief of Staff and Deputy Commander for Administration of Brooke Army Medical Center, at Fort Sam Houston, Texas. Dr. Swofford has over 23 years of professional experience providing health services administration and operational expertise to the Army Medical Department and its subordinate organizations. His assignments have included the direct provision of health services to combat units, the administration of hospitals/health clinics, the direction of clinical services at the regional level, and the analysis of financial and clinical data for the entire Army healthcare system. His educational background includes a PhD in Health Services Organization Research and Methods from Virginia Commonwealth University, Richmond, Virginia; a Master of Healthcare Administration from Baylor University, Waco, Texas; and a Bachelor of Science Degree from Davidson College, Davidson, North Carolina. He has been recognized with several academic honors and military honors, including the James W. Begun Award for Excellence in Doctoral Research from Virginia Commonwealth University, an American College of Healthcare Executives Regent's Award in 2004, the Boone Powell Award for Excellence in Research from the U.S. Army Baylor Program, and the Order of Military Medical Merit from Army Medical Department Regiment. He is currently an adjunct faculty member for both Webster University and Baylor University, and a Fellow in the American College of Healthcare Executives. He resides in San Antonio, Texas with his wife and three children.

Mamas Theodorou has studied Economics at the University of Athens, Economic Development at the North London Polytechnic, Health Care Management at the Athens National School of Public Health and got his doctoral degree from the Nursing Department of the University of Athens. He has worked as an Adjunct

Professor at the Technological Institute of Athens, the National School of Public Administration and the Open University of Patras. In August 2006 he was elected Associate Professor on Health Care Management and Health Policy at the Open University of Cyprus. His research interests are mainly focused on the fields of evaluating the efficiency and organization of health units, the financing of health services, the measurement of health systems performance and the quality of the care provided. He has authored and published individually or with others more than 90 articles, books and chapters in collective volumes on issues of health policy, financing and quality of health services, patient satisfaction etc.

Ashish Upadhyay is a GIS Manager in Indian Institute of Public Health – Gandhinagar. He holds a Master of Science in Geomatics from CEPT University, Faculty of Technology in Ahmedabad 2012. He also holds a Certificate Course on Remote Sensing Technology and its Applications including Image Processing, Pattern Recognition and GIS from National Remote Sensing Agency (NRSA), Hyderabad, India in July to September. 2002. Before joining IIPHG in 2012, he was a Research Associate playing the role of GIS Analyst and delivering courses of GIS and Remote Sensing and its applications in the CEPT University. Currently, he works in the many international and national projects in the field of GIS and Remote Sensing. His research interests are geospatial coordination in government, public health, Health system studies, social implications of spatial data infrastructures and the use of geo-information in policy processes.

Kranti Suresh Vora is working as an associate professor at IIPH, Gandhinagar since October, 2012 and is faculty coordinator for an EU funded project. Dr Vora has done MD (ObGyn) from Gujarat University, MPH from Johns Hopkins School of Public Health, USA and PhD from University of Maryland, USA. Her experience extends from private practice specializing in infertility to working in UNFPA led government of Gujarat project. Highlights of her public health career are establishing emergency obstetric care centers in Gujarat for the first time and Bill and Melinda Gates Foundation scholarship to pursue MPH at Johns Hopkins School of Public Health.

Athanassios Vozikis is a Lecturer at the Department of Economics of the University of Piraeus. He holds a degree in Public Administration from the Panteion University, a M.Sc. in Health Informatics from Kapodistriako University of Athens and a Ph.D. in Health Economics and Information Systems from the University of Piraeus. He has been an I.K.Y. (State Scholarships Foundation) scholar for his M.SC. and Ph.D. studies. He is member of the National Council of Public Health, member of several scientific associations and organizations and reviewer of academic journals. He has participated in several research projects related to the analysis–development and implementation of Information Systems, Business and Economic Re-engineering Processes in the Health Care Sector, as well as in various other sectors in Public and Private Organizations. He has participated in several Conferences and a number of his articles have been published in academic journals, academic issues and scientific conferences proceedings. He teaches Health Economics, Environmental Economics, Information Systems and Digital Economy courses at an undergraduate level and Health Economics, Health Information Systems and Strategic Information Systems courses at a postgraduate level. He has been Supervisor and referee of several dissertations of postgraduate students. His research interests are in the field of Health Economics, Public Health, E.R.P. Systems, Health Information Systems and Digital Economy.

Sofia Xesfingi is a Post-Doc Researcher at the Department of Economics, University of Piraeus, Greece, and holds a Ph.D. from the same department. She received the diploma in Biology from the Aristoteles University of Thessaloniki, in 2007 and the M.Sc. in Healthcare Management from the Department of Economics of the University of Piraeus, in 2010. Her research interests are in Health Economics, Patient Satisfaction and Service Quality, and Econometric Analysis. She speaks fluently four languages and has participated in several conferences to promote her working papers.

Denis Yannacopoulos is Professor of Management Information Systems in the Business Administration Department of the TPiraeus University of Applied Sciences. He holds a BSc in Chemistry, a MSc and a PhD in Information Systems. His research interests are in Operational Research, Multicriteria Analysis and Decision Support Systems. His expertise in training issues and EU projects is utilized by the Ministry of Employment and Education and he has been a consultant of numerous public and private organisations in Greece and Cyprus. He is an active member of editorial boards and a referee of many scientific journals. He was Dean of the Administration and Economy School of the TEI of Piraeus from 2006 to 2010 and 2014 to 2016 and also President of the Hellenic Operational Research Society (HELORS) from 2005 to 2009.

Sandul Yasobant is a public health researcher, currently involved in large scale community based health system evaluation projects at Indian Institute of Public Health- Gandhinagar (IIPHG), India. Dr. Yasobant earned his Master in Public Health (MPH) from WHO collaborating Centre of Occupational Health, Sri Ramachandra Medical College & Research Institute, India. He also has experience in Ergonomics Consultancy & Occupational Health Promotion in various industries for decades. Prior to this he was serving as an academician for health science graduate at Utkal University, Odisha, India. He also earned Health promotion certification from National Institute of Health & Family Welfare (NIHFW), New Delhi, India and Health Education certification from IGNOU, India. He is actively serving as an editorial board member/ reviewer for many national and international journals.

Stelios Zimeras holds a BSc. (Hons) on Statistics and Insurance Sciences from University of Piraeus (5fth in the rank) and Ph.D. on Statistics from the University of Leeds, U.K. He had received a full scholarship (fees and maintenance) during his research studies (1993- 1997) from the University of Leeds. Since 2008, he is a full time staff member (Assistant Prof) on statistics and probabilities at the Department of Mathematics, Division of Statistics and Financial-Actuarial Mathematics, University of the Aegean, Samos, Greece. He had worked as post-doc at University of Leeds, Department of Electrical Engineering (funded by EPSRC), at IRISA/INRIA-VISTA PROJECT institute, France (funded by EUMETSATESA) and at MedCom GmbH, Germany (funded by Marie-Curie grants). Finally 2011-2012 he had worked during his sabbatical in University of Piraeus, Department of Digital Systems, in computer virus modelling. In 2011 he has nominated the Best Paper for the 5th International Conference on Energy and Development - Environment - Biomedicine 2011 (EDEB '11) with title "Spatial Uncertainty", pp. 203-208, by S. Zimeras, Y. Matsinos. He has involved in national and international projects (FP7, ESPA, Marie-Curie). His published material and presentations are on a number of topics of Data Processing, Statistical Simulations, Image analysis, Medical Image analysis, Spatial Statistics, Telemedicine, and Statistical Modelling with applications in biology, ecology, and medicine, statistical epidemiology, and Bayesian statistics. He has been a member of a number of professional and scientific societies and associations; while he is a reviewer for a number of conferences.

Index

A

access 4, 11-12, 19, 64, 67, 103-104, 115, 117-119, 125, 128, 142, 145, 152-155, 158-159, 161, 163-164, 166, 168-170, 173, 175, 180, 187, 189, 196, 198-199, 204, 211, 218, 221, 225, 229-231, 233-235, 239-240, 244-246, 249, 251-252
Accountable Care Organization 110, 113
analytics 46-48, 50, 52, 55, 65, 68-71, 73, 123-125, 127, 130, 133

C

Compensation and Benefits 16, 25, 43
conflict 202-203, 205-209, 212-219, 221-227
contact 46, 144, 169, 174, 188, 202, 227
cooperation 172-173, 202-203, 205, 210, 214, 217-218, 225, 227, 231, 242

D

decision support 45, 47-48, 50, 55-56, 66, 68, 73, 114, 116-118, 127, 131-133, 139, 161, 199
Decision Support Techniques 45
drug-related problems 172, 177, 181, 190, 194, 200-201

E

elective surgery scheduling 90, 93, 95, 103, 105, 107
Electronic Health Record 69-70, 110, 113, 115, 117, 128, 131, 133
Electronic Medical Record 110, 116, 130, 132
Emotional Intelligence 202, 206, 218, 220, 222, 224, 227
Empathy 67, 202, 227
employee outcomes 18, 21-22, 28-29, 44
Employee Relations 16, 27, 32
Equity 161, 165, 171, 229-231, 239, 245, 250, 254-255
Europe 204, 210, 226, 229-233, 235-236, 238-239, 244, 246-255

G

gender 124, 160, 226, 229, 239-242, 253-254, 256
GIS 137-146, 149-166
group 25, 36, 41, 44, 48, 60-62, 113, 123, 145, 157, 179-180, 184, 187, 190, 205, 209, 227, 239, 246

H

Health Care Reform 111, 128, 133, 221
healthcare sector 5, 16, 37
Health Facility Administration 45
Health Insurance Portability and Accountability Act 119, 122
health planning 160
health research 131, 137-139, 144-145, 150, 164
Health Services Quality 1
Health Services Research 7, 38, 107, 129

high-performance work practices 16-17, 36, 44
Human Resource Management 16-18, 20, 22, 24, 26-27, 30, 32-38, 40-44, 224
Human Resource Management Policy 27, 44
Human Resource Management Practice 44

I

improvement 1, 3-4, 54, 59-60, 64-66, 71, 73, 91, 104, 125, 128, 159, 163, 168, 171, 173-174, 192, 204, 213, 215, 219-220, 234-236, 248
inequalities 12, 154, 164, 229-239, 241, 245, 248-250, 252-254
integration 25, 45-48, 52, 55, 62-63, 65-69, 71, 73, 107, 110, 143, 157, 231, 239, 249
Interdependency 73

J

job and work design 20

L

linear programming 90, 93-94, 100

M

Mediator 44
mixed integer nonlinear programming 90, 94
models 7, 53, 65, 76-78, 81-83, 85, 87, 89-90, 92, 94, 105, 108, 128, 131, 137, 149, 154-155, 157, 162, 164, 166, 220, 231-232
Moderator 34, 44

O

optimization 53, 92-95, 106, 126, 220
organizational 5, 16-34, 36-70, 73, 207-208, 211-214, 218-227
organizational innovation 39
organizational outcomes 16-18, 28-33, 44, 68

P

Patient Centered Medical Home 114-115
Patient Protection and Affordable Care Act 111-112, 132
patient satisfaction 1-7, 9-14, 29, 33, 187, 195, 198, 214
Performance Management and Appraisal 26
pharmaceutical care 171, 190-199, 201
pharmaceutical consultations 171-172, 175, 201
Pharmaceutical Counseling 201
Pharmaceutical Enterprise 189, 201
pharmaceutical services 168-171, 174, 180, 186-188, 190, 200-201
Pharmacist 168-175, 177-179, 186-191, 193-194, 196, 198, 200-201
Phytotherapics 170, 201
primary care 2, 114, 116, 118, 130-132, 161, 197, 229, 247-249, 255
Project 53, 58, 61-66, 71, 73, 129, 146-149, 157, 166, 192, 219, 253
Project Prioritization 64, 73
public health 116, 132, 134, 137-139, 141-142, 144, 146, 149-153, 155-157, 159-162, 164, 166, 179, 196, 200, 204, 216, 223, 229, 232, 235-237, 239, 244, 249-252

Q

Quality Assurance 1, 3-4, 12, 15
quality improvement 1, 3, 66, 71, 163, 173
quality of care 1-5, 8, 10, 14-15, 29, 34, 70, 72, 92, 115, 127, 158-159, 169

R

recruiting and selection 22

S

scheduling 90-99, 101-108
secondary care 249
sequencing 92, 94, 106

services 1-2, 4-5, 7-9, 11-15, 33, 38, 45, 48, 62, 67, 69, 90-91, 94, 104, 107-108, 113-115, 119, 122, 129, 131, 133-135, 138, 145, 152-155, 157-158, 160, 162-166, 168-175, 179-181, 186-192, 196-198, 200-201, 203-204, 210, 219-220, 223, 230-232, 234-235, 238-239, 241-242, 244-247, 249, 251
side effects 170, 175, 180-181, 186, 201
simulation 78, 85-86, 88-89, 92-94, 105, 108, 145, 198
Social Skills 227
stochastic 77-78, 86, 92-95, 107
surgery 60, 90-108

T

training and development 18, 24, 32, 135

W

Web GIS 137, 146

www.ingramcontent.com/pod-product-compliance
Lightning Source LLC
LaVergne TN
LVHW061546290926
849162LV00004B/924